Textbook of Family Medicine

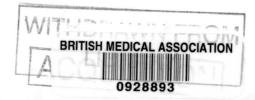

TEXTBOOK OF FAMILY MEDICINE

THIRD EDITION

Ian R. McWhinney

Professor Emeritus
Department of Family Medicine
Schulich School of Medicine and Dentistry
The University of Western Ontario

Thomas Freeman

Chair
Department of Family Medicine
Schulich School of Medicine and Dentistry
The University of Western Ontario

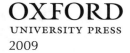

UNIVERSITY PRESS
2009

Oxford University Press, Inc., publishes works that further
Oxford University's objective of excellence
in research, scholarship, and education.

Oxford New York
Auckland Cape Town Dar es Salaam Hong Kong Karachi
Kuala Lumpur Madrid Melbourne Mexico City Nairobi
New Delhi Shanghai Taipei Toronto

With offices in
Argentina Austria Brazil Chile Czech Republic France Greece
Guatemala Hungary Italy Japan Poland Portugal Singapore
South Korea Switzerland Thailand Turkey Ukraine Vietnam

Copyright © 2009 by Oxford University Press, Inc.

Published by Oxford University Press, Inc.
198 Madison Avenue, New York, New York 10016
www.oup.com

Oxford is a registered trademark of Oxford University Press

Library of Congress Cataloging-in-Publication Data

McWhinney, Ian R.
Textbook of family medicine / Ian R. McWhinney, Thomas Freeman. — 3rd ed.
p. ; cm.
Includes bibliographical references and index.
ISBN 978-0-19-536985-4
1. Family medicine—Textbooks.   I. Freeman, Thomas, 1948–   II. Title.
[DNLM: 1. Family Practice.   WB 110 M4787t 2009]
RC46.M258 2009
610—dc22   2008033966

9 8 7 6 5 4 3 2 1
Printed in the United States of America
on acid-free paper

To the memory of Betty and to Heather and Julie
and
To Moira, Kate and Amy

Preface

There are two kinds of textbooks: those that aim to cover a field of knowledge and those that aim to define and conceptualize it. This book is of the second kind. Most textbooks in clinical disciplines are structured in accordance with the conventional system for classifying diseases. A family medicine text that adopts this structure faces two difficulties. Family physicians encounter clinical problems before they have been classified into disease categories. In principle, family physicians are available for any type of problem. There is thus no disease, however rare, that may not be encountered in family practice. If a text tries to cover the whole field, it risks becoming a watered-down textbook of internal medicine. More seriously, family medicine differs from most other disciplines in such fundamental ways that the conventional structure, though used in family medicine when appropriate, is at a variance with the organismic thinking that is natural to our discipline.

The third edition breaks new ground by having two authors. Professor Ian McWhinney, who was author of the first two editions of this textbook, graduated from Cambridge University in 1949 and entered practice in Stratford-on-Avon after internships in St Bartholomew's Hospital, London, and a year of internal medicine at Warwick Hospital. In 1968, he became the first professor of Family Medicine at The University of Western Ontario. Thomas Freeman, professor of the Department of Family Medicine at the Schulich School of Medicine and Dentistry, The University of Western Ontario, graduated from The University of Western Ontario in 1976 and completed training in family medicine at Dalhousie University, Halifax, Nova Scotia. After practicing in Woodstock Ontario for 11 years, he became a full-time member of the Department of Family Medicine at Western in 1989.

The long time that McWhinney and Freeman have worked together and the closeness of their views on family medicine have played an important part in the new edition. For more than a year, they have met together every week to read every page of the 2nd edition. Parts that they agree were out of date were removed. New items were discussed and written between them and entered into the 3rd edition. Every chapter was scrutinized and altered accordingly. Considerable new material was added. The effects of new technologies were discussed together, and the affected chapters altered. For example, the advances in electronic communication have made superfluous the long alphabetical list of procedures for special conditions, which covered many pages in Chapter 9 in the second edition.

The five clinical chapters (11–15) were in the second edition to illustrate the section on basic principles (Chapters 1–10). The book does not set out to cover the whole field of clinical family medicine. Three of them are devoted to symptoms (sore throat, headache, and fatigue), one to a conventional disease category (diabetes), and one to a physiological variable/risk factor (hypertension). The five chapters have become out of date in 10 years, so these were all examined and updated, as well as the chapter on alternative, or complementary, medicine. Major advances have been made in records, home care, shared care, and practice management: major changes have been made in these chapters.

In therapeutics, the recommendations are in accordance with authoritative opinion at the time of writing. As time passes, these inevitably become outdated, and more current recommendations will need to be consulted. It is doubtful nowadays whether any textbook can be considered an appropriate source for information on pharmacotherapy. Drug dosages are not given unless they are of special significance.

This is actually the third edition of a book that began life as *An Introduction to Family Medicine* in 1981. The clinical chapters and the section on the practice of family medicine were added in the edition of 1989. The book and the ideas it presents have grown with the development of the discipline. Important themes run right through the book. For example, the process of clinical reasoning and narratives of illness emerge in many chapters, with cross-references to other chapters and to case reports. We have visualized the book as a whole, rather than as a series of disconnected chapters, so it is intended to be read as a whole. Since we have tried to anchor it to some fundamental ideas, we hope readers will find it an aid to reflection.

London, Ontario   Ian R. McWhinney
2008   Thomas Freeman

Acknowledgments

Many people helped us with this edition of the Textbook of Family Medicine. Sandra Richard-Mohamed organized and prepared the manuscript, and acted throughout as the liaison between us. As the book reached its final stages, Andrea Burt, Leslie Meredith, and Nicole Robinson helped in the last touches to the manuscript and Nuala Marshall did work on the tables. Judith Belle Brown, John Feightner, Stewart Harris, Rob Petrella, and Eric Wong read and critiqued chapters. Moira Stewart provided important contributions to the chapter on Clinical Method and in numerous other ways. Lynn Dunikowski and her staff at the Library of the College of Family Physicians of Canada were invaluable support in locating needed reference material. Michelle Homer sat in on our meetings during the first summer helping in research and adding much to our discussions.

As before we are much obliged to John Biehn, Dorothy Haswell, Eric McCracken, and John Sangster for providing us with case reports.

We thank Bill Lamsback, Editor for Medicine, Oxford University Press; Ciara Vincent, Assistant Editor, Clinical Medicine; and Anupama Gopinath.

Contents

Part III   The Practice of Family Medicine

Part IV   Education and Research

Part I

Basic Principles

The Origins of Family Medicine

The profound changes now occurring in medicine can only be fully understood if they are viewed from the perspective of history. There is nothing new about change: medicine has been changing constantly since its beginnings. Only the pace is different.

Medicine changes in response to many influences, some scientific and technological, some social. Family medicine is only one of many new disciplines that have developed in the course of medical history. New disciplines arise in a number of ways: some—such as surgery and obstetrics—have developed from ancient craft skills; some have grown up around new techniques, such as otolaryngology in the nineteenth century and anesthesiology in the twentieth; others have been formed because some area of need, such as child health, was being neglected by existing disciplines. All these influences have played their part in the recent growth of family medicine. Social changes, specialization, and a new pattern of illness have demanded a new type of physician; science has given us new insights into some old problems; and existing disciplines have tended to neglect the problems encountered in family practice.

New disciplines can begin in three ways: by transformation from an older discipline, de novo, or by fragmentation from a larger discipline. Family medicine has evolved from an older branch of medicine—general practice. The relationship, however, is not a simple one; we will be returning to it later. Let us now look in more detail at some modern trends that have influenced the development of family medicine.

Changes in Mortality and Morbidity

The successful control of the major infectious diseases, which ravaged even the most advanced countries up to the earlier years of this century, has been followed in countries with a high standard of living by the emergence of a new pattern of disease. Instead of severe acute illnesses such as typhoid, lobar pneumonia, and diphtheria, the physician[1] is now faced mostly with chronic diseases, developmental disorders, behavioral disorders, accidents, and a different range of infectious diseases. The reduced mortality in children and adults has, with each succeeding generation, increased the proportion of elderly people in society.

This new pattern has produced a gradual change in the role of the practitioner. A person afflicted with one of the great mortal infections either died or recovered in a comparatively short period of time. A person afflicted with a chronic disorder is often engaged in a prolonged struggle to adapt to his or her environment. Rather than dealing with acute life-or-death situations, therefore, today's practitioners are more likely to find themselves helping patients to achieve a new equilibrium with their environment in the face of chronic illness and disability.

Management of chronic disorders calls for an understanding of both the patient and the environment. Because many of the situations facing the physician are complex combinations of physical and behavioral factors, the conventional separation of physical and mental illness becomes unrealistic. The practice of preventive medicine has also changed. In a sense, we have moved from an era of public health to one of private health. The health of society depends less on new legislation than on millions of private decisions about matters as diverse as smoking, family planning, and immunization. In influencing these decisions, the physician's educational role has assumed new importance.

This is not to say that public health has ceased to be important. Clean water, a balanced diet, and good housing are still major determinants of health. There is still scope for improving public health by legislation in such areas as industrial hazards, smoking, environmental pollution, and traffic accidents. Many of our present threats to health, however, are out of reach of legislation.

The above remarks apply only to developed, industrial societies. Most of the world's population still lives under conditions that have not existed in advanced countries since the nineteenth century. This means that the role of the family physician in such societies is different from his role in developed societies. The differences are discussed in more detail later.

The Growth of Specialization

A brief review of the development of the modern medical profession will help put our present position in perspective. The profession as we know it has existed only since the nineteenth century. Before that time, society was served by a variety of healers, only a small proportion of whom were physicians. In the seventeenth and eighteenth centuries, physicians were a small and elite group of learned men, educated in the few universities. They practiced in towns among the rich and influential, did not perform surgery or dispense drugs, and did not associate, either professionally or socially, with the craftsmen and tradesmen who ministered to the medical needs of poorer and rural people. Surgeons were craftsmen who were trained by apprenticeship; apothecaries were tradesmen who originally dispensed and sold drugs but who, in response to need, gradually took on the role of medical practitioner.

Although some physicians were among the early immigrants to North America, there were not nearly enough to meet the needs of the population. The early colonies were served, therefore, by a great variety of practitioners. Because there were no medical schools until the founding of the school at Philadelphia in the 1760s, those who wished to become physicians had to study in Europe. Their numbers were not enough for the growing population: in eighteenth-century Virginia, for example, only one in nine practitioners had been trained as a physician (Boorstin, 1958).

For a long time, graduates returning from their studies in Europe tried to maintain their distinctiveness by refusing to practice surgery or dispense drugs. The American students at Edinburgh formed the Virginia Club, one of whose articles was "that every member of this club shall make it his endeavour, if possible, for the honour of his profession, not to degrade it by hereafter mingling the trade of an apothecary or surgeon with it." However, the heavy demand for services and the breakdown of old social barriers in the new colonies soon made these aspirations impossible to fulfill. Before long all practitioners, whether graduates or not, were practicing as general practitioners. Thus was the general practitioner born in eighteenth-century America.

In Britain, meanwhile, the same historical process was going on. By the beginning of the nineteenth century, the status of surgeons and apothecaries had risen substantially and their work had become increasingly medical. Edward Jenner (1749–1823), the discoverer of vaccination, was a country surgeon in the west of England. By the nineteenth century, surgical training had been improved, and surgeons took the examination for membership in the Royal College of Surgeons (MRCS) after a combination of apprenticeship and hospital training.

In 1815, the Apothecaries Act gave legal recognition to the right of apothecaries in Britain to give medical advice as well as to supply drugs. The Act made it compulsory for apothecaries to undergo a five-year apprenticeship and to take courses in anatomy, physiology, the practice of medicine, and *materia medica*. It also established a qualifying examination, the Licentiate of the Society of Apothecaries (LSA). It soon became customary for practitioners to take the double qualification (LSA and MRCS) and, when an examination in midwifery was added, the graduate was qualified to practice medicine, surgery, and midwifery.[2] The term general practitioner was first used in the *Lancet* early in the nineteenth century. Thus, the general practitioner, born in eighteenth-century America, was named in nineteenth-century Britain. By a slow process of response to social demands, surgeons and apothecaries were gradually integrated with physicians to form the modern medical profession. The process took many years to complete, and even in Victorian times, remnants of the old distinctions were clearly evident. George Eliot's *Middlemarch* and Anthony Trollope's *Dr. Thorne* provide fascinating glimpses of the life and work of a general practitioner in nineteenth-century England.

These historical events are not irrelevant to the position of the medical profession today. Two lessons we would do well to ponder:

1. If the profession is failing to meet a public need, society will find some way of meeting the need, if necessary by turning to a group outside the profession.[3]
2. Professions evolve in response to social pressures, sometimes in ways that conflict with the expressed intentions of their members.

The Age of the General Practitioner

In Europe and North America, the nineteenth century was the age of the general practitioner. On both continents, most members of the profession were general practitioners and there was little differentiation of function, even among the faculties of medical schools. Toward the end of the century, however, the major specialties began to emerge. Osler's address "Remarks on Specialism" (1892) was given to mark the origin of pediatrics as a separate discipline. At the same time, progress in the sciences—chemistry, physics, physiology, and bacteriology—was beginning to have an impact on medicine. Medical education, especially in North America, was divorced from the scientific foundations of medicine, and much of it was of very poor quality. In his report in 1910, Abraham Flexner described appalling conditions in many of the hundreds of small medical schools that existed in the United States and Canada. Even the time-honored apprenticeship system had fallen into abeyance. North America had an ample supply of doctors both in town and country, but they were little prepared for the technological revolution that was about to transform medicine.

The founding of Johns Hopkins in 1889 was a landmark in the development of medicine in North America. The aim of the founding fathers—Osler, Halsted, Hurd, Welch, and Kelly—was to place medical education on a firm scientific foundation. From the beginning, the faculty consisted entirely of specialists. In his proposals for reform, Flexner used Johns Hopkins and the German medical schools as his models. The Flexner reforms in the years between 1910 and 1930 paved the way for the next stage: the age of specialization.

The Age of Specialization

The first half of the twentieth century saw the emergence of the major specialties of medicine, each with its defined training program and its qualifying examination. Technological progress was rapid and investment in research produced good dividends. Medical education became increasingly oriented toward laboratory science and the technology of medicine. The increasing prestige accorded to specialists and the valuation of technical and research skills over personal care made general practice unpopular as a career.

The number of general practitioners declined steadily from the 1930s, both in absolute terms and as a proportion of the profession as a whole. The process was accelerated by the virtual disappearance of general practitioners from medical faculties after World War II and by the fragmentation of the major specialties that began to occur in the 1950s.

Since the 1960s, it has become customary to distinguish between three kinds of service provided by physicians, corresponding to three levels of health care. At the primary level, generalist physicians provide continuing personal and comprehensive care. The physicians may be general practitioners or physicians limiting their practice to adults or children. At the secondary level, specialists provide care only to patients with disorders in their field of expertise, usually by referral from primary physicians. The tertiary level comprises highly specialized services often available only in regional centers.

The fragmentation of the profession and the emphasis on technology have had one other serious effect: a deterioration of the doctor–patient relationship. More than 60 years ago, Flexner (1930) realized that something had been lost as well as gained by the reform of medical education. In his book *Universities, American, English and German*, he wrote: "the very intensity with which scientific medicine is cultivated threatens to cost us at times the mellow judgement and broad culture of the older generation at its best. Osler, Janeway, and Halsted have not been replaced." This neglect of the caring and personal aspects of medicine is now beginning to have consequences such as the increase in malpractice suits and a growing disenchantment with technology.

As the age of specialization reaches its culmination, therefore, we can see the need for a new kind of generalist. The new generalists, however, must be different from the old general practitioners. Instead of being the undifferentiated bulk of the profession, defined chiefly by lack of special training and qualifications, they now have a well-differentiated role and a defined set of skills. In the United States, the requirements for the new generalist were set out in two key reports: The Graduate Education of Physicians (Millis, 1966) and Meeting the Challenge of Family Practice (Willard, 1966). It is no coincidence that parallel changes have taken place in Canada, the United Kingdom, Holland, Australia, and other industrialized countries.

One response to the decline in general practice was the formation in the 1950s and 1960s of colleges and academies of general practice in a number of countries. The first postgraduate training programs[4] were established and much progress was made in defining the curriculum and designing examinations. At this time, the first academic chairs were established in Britain, Canada, the Netherlands, and the United States, and family medicine was introduced into the undergraduate curriculum. In 1972 the World Organization of National Colleges and Academies of General Practice/Family Medicine (WONCA) was formed.[5]

New Developments in the Behavioral Sciences

The study of human behavior has always been important to general practitioners. In the past, however, insights have been gained intuitively rather than by an organized approach to problems. Recent developments in behavioral and social science have been important to medicine as a whole, but particularly to family medicine.

Behavioral science has directed our attention to the process by which people seek medical care, a crucial area for all primary physicians. It has made physicians themselves the objects of study, thus making us more aware of the importance of our own behavior in determining the quality of care, for example, in decision making and prescribing. It has increased our insights into the doctor–patient relationship, family relationships, and the behavioral aspects of illness. It has made us think about some of the fundamental aspects of medicine, such as our concepts of health, disease, and illness, the role of the physician, and the ethics of medicine. It has brought to our attention the large portion of the iceberg of hidden illness normally not seen by the medical profession. Finally, it has increased our knowledge of behavioral and social factors involved in the causation of disease.

The situation with behavioral science is analogous to that of chemistry and physiology a century ago. A new body of knowledge demanded integration with medicine, and integration was eventually achieved, partly by changes in curriculum, but mainly by changes in clinical practice introduced by clinicians who had mastered the new knowledge. In the same way, new knowledge from the behavioral sciences will be integrated with medicine through changes in clinical practice. As generalist clinicians practicing a patient-centered clinical method, family physicians are in a key position to make this synthesis.

The Changing Role of the Hospital

Another factor in the development of family medicine has been the resurgence of interest in health care outside the hospital. The cost of inpatient care has become so prohibitive that criteria for admission to hospitals have become increasingly strict. The acute care hospital seems to be evolving into an institution where only those patients needing highly technical and specialized care are treated, either as inpatients or as outpatients in specialized clinics. For those who need care for a variety of problems over a long period of time, the hospital is a much less satisfactory form of care. A large institution can hardly avoid the fragmentation of care and frequent changes of personnel that are the antithesis of integrated, personal medicine. There are also some risks associated with hospitalization, especially for the elderly.

The practice of medicine outside the hospital, particularly at the neighborhood level, has assumed a new importance. We can now see that the overwhelming concentration of care in the hospital during the past few decades has been a mistake of emphasis. The need during the next few decades is for a balanced system in which personal and continuing care will be available for all at the neighborhood level, while the hospital provides specialized support when it is needed. In some health-care systems, including some managed care organizations in the United States, primary physicians do not have responsibility for inpatient care, except in a supportive role.

Managed Care and the Age of Integration

In the present age we are seeing the rapid reorganization of health care in response to economic forces. The division of services into three levels—primary, secondary, and tertiary—has proved to be highly effective, validating the work done on vocational training for family medicine in the preceding decades. At its 1978 conference in Alma-Ata, the World Health Organization recognized the fundamental importance of primary care (World Health Organization, 1978).

The well-trained family doctor has become a key figure, and often a leader, in the organization of health care. At the same time, integration of services has become essential to conserve resources and eliminate waste. Horizontally, integration is achieved by family doctors working as team members with other health professionals and in collaboration with community support services. Vertical integration is achieved by collaboration between the three levels of care, as in hospital discharge planning.

The reorganization of health care is being carried out by managed care in its various forms. A managed care organization is one that takes on the financial budget and is responsible for coordinating a full spectrum of clinical services. Health service or maintenance organizations (HMOs) and groups organized by physicians are examples of managed care in the United States. In countries with national health services, such as Canada and Britain, responsibility for financing and providing services rests with government. Within an organization some of the risk may be transferred to smaller groups of physicians caring for defined populations.[6]

In the United States, the role of the family physician in HMOs is sometimes described as that of gatekeeper. The name has taken on the negative connotation of a person who tries to keep people out. There are, however, many positive aspects of the role. The gatekeeper can also be described as the person who makes others welcome, meets many of their needs, and guides them through the system. The division of function between primary and secondary care physicians enables both groups to do what they do best. Primary-care physicians help specialists to maintain their skills by concentrating their experience on the patients whose problems come within their field of expertise.

Although managed care provides primary-care physicians with great opportunities, the rapid pace of change and the loss of independence can be very unsettling. As physicians become more involved in financial management, they may find themselves in conflicts of interest between the needs of their patients and the requirements of the organization.

Because clinical education must follow the patient, this shift toward care in the community must lead eventually to a change in the clinical curriculum. Logically, medical students should be based in primary-care institutions, where they can experience the long-term care of patients near where they and their families live and work. Some of their specialty experience can be obtained in the same setting, where family physicians, specialists, and other health professionals are increasingly collaborating. For other aspects of their education in the specialties, students can be seconded to the acute care hospital.[7]

General Practice or Family Medicine

At the time of the revival of general practice, there was a move to change its name to family practice or to family medicine, and to refer to general practitioners as family physicians. Thus, the new Board in the United States was named the Board of Family Practice. The Academy of General Practice became the Academy of Family Practice. In Canada, the College of General Practitioners changed its name to the College of Family Physicians.

The reasons for this change were mixed. On the one hand was the feeling that the name general practice had become associated with an obsolete type of medicine. On the other hand was a wish to emphasize that family practice was something new and different from general practice. Also, there was the need to find a name for the body of knowledge, the new clinical discipline that was being defined.

The change of name did have some repercussions. Many general practitioners had been providing exemplary care and were functioning in precisely the way expected of the new family physicians. Family medicine was based on the best of general practice. It was sometimes difficult to explain exactly what was different about family medicine. Some existing general practitioners also felt offended by the implication that what they were doing was somehow inferior.

In the new academic departments the change of name was viewed differently by different people. To some, using the term *family* meant that the new body of knowledge was about the family and health, and that this was what made family practice unique among clinical disciplines. To others, family physician was the revival of a time-honored title, used for many years as an alternative to general practitioner. The term *family medicine* then became the name of the body of knowledge on which family practice is based, a body of knowledge that includes the family, but much else besides. The latter is the point of view we have taken, and in this book we have used the terms family physician and general practitioner interchangeably. Family medicine is the term we use for the body of knowledge on which their practice is based.

Family Medicine as a Clinical and Academic Discipline

Clinical disciplines in medicine are based on a number of factors, some epistemological, some practical and administrative. An epistemological basis for a discipline is a consensus among its members about the important problems confronting the discipline, and the knowledge appropriate for dealing with them (from Greek episteme, "knowledge"). In a clinical discipline this will include a common experience of clinical problems and an agreed clinical method, as well as an agreement about an agenda for research. For a discipline to be truly independent, there should be some research questions that can only be addressed from inside the discipline. Even if methods are borrowed from other disciplines, only somebody inside the discipline can know the context in which the methods are applied, especially the methodological pitfalls. An epistemological basis also implies an agreement about what knowledge of the discipline is, and how it is acquired. As Kuhn (1970) has observed, members of a discipline also share a worldview, much of it at the unconscious level.

We believe that family medicine is a clinical discipline as we have described it. It would not be true to say that there is complete agreement on all the above questions. As Kuhn, again, has observed, disagreements do occur at certain stages in a discipline's development. Psychiatry has become a major clinical discipline without ever having resolved some fundamental issues. Even allowing for these disagreements, we are impressed, in talking to family physicians from many parts of the world, how much they do share the same worldview, molded by the same experience of medicine.

Some have doubted whether family medicine is a discipline in its own right, because it shares so much with other primary-care disciplines, notably primary-care internal medicine. These doubts have prompted a search for uniqueness in the idea of "the family as patient." The fact that we share a worldview with another discipline need not concern us. If an internist is providing primary, comprehensive, and continuing care to adult families, with the same epistemological base as a family physician, then he is, to all intents and purposes, a family physician. We must not confuse things with the names we call them by. Our own view is that primary-care internal medicine and family medicine in the United States are now so close that they could come together as a single discipline. The obstacles to this are not epistemological but administrative and political. It is not unusual in medicine for divisions between disciplines to be administrative rather than epistemological. Whether pediatric cardiology belongs to pediatrics or cardiology and whether psychogeriatrics belongs to psychiatry or geriatrics are questions likely to be resolved on administrative grounds, perhaps differently in different institutions. We should not make too much of the divisions between disciplines, in medicine or in any other field. On this subject Karl Popper (1972), the philosopher of science, has written:

But subject matter, or kinds of things, do not, I hold, constitute a basis for distinguishing disciplines. Disciplines are distinguished partly for historical reasons and reasons of administrative convenience...and partly because the theories we construct to solve our problems have a tendency to grow into unified systems. But all this classification and distinction is a comparatively superficial affair. We are not students of some subject matter but students of problems. And problems may cut right across the borders of any subject matter or discipline.

Family medicine could have developed as a division of internal medicine. The reasons why it did not are as much historical and administrative as they are epistemological. By the early decades of the twentieth century, internists had ceased to see children and to do gynecology. At the same time, in many countries, internal medicine had become functionally differentiated from general practice. By the 1950s, when family medicine began to develop as a discipline, the leadership of academic internal medicine, with few exceptions, did not see the problems raised by family medicine as important. Internal medicine at that time was focusing its attention on the laboratory, rather than on purely clinical observation or on behavioral and population studies. There is no reason for thinking that this direction for internal medicine was inappropriate. It did, however, leave a whole range of problems unattended to, and family medicine was the appropriate discipline to attend to them.

References

Boorstin DJ. 1958. *The Americans: The Colonial Experience*. New York: Random House.

Flexner A. 1910. Medical education in the United States and Canada: A report to the Carnegie Foundation for the Advancement of Teaching. New York.

——. 1930. *Universities, American, English and German*. New York: Oxford University Press.

Kuhn TS. 1970. *The Structure of Scientific Revolutions*. Chicago, IL: University of Chicago Press.

Millis JS (chairman). 1966. The graduate education of physicians: Report of the Citizens Committee on Graduate Medical Education. American Medical Association.

Osler W. 1892. Remarks on specialism. *Archives of Paediatrics* 9:481.

Popper KR. 1972. *Conjectures and Refutations*, 4th edn. London: Routledge and Kegan Paul.

Willard RD (chairman). 1966. Meeting the challenges of family practice: Report of the Ad Hoc Committee on Education for Family Practice of the Council on Medical Education. American Medical Association.

World Health Organization. 1978. *Alma-Ata 1978: Primary Health Care*. Geneva: World Health Organization.

Notes

1. In Britain, Australia, New Zealand, and South Africa the term physician is equivalent to internist in North America. In the United States and Canada, physician is a generic term for all medical practitioners. In this book we have used it in its generic sense.

2. The gradual absorption of apothecaries into the medical profession could conceivably have a modern parallel. If nurse practitioners assume more functions at present regarded as "medical," they may eventually be redefined as physicians.

3. The growing use of alternative medicine could be interpreted as a response to some of medicine's shortcomings.

4. An early pioneer of postgraduate training for general practice was Dr. Andrija Stamper of the former Yugoslavia.

5. WONCA has advanced the international development of family medicine and primary care in projects such as the International Classification of Primary Care (1987) and its Statement on the Role of the Family/General Practitioner in Health Care Systems (1988).

6. For a more detailed discussion of managed care, see Chapter 22.

7. A vision of the future medical school is provided by the report of the Pew-Fetzer Task Force (Tresolini CP and the Pew-Fetzer Task Force. 1994. *Health Professions Education and Relationship-centered Care*; San Francisco, CA: Pew Health Professions Commission).

2

Principles of Family Medicine

Family medicine can be described as a body of knowledge about the problems encountered by family physicians. This is, of course, a tautology, but then so are the descriptions of all applied subjects. As in other practical disciplines, the body of knowledge encompassed by family medicine includes not only factual knowledge but also skills and techniques. Members of a clinical discipline are identifiable not so much by what they know as by what they do. Surgeons, for example, are identifiable more by their skill in diagnosing and treating "surgical" diseases than by any particular knowledge of anatomy, pathology, or clinical medicine. What they do is a matter of their mind set, their values and attitudes, and the principles that govern their actions.

In describing family medicine, therefore, it is best to start with the principles that govern our actions. We will describe nine of them. None is unique to family medicine. Not all family physicians exemplify the whole nine. Nevertheless, when taken together, they do represent a distinctive worldview—a system of values and an approach to problems—that is identifiably different from that of other disciplines.

1. Family physicians are committed to the person rather than to a particular body of knowledge, group of diseases, or special technique. The commitment is open-ended in two senses. First, it is not limited by the type of health problem. Family physicians are available for any health problem in a person of either sex and of any age. Their practice is not even limited to strictly defined health problems: the patient defines the problem. This means that a family physician can never say: "I am sorry, but your illness is not in my field." Any health problem in one of our patients is in our field. We may have to refer the patient for specialized treatment, but we are still responsible for the initial assessment and for coordination and continuity of care. Second, the commitment has no

defined end point. It is not terminated by cure of an illness, the end of a course of treatment, or the incurability of an illness. In many cases the commitment is made while the person is healthy, before any problem has developed. In other words, family medicine defines itself in terms of relationships, making it unique among major fields of clinical medicine. The full implications of this difference are discussed on pages 16 and 17.

2. The family physician seeks to understand the context of the illness. "To understand a thing rightly, we need to see it both out of its environment and in it, and to have acquaintance with the whole range of its variations," wrote the American philosopher William James (1958). Many illnesses cannot be fully understood unless they are seen in their personal, family, and social context. When a patient is admitted to the hospital, much of the context of the illness is removed or obscured. Attention seems to be focused on the foreground rather than the background, often resulting in a limited picture of the illness.

3. The family physician sees every contact with his or her patients as an opportunity for prevention of disease or promotion of health. Because family physicians, on the average, see each of their patients about four times a year, this is a rich source of opportunities for practicing preventive medicine.

4. The family physician views his or her practice as a "population at risk." Clinicians think normally in terms of single patients rather than population groups. Family physicians have to think in terms of both. This means that patients who have not attended for such procedures as immunization, papanicolaou smears, or blood pressure test are as much a concern as those who are attending regularly. Electronic records make it very easy to maintain up-to-date attendance records of the whole practice population.

5. The family physician sees himself or herself as part of a communitywide network of supportive and health-care agencies. All communities have a network of social supports, official and unofficial, formal and informal. The word network suggests a coordinated system. Up to recently this has often not been the case. Too often, family physicians, hospital doctors, medical officers of health, home care nurses, social workers, and others have worked in watertight compartments without a grasp of the system as a whole. At the time of writing, many jurisdictions are in the process of reforming general practice as a key link in the network, which will enable patients to benefit from whichever provider they require.

6. Ideally, family physicians should share the same habitat as their patients. In recent years, this has become less common, except in rural areas. Even here, the commuting doctor has made an appearance. In some communities, notably the central areas of large cities, doctors have virtually disappeared. This has all been part of the recent trend toward the separation of life and work. To Wendell Berry (1978) this is the cause of many modern ills: "If we do not live where we work, and when we work," he writes, "we are wasting our lives, and our work too." The Love Canal disaster in Niagara Falls provides a vivid illustration of what can happen when physicians are remote from the environment

of their patients. This abandoned canal had been used by a local industry for the disposal of toxic waste products. The canal was then covered over and, some years later, houses were built on the site. During the 1960s, householders began to notice that chemical sludge was seeping into their basements and gardens. Trees and shrubs died, and the atmosphere became polluted by malodorous fumes. About the same time, residents in the neighborhood began to suffer from illnesses caused by the toxic chemicals. It was not, however, until a local journalist did a health survey in the area that an official health study was done. This showed rates of illness, miscarriage, and birth defects far in excess of the norm (Brown, 1979). How did the cluster of illnesses in an obviously polluted environment escape the notice of local physicians? One can only assume that they treated patients without seeing them in their home environment. It is difficult to believe that a neighborhood family physician, visiting patients in their homes and interested in their environment, would have remained unaware of the problem for so long. To be fully effective, a family physician still needs to be a visible presence in the neighborhood.

7. The family physician sees patients in their homes. Until modern times, attending physicians in their homes was one of the deepest experiences of family practice. It was in the home that many of the great events of life took place: being born, dying, enduring or recovering from serious illness. Being present with the family at these events gave family doctors much of their knowledge of patients and their families. Knowing the home gave us a tacit understanding of the context or ecology of illness. Ecology, derived from two Greek words, oikos (home) and logos, means literally "study of the home." The rise of the modern hospital removed much of this experience from the home. There were technical advantages and gains in efficiency, but the price was some impoverishment of the experience of family practice. The current redefinition of the hospital's role is now changing the balance again and we have the opportunity to restore home care as one of the defining experiences and essential skills of family medicine. The family physician should be a natural ecologist (see Chapter 16). At the time of writing, a shortage of general practitioners (GPs) has made it difficult for practices to visit their patients in their need. At the same time, there are new reasons for attending housebound patients. Hospitals are dangerous for the elderly, from hospital infections and rapid deterioration from the change of environment. Attending patients with short-term illnesses prevents patients spreading or acquiring diseases in emergency rooms, and doctors' offices. Advances in technology have made diagnosis and therapy much easier than before.

8. The family physician attaches importance to the subjective aspects of medicine. For many years, medicine has been dominated by a strictly objective and positivistic approach to health problems. For family physicians, this has always had to be reconciled with a sensitivity to feelings and an insight into relationships. Insight into relationships requires knowledge of emotions, including our own emotions. Hence, family medicine should be a self-reflective practice (see pp. 81 to 85, Chapter 5).

9. The family physician is a manager of resources. As generalists and first-contact physicians, they have control of large resources and are able, within certain limits, to control admission to hospital, use of investigations, prescription of treatment, and referral to specialists. In all parts of the world, resources are limited, sometimes severely limited. It is, therefore, the responsibility of family physicians to manage these resources for the benefit of their patients and for the community as a whole. In certain cases, the interests of an individual patient may conflict with those of the community as a whole, and this can raise ethical issues.

Implications of the Principles

Defining our discipline in terms of relationships sets it apart from most other fields of medicine. It is more usual to define a field in terms of content—diseases, organ systems, or technologies. Clinicians in other fields form relationships with patients, but in general practice the relationship is usually *prior* to content. We know people before we know what their illnesses will be. It is, of course, possible to define a content of general practice, based on the common conditions presented to family physicians at a particular time and place. But strictly speaking, the content for a particular doctor is whatever conditions his or her patients happen to have. *One of the consequences of this is that family physicians' practices frequently have a low prevalence of many rare diseases (e.g., Charcot-Marie-Tooth disease, myasthenia gravis). This means that sometimes an individual practitioner will become knowledgeable about individual rare diseases, especially in the way that they affect his/her patients.* Other relationships also define our work. By caring for members of a family, the family doctor may become part of the complex of family relationships, and many of us share with our patients the same community and habitat.

Defining our field in these terms has consequences, both positive and negative. Not to be tied to a particular technology or set of diseases is liberating. It gives general practice a quality of unexpectedness and flexibility in adapting to change. On the other hand, it is poorly understood in a society that seems to place less and less value on relationships and emphasizes brief episodic encounters. In current society many equate the idea of specialization with progress itself, though not without its critics. According to Wright, "As cultures grow more elaborate, and technologies more powerful, they themselves become ponderous specializations—vulnerable and, in extreme cases, deadly."[1] One major consequence of the family medicine worldview is that we cannot be comfortable with the mechanical metaphor that dominates medicine, or with the mind/body dualism derived from it. Another is that the value we place on relationships influences our valuation of knowledge. Those who value relationships tend to know the world by experience rather than by what Charles Taylor (1991) calls "instrumental" and "disengaged" reason. Experience engages our feelings as well as our intellect. The emotions play a very significant part in family practice.

Long-term relationships lead to a buildup of particular knowledge about patients, much of it at the tacit level. Because caring for patients is about attention to detail, this knowledge of particulars is of great value when it comes to care. On the other hand, it can make us somewhat ambivalent about classifying patients into disease categories. "Yes," we might say, "this patient has borderline personality disorder but he is also John Smith, who I have cared for for fifteen years." On the whole, our tendency to think in terms of individual patients more than abstractions is a strength, though it can lead us astray if it diverts us from the appropriate pursuit of diagnostic precision. Our valuation of particular knowledge, however, can make it difficult for us to feel comfortable in the modern academic milieu, where diagnosis and management are more usually seen in terms of generalizations than particulars. The risk of living too much in a world of generalizations and abstractions is detachment from the patient's experience and a lack of feeling for his suffering. Abstraction produces accounts of experience that, for all their generalizing power, are stripped of their affective coloring and far removed from the realities of life. The ideal for all physicians is an integration of the two kinds of knowledge: an ability to see the universal in the particular.

The most significant difference between family medicine and most other clinical disciplines is that it transcends the mind/body division that runs through medicine like a geological fault line. Most clinical disciplines lie on one side or the other: internal medicine, surgery, and pediatrics on one side; psychiatry, child psychiatry, and psychogeriatrics on the other. Separate taxonomies of disease lie on either side: textbooks of medicine and surgery on one, the *Diagnostic and Statistical Manual of Mental Disorders* on the other. Therapies are divided into the physical and the psychological. In clinical practice, internists and surgeons do not normally explore the emotions, psychiatrists do not usually examine the body. Because family medicine defines itself in terms of relationships, it cannot divide in this way.[2]

One of the legacies of the mind/body division is a clinical method that excludes attention to the emotions as an essential feature of diagnosis and management. Another is the neglect in medical education of the emotional development of physicians. A contemporary writer has referred to the "stunted emotions" of physicians (Price, 1994). We may be seeing the consequences of this neglect in the alienation of patients from physicians, the widespread criticism of medical care, and the high levels of emotional distress among physicians.

Because family medicine transcends the "fault line," the conventional clinical method has never been well suited to family practice. Perhaps this is why the moves to reform the clinical method have often come from family medicine. The most important difference about the patient-centered clinical method is that attention to the emotions is a requirement. Family medicine has also emerged as one of the most self-reflective of disciplines.

With developments in cognitive science and psychoneuroimmunology, and the high prevalence of illness that does not lie on one side or the other, the fault line is likely to become increasingly redundant. As medicine strives to achieve a new synthesis, it could learn much from our experience.

Conflicting Roles

Hidden among the principles are some potential conflicts between the family doctor's roles and responsibilities. The first principle is one of commitment to the individual patient, to respond to any problem the patient may bring. It is the patient who defines the problem. According to the third principle (responsibility for prevention), it is usually the doctor who defines the problem, often in situations where the patient has come for an entirely different purpose. It may be argued that anticipatory medicine is part of good clinical practice. Taking the blood pressure is part of the general clinical assessment, and if the diastolic pressure is 120 mm Hg, good preventive and clinical practice requires that the problem be attended to, even if the patient has no symptoms related to high blood pressure and has only come because of a tension headache.

The issue becomes more complex as one moves along the continuum from the presymptomatic detection of disease to the identification of risk factors arising from a patient's habits and way of life. The number of risk factors increases and the reduction of risk involves behavioral changes that may be very difficult to attain. All this may be successfully integrated with clinical practice, and may actually be demanded by a public who are educated to expect anticipatory care. At some point, however, an emphasis on anticipatory care may compete for time and resources with care based on responding to problems identified by patients. Striking the right balance may be difficult if physicians are constrained either by requirements of managed care or by funding arrangements designed to emphasize anticipatory care.

The fourth principle (the practice as a population at risk) adds another dimension. Here, the focus is switched from the individual to the group. The measure of success is statistical. The motivation may be to extend effective care to all patients in the practice, especially those who may not be aware of its availability. The other extreme, however, is to judge success by the magnitude of adherence in the practice population. If funding is dependent on certain targets, outreach to the practice population may compete for time and resources with other practice services, and there may be pressure on patients to adhere to recommendations. The demand on practice resources may be increased by approaches aimed at identifying unmet needs in the geographic area of the practice, and of conducting audits requiring expensive epidemiological methods. Too much emphasis on the population approach, at the expense of meeting the needs of individual patients, may, as Toon (1994) suggests, have an effect on the orientation and thought patterns of the physicians. Rather than thinking about their patients, they may find themselves preoccupied with their figures.

The ninth principle (management of resources) may also become the source of conflict if a practice becomes responsible for managing and paying for all the services needed by its enrolled patients. The time necessary for management may reduce the time for patient care, and conflicts of interest may arise when an individual patient's interest conflicts with the interests of the group, or if the doctor stands to gain from economies in expenditure.

Conflicting ideas on the roles of the family physician can make it difficult to agree on criteria of quality, especially at times of rapid social change like the present. Toon (1994) suggests that where there is already a strong tradition of general medical practice there may be an intuitive concept of good general practice that will eventually lead to a synthesis. The path to a synthesis will be easier if administrators and managers tread lightly in making changes that alter the balance between the doctors' responsibilities, especially those changes that can divert us from our traditional responsibilities to individual patients.

Continuity of Care

For a discipline that defines itself in terms of relationships, continuity in the sense of an enduring relationship between doctor and patient is fundamental. Hennen (1975) has described five dimensions of continuity: interpersonal, chronological, geographic (continuity between sites: home, hospital, office), interdisciplinary (continuity in meeting a variety of needs, e.g., for obstetric care, surgical procedures), and informational (continuity through the medical records). We use continuity here in the sense of overall, direct, or coordinative responsibility for the different medical needs of the patient (Hjortdahl, 1992a). The key word here is *responsibility*. Obviously the physician cannot be available at all times, nor can he or she carry out all the care a patient may need. The doctor is responsible for ensuring continuity of service by a competent deputy and for following through when some aspect of care is delegated to a consultant. Responsibility is the key in all important relationships.

On the basis of a sequence of studies from a number of perspectives, Veale (1995, 1996)[3] has described four types of general practice utilization. In the first, a consumer visits only one GP. In the second, all the visits are to one practice. In the third type, the consumer visits a variety of GPs for different purposes. One doctor may be seen because of proximity to place of work, another for proximity to home, or the selection of GP may depend on the nature and severity of the problem and the doctor's expertise. This type of utilization appeared to work well for consumers who take responsibility for coordinating their own care. In the fourth type of utilization, the consumers decide which doctor they will see on a visit-by-visit basis, with no expectation that there will be continuity of care from any of them.

There was strong preference, by both consumers and doctors, for the first type of utilization. Three benefits were associated with visits to one GP: coordination of care, familiarity and openness in the therapeutic relationship, and the opportunity for monitoring of treatment and mutual agreement about management. However, consumers who had all their visits to one GP did not necessarily reap the benefits of continuity. Nor did visits to several GPs in the same practice, or to GPs in different practices, preclude continuity.

Brown et al. (1997) have shown that continuity of care can be experienced by patients even in a university group teaching practice with frequent changes of trainees.[4] Long-term patients of the practice, recruited to focus groups, identified four factors contributing to their experience of continuity: the sense of being known as a person by the doctors, nurses, and receptionists; the relationship with a team of doctor–nurse–trainee–receptionist; the sense of responsibility demonstrated by the physicians, including their openness and honesty in dealing with uncertainty; and the comprehensiveness and availability of the services provided, including a 24-hour on-call service and willingness to see patients at home and in the hospital.

Continuity in the doctor–patient relationship is a mutual commitment. Veale concludes that it is best understood, "not as an entity provided by doctors, but rather as an interaction over time, constructed jointly by consumers and their G.P.s." Continuity "cannot be delivered to a passive recipient by the G.P., however skillful." The essential preconditions of continuity were ready access, competence of the doctor, good communication, and a mechanism for bridging from one consultation to the next. There was a tendency for young and healthy people to prefer the visit-by-visit approach, for people with young children to have continuity with a practice, for those with several distinct problems to visit a variety of GPs, and for the elderly and people with serious illness to prefer continuity with one doctor. Attitudes to continuity may therefore change as people grow older and experience different needs (Veale, 1996).

It is difficult for a doctor to feel continuing responsibility for a patient who does not value it. Some experience of a continuing commitment is required for a sense of responsibility to grow. Hjortdahl (1992a) found that duration of the relationship and frequency of contacts (density) were important in developing the sense of responsibility. After one year, the odds of the doctor feeling this sense doubled, and after five years they increased 16-fold. If there were four or five contacts over the previous year there was a 10-fold increase in the sense of continuing responsibility, compared with only one visit.

Once this mutual commitment has developed, failure to honor the commitment may be seen as a betrayal of trust: if, for example, the doctor terminates the relationship when a patient develops AIDS or is too ill to leave home.

A commitment of this nature carries with it a sense of loyalty. Spiro, quoting Royce reminds us that loyalty is: "the willing and practical and thoroughgoing devotion of a person to a cause. A man [or woman] is loyal when, first, he has some cause to which he is loyal; when, secondly, he willingly and thoroughly devotes himself to this cause; and when, thirdly, he expresses his devotion in some sustained and practical way, by acting steadily in the service of his cause" (Spiro, 1998). Loyalty is a virtue if it is directed at something greater than self-interest or group interest. The proper application of any virtue such as loyalty requires constant attention to the ever changing context and a sense of proportionality. It is tied to the old concept of justice as the sense of giving anything or anyone their just "due" (Grant, 1986). This exercise requires self-discipline and sometimes is referred to as mindfulness. "If I am loyal, my cause must from moment to moment fascinate me, awaken my muscular vigor, stir me with some eagerness for work, even if this be painful work. I cannot be loyal to barren abstractions. I can only be loyal to what my life can interpret in bodily deeds." In the words of George Grant: "In the traditional teaching about justice it was recognized that human nature was so constituted that any desire which has not passed through the flesh by way of actions and settled dispositions appropriate to it is not finally real in the soul."

The value placed on continuity of personal care is reflected in the way a practice is organized. Reception staff can make every effort to book patients with their chosen physician. The practice's philosophy of continuity can be clarified and conveyed to staff and patients. Individual patients' preferences with regard to continuity can be noted, and if possible, accommodated. The on-call system can be organized so that patients see a doctor who communicates with their own doctor, has access to their medical record, and can make a home visit when required. Dying patients, and others with special needs, can be kept out of the on-call system. Continuity can be enhanced by having the patient's record available at all times to those providing care.

The Doctor's Work

Continuity of care is based on the idea that physicians cannot be substituted for one another like replaceable parts of a machine. What kind of people will physicians become if they treat themselves as replaceable parts? In his book *The Transformations of Man*, Lewis Mumford (1972) describes work as an educative process. He quotes Le Play as saying, "The most important product that comes out of the mine is the miner." In his book *Good Work*, Schumacher (1979) describes work as "one of the most decisive influences on (a person's) character and personality." Yet, he writes, "The question of what the work does to the worker is hardly ever asked."

Hannah Arendt differentiated between three types of activity: action, work, and labor (Graner, 1987). Action, the highest of human activities, is self-expression; it has no product to which it is secondary; the activity is good in its own right. Work has an end or product, but still has an element of self-expression in that the worker—a craftsman or artist—can put something of himself or herself into the product. The products are not standardized; each one is unique. In his book *Akenfield*, about the changing life of an English village, Ronald Blythe (1969) describes how plowmen used to work in the old days:

Each man ploughed in his own fashion and with his own mark. It looked all the same if you didn't know about ploughing, but a farmer could walk on a field ploughed by the different teams and tell which bit was ploughed by which. Sometimes he would pay a penny an acre extra for perfect ploughing.... The men worked perfectly to get this, but they also worked perfectly because it was their work. It belonged to them. It was theirs.

In labor, man has the least opportunity for self-expression and he produces nothing that is his own. The production line is a modern example of labor, but history has many others. (One laborer is indeed replaceable by any other.) Even labor can be redeemed, but only by making it an opportunity for fellowship, as when laborers share danger, or sing together as they work.

Some historic trends have been moving medicine away from action toward labor. The whole aim of technology is to turn out a standardized product of high quality and consistency. This is not an ignoble aim and, wherever it is attainable in medicine, is to be welcomed. Sometimes new technologies replace human activities that have become drudgery. At the time when the printing press was introduced, hand copying had become a standardized, repetitive activity. In medicine, however, the opportunities for standardization are limited. Human variability is such that for a seriously ill person, the physician cannot be entirely replaced by a machine. If we insist on treating ourselves as such, we should not be surprised if society treats us as laborers rather than as professionals. We should also not be surprised if it does something to us as people. As we withdraw from our patients we will be the poorer for it. Our professional lives will be less satisfying and we will lose much of the depth of experience that medicine can give us.

Changes in the organization of the practice can interfere with the patient–doctor relationship. Difficulty in getting appointments can divert patients with acute illness to the Emergency Room or walk-in clinic, or to another doctor in the practice. Keeping some gaps in the schedule for patients with acute illnesses does not take much time and will maintain the doctor's experience in this branch of medicine. A practice that opts out of home or hospital visits, or out of hours service, will cut itself off from many of their patients.

Robert Louis Stevenson thought that the physician, like the soldier, the sailor, and the shepherd, stood above the common herd. In all generations up to our own, the people who followed these callings were brought face-to-face with the fundamental data of human existence. For the physician, it was the daily confrontation with disease and death. Our technology now makes it possible to experience disease more as a computer printout, a scan, or monitor reading, and to distance ourselves from the dying. Because our work has a great influence on the kind of people we become, the implications for our profession are profound. Susanne Langer (1979) also wrote of how we find meaning in our work:

Men who follow the sea have often a deep love for that hard life.... Waters and ships, heaven and storm and harbour, somehow contain the symbols through which they see meaning and sense in the world...a unified conception of life whereby it can be rationally lived. Any man who loves his calling loves it for more than its use; he loves it because it seems to have 'meaning'.

Unfortunately, we do not always have the choice of how we will work. There is a strong trend toward managed care, either in the form of large corporations, or in state-controlled health services. Much of this is the inevitable result of the increasing complexity of medicine, the need to control costs, and the desire for equality of access to care. The drive by managers for efficiency can place stresses on relationships between doctors and patients and between professional colleagues. The rigid application of clinical guidelines, and the enforcement of sharply defined professional roles, can be a threat to clinical judgment and professional morale. The fragmentation of medicine makes it necessary to distinguish the roles of primary care physician and referral specialist. But the types of collaboration between family physician and specialist vary from patient to patient and condition to condition. It is better to leave room for clinical judgment and some flexibility of professional roles. Tight control can become soul destroying, with an ultimate reduction, rather than improvement, in efficiency and quality.

Cumulative Knowledge of Patients

Continuous and comprehensive care allows the family physician to build up, piece by piece, a "capital" of knowledge about patients and families. This is one of the family physician's most precious assets. Hjortdahl (1992a) found a strong link between continuity of personal care and accumulated knowledge. Knowledge accumulates slowly during the first few months of the relationship, increases sharply between 3 and 12 months, then flattens out somewhat, but still increases steadily during the next few years. The frequency of contact also contributes to the accumulation of knowledge, the major impact being at four to five visits a year. Much of this knowledge is at the tacit level. Prior knowledge reduced the duration of the consultations in 40 percent of visits and was associated with fewer tests, more use of expectant management, fewer prescriptions, more use of sickness certification, and more referrals (Hjortdahl and Borchgrevink 1991; Hjortdahl 1992b). Doctors felt that prior knowledge contributed more to management than diagnosis, and more to chronic problems than to minor infections and injuries. The contribution of personal knowledge to our work accounts for the nakedness we feel when seeing a patient for the first time and, most poignantly, when we leave our practice and find that there is a whole body of knowledge we cannot take with us. It is a fallacy to assume that we have a comprehensive knowledge of all our patients, however, even after many years. The knowledge is acquired only as the opportunity arises and when it is needed. Often it is acquired only when the patient is ready to give it. Only in a minority of patients does this knowledge amount to a full picture.

The Role of Generalist

The family physician is, by nature and function, a generalist. If any organization is to remain healthy, it must have a balance between generalists and specialists. If this seems like a statement of the obvious, let us remember that until very recently, many influential voices in medicine questioned the value of a medical generalist. The explosion of knowledge, this argument ran, has made it impossible for any individual to cover the whole field: it is inevitable, therefore, that medicine will fragment into specialties as it advances. The fallacy in the argument is the assumption that knowledge is a quantity—a lump of material that grows by accretion. We call it "the lump fallacy." The naivete of the assumption can be demonstrated by following the argument to its conclusion. Let us assume that the knowledge of one branch—pediatrics, for example—is at present of a quantity that can be covered by one physician. If knowledge is exploding, then after *n* years, it will have to fragment into pediatric subspecialties, and after another interval each subspecialty will have to fragment again, and so on. If the original assumption is correct, then there is no reason why the process should stop at any time, for further fragmentation is always possible. What we end with, of course, is a *reductio ad absurdum*. Nevertheless, the prospect of being a generalist is one that many students and residents find daunting. It may be helpful, therefore, to examine the role of generalist in medicine and other walks of life, for the generalist/specialist problem runs through the whole of modern society.

The role of generalists in any organization—whether it be a business, a university, or an orchestra—can be described as follows: They have a perspective of the whole organization—its history and traditions, its general structure, its goals and objectives, and its relationships with the outside world. They understand how each part functions within the whole. They act as a communication center: information flows to them from all parts of the organization and from the outside world; information flows from them in both these directions. They help the organization adapt to changes, both internal and external. Problems arising within the organization, or between the organization and its environment, come to the generalist for assessment. Having defined the problem, the generalist may either deal with it or refer it to a specialist.

Once the problem has been defined as lying in his or her field, the specialist may then take on a decision-making role, with the generalist maintaining overall responsibility for ensuring that the problem is dealt with in the best interests of the whole organization. If the specialist finds that the problem is not in his or her field, it is referred back to the generalist. If we substitute the word organism, person, or family for organization, it is not difficult to see how these functions are carried out by the family physician.

Much of the apprehension about becoming a generalist is based on six misconceptions about the roles of generalist and specialist in medicine:

1. *The generalist has to cover the whole field of medical knowledge.* The generalist's knowledge is just as selective as the specialist's. Like specialists, generalists select the knowledge they need to fulfill their role. In subarachnoid hemorrhage, for example, the family physician needs to know the presenting symptoms and the cues that enable him or her to make an early diagnosis and referral. The neurosurgeon, on the other hand, needs to know the detailed pathology and the techniques of investigation and surgical treatment. I have chosen as an example a condition in which the generalist's role is chiefly early identification of the problem. In other conditions, of course, the generalist will retain total responsibility for management, and the knowledge required will differ accordingly.

2. *In any given field of medicine, the specialist always knows more than the generalist.* This statement expresses the feeling of generalists that when they survey the field of medical knowledge, there is no area they can call their own. Wherever they look, there is some specialist whose knowledge is greater than theirs. But this is not true. We become knowledgeable about the problems we commonly encounter. Specialists become knowledgeable about rarer variants of disease because they are selected for them by generalists. Generalists become knowledgeable about the common conditions that rarely reach the specialists. Family physicians sometimes encounter this when, under pressure from a patient or his family, they consult a specialist even though they know that they are in full command of the situation. They then find to their surprise that the specialist is out of his or her depth, because it is a common variant of the disease that he or she has rarely encountered. Note that the two domains complement each other. Specialists can become knowledgeable about the rare variants only because their experience is concentrated for them by generalists.

3. *By specializing, one can eliminate uncertainty.* The only way to eliminate uncertainty is, as Gayle Stephens (1975) pointed out, to reduce problems to their simplest elements and isolate them from their surroundings. Any clinical specialty that did this would soon cease to be of value.

4. *Only by specializing can one attain depth of knowledge.* This fallacy confuses depth with detail. Depth of knowledge depends on the quality of the mind, not on its information content. The difference between depth and detail is illustrated in a story told of the Vietnam War by Peer de Silva (1978). De Silva was listening to a briefing for Robert McNamara during one of his visits to Saigon. McNamara was bombarding the briefing officers with questions about yards of barbed wire and gallons of gasoline. "I sat there amazed," wrote de Silva, "and thought to myself, what in the world is this man thinking about? This is not a problem of logistics. . . . This is a war that needs discussion of strategic purpose and of strategy itself. What is he talking about?" McNamara was, of course, a generalist and an able one. But in this case he was confusing depth with detail, thus failing to identify the main problem.

5. *As science advances, the load of information increases.* The contrary is true. It is the immature branches of science that have the greatest load of information: "The factual burden of a science varies inversely with its level of maturity," wrote Sir Peter Medawar (1967). "As science advances, particular facts are comprehended within, and therefore, in a sense annihilated by, general statements of steadily increasing power and compass—whereupon the facts need no longer be known explicitly, that is, spelled out and kept in mind." Imagine what it must have been like to learn about infectious diseases before the days of Koch and Pasteur! It is true, of course, that information, as measured by publications, is increasing exponentially. We must not make the mistake, however, of equating this information with knowledge. Much of it is of little value, much of it ephemeral, much of technical interest to specialists only, and much of it related to the testing of hypotheses that will eventually be rejected or incorporated into the main body of medical knowledge.

6. *Error in medicine is usually caused by lack of information.* Very little medical error is caused by physicians being ill informed. Much more is caused by carelessness, insensitivity, failure to listen, administrative inefficiency, failure of communication, and many other factors that have more to do with the attitudes and skill of the physician than his lack of factual knowledge. Naturally, we want physicians to be well-informed, but this will not guarantee medical care of high quality. The physician must also know how to obtain information and how to use it.

Society's attitude to generalists, like its attitude to work, has implications for the development of the human personality. In his book *The Conduct of Life*, Lewis Mumford (1951) describes the effects of the fragmentation produced by our mechanistic culture: "In accepting this partition of functions and this overemphasis of a single narrow skill, men were content, not merely to become fragments of men, but to become fragments of fragments: the physician ceased to deal with the body as a whole and looked after a single organ. . . ."

"As a result," Mumford goes on, "the apparently simple notion of the balanced person...almost dropped out of existence: repressed in life, rejected in thought. Even groups and classes that had once espoused the aristocratic ideal of living a full and rounded life,...dropped their traditional aspirations and made themselves over into specialists, those people Nietzsche called *inverted cripples*, handicapped not because they have lost a single organ, but because they have over-magnified it."

To Alfred North Whitehead (1926), wisdom is the fruit of a balanced development of the personality. His criticism of professional education in his day (the 1920s) was that it lacked balance. The student was expected to master a set of abstractions, but there was no balancing emotional and moral development. If anything, professional education in our own day is even more unbalanced. Perhaps this explains the decline of wisdom that has been a notable feature of the last century.

Many of us live in societies that value excellence. The idea of excellence, however, is the development of a single talent to its utmost limit, whether it is in sport, business, or professional life. Little attention is given to the price that may be paid for this excellence in stunted, one-sided personalities, or to the effects on society as a whole of fostering in its members only one type of excellence. In deciding to be generalists, family physicians have renounced one-sided development in favor of balance and wholeness. They do pay a price for this: in lack of recognition by a society that is itself unbalanced; and in sacrificing special talents in favor of overall excellence. The personal rewards, however, are great. "Only men who are themselves whole," wrote Mumford, "can understand the needs and desires of other men."

Two final points should be made. Because the family physician is a generalist, this does not mean that all family physicians have identical knowledge and skills. All of them share the same commitment to patients. By virtue of special interest or training, however, a physician may have knowledge that is not shared by colleagues. In any group of family physicians, this can be a source of enrichment. One may be skilled in reading ECGs, another may have a special interest in child health or the care of elderly patients. This distinction sometimes becomes blurred in debates between rural and urban physicians, whose workloads differ. Both have become adapted to the needs of their patients and the resources available in the community in which they practice. The rural family physician may be required to do more procedures, including surgery, while the urban family physician may develop greater knowledge and expertise in management of drug dependency for example. Though their practice profiles differ, they are both family physicians who are attending in a comprehensive way to their practice population and the needs of their community. The important point is that this should not lead to fragmentation. Family physicians may be differentiated, but family medicine should not fragment. If it were to do so, the role of generalist would be lost.

The family physician acts not only across clinical boundaries, but across that very difficult one: the boundary between medical and social problems. The boundary is difficult because it is seldom clear-cut. Patients' problems have a way of bestriding it. To the family physician, therefore, falls the responsibility of managing the interface between clinical practice and the counseling professions.

The Human Scale

General practice has traditionally been based in small, widely dispersed units rather than large institutions. This has been important in providing an environment on the human scale, where patients can feel at home in familiar surroundings, close to their own neighborhood. If this sense of intimacy is to be preserved, it is important that these small units continue to be the basic organization of general practice. In former times, the office or surgery was often in the doctor's home, which itself was part of the community served by the practice. Now, the more usual setting is a medical center where family physicians work in a team with other professions. There are many benefits to this type of organization, but there are also risks. The larger the organization, and the more people involved, the more difficult it becomes to preserve the sense of the practice as a welcoming and familiar place.

One disadvantage of the dispersal of general practice in small units is the difficulty we have in organizing ourselves for activities that go beyond the individual practice. This may be needed, for example, when tackling some communitywide health problem, negotiating shared care with specialized services, or arranging deputizing services. The funding of Divisions of General Practice by the Australian government is an approach to meeting this need. Grants are provided to groups of GPs who wish to organize themselves to address issues in their local health services. In the United States, the growth of managed care has stimulated the development of primary care physicians' organizations. In the developed world there are many new versions of primary care renewal. One characteristic common to many of them is the concept of a team approach to delivery of care in the community (Institute of Medicine, 2001). Teams that function effectively have been found to improve access to care, continuity of care, patient satisfaction, and better processes of care for specific diseases (Grumbach and Bodenheimer, 2004). Nevertheless, organizing interdisciplinary teams for the family medicine setting is a challenging task and may involve some drawbacks. The family physician may feel that some of the most important positive interactions with their patients are taken away from them and delegated to other team members, thereby reducing satisfaction with work. The optimal make up of teams that meet the variety of problems common in family medicine will differ from one area to another. There is a move toward a disease management approach in primary care, but patients do not come with a single disease.

Is Family Medicine Universal?

If the principles set out in this chapter have an enduring value, they should be applicable to all cultures and all social groups. If family medicine were to become a service available only to the affluent members of industrialized societies, it would soon lose adherents. Yet there are those who see the problems of poor countries and poor communities as so different that they require a different and more basic approach. Their needs, it is argued, are for clean water, better housing, sanitation, and immunization, rather than for the type of personal care provided by family physicians.

There is some truth in this. Elementary public health measures are still the first need in many societies. But they are not the only need. Other problems will yield only to the personal, family-centered approach. Dr. Cicely Williams (1973), well known for her description of kwashiorkor, became convinced that the answer to malnutrition was family-based health care.

We believe firmly that these principles have universal application. How they are applied, however, will vary according to circumstances. If there is only one physician for 50,000 people, it is obvious that his or her role as a manager of resources, leader, teacher, and resource for difficult problems will be predominant. The application of the principles on the personal level will be the responsibility of other personnel working under his or her supervision. With cities in some countries growing in population up to 14 million, the public health services can be overwhelmed, especially when many areas are covered with slums without sewage and garbage disposal and basic communications. In these cases, the task of maintaining health may fall on organizations with physicians who have a generalist orientation.

References

Berry W. 1978. *The Unsettling of America: Culture and Agriculture.* New York: Avon Books.

Blythe R. 1969. *Akenfield: Portrait of an English Village.* London: Allen Lane, Penguin Press.

Brown JB, Dickie I, Brown L, Biehn J. 1997. Long-term attendance at a family practice teaching unit. *Canadian Family Physician,* 43 (May):901.rown MH. 1979. Love Canal and the poisoning of America. Atlantic Monthly, December.

De Silva P. 1978. *Sub rosa: The C.I.A. and the Uses of Intelligence.* New York: Times Books.

Graner JL. 1987. The primary care crisis, part II: The physician as labourer. *Humane Medicine* 3:20.

Grant G. 1986. *Technology and Justice.* Toronto: Anansi Press.

Grumbach K, Bodenheimer T. 2004. Can health care teams improve primary care practice? *Journal of the American Medical Association* 291(10).

Hennen BKE. 1975. Continuity of care in family practice, part 1: Dimensions of continuity. *Journal of Family Practice* 2(5):371.

Hjortdahl P, Borchgrevink CF. 1991. Continuity of care: Influence of general practitioners' knowledge about their patients on use of resources in consultations. *British Medical Journal* 303:1181.

Hjortdahl P. 1992a. Continuity of care: General practitioners' knowledge about, and sense of responsibility towards their patients. *Family Practice* 9(1):3.

Hjortdahl P. 1992b. The influence of general practitioner's knowledge about their patients on the clinical decision-making process. *Scandinavian Journal of Primary Health Care* 10(4):290.

Institute of Medicine. 2001. *Crossing the Quality Chasm: New Health System for the 21st Century.* Washington, DC: Naitonal Academy Press.

James W. 1958. *The Varieties of Religious Experience.* New York: Penguin Books.

Langer SK. 1979. *Philosophy in a New Key.* Cambridge, MA: Harvard University Press.

Medawar PB. 1967. *The Art of the Soluble.* London: Methuen.

Mumford L. 1951. *The Conduct of Life.* New York: Harcourt Brace and World.

———. 1972. *The Transformations of Man.* New York: Harper Torchbooks.

Price R. 1994. *A Whole New Life.* New York: Atheneum Macmillan.

Schumacher EF. 1979. *Good Work.* New York: Harper and Row.

Spiro H. 1998. *The Power of Hope*: A Doctor's Perspective. New Haven, CT and London: Yale University Press.

Stephens GG. 1975. The intellectual basis of family practice. *Journal of Family Practice* 2:423.

Taylor C. 1991. *The Malaise of Modernity.* Concord, Ontario: Anansi Press.

Toon PD. 1994. What is good general practice? Occasional Paper 65. Royal College of General Practitioners.

Veale BM, McCallum J, Saltman DC, Lonesgan J, Wadsworth YJ, Douglas RM. 1995. Consumer use of multiple general practitioners: An Australian epidemiological study. *Family Practice* 12:303.

Veale BM. 1996. Continuity of care and general practice utilization in Australia. Ph.D. thesis, Australian National University.

Whitehead AN. 1926. *Science and the Modern World.* Cambridge: Cambridge University Press.

Williams C. 1973. Pediatric perceptions: Health services in the home. *Pediatrics* 52:773.

Notes

1. Wright R. 2004. *A Short History of Progress.* Toronto. House of Anansi Press, p. 29.

2. For a fuller discussion of these implications, see article by McWhinney IR.1996. "The Importance of Being Different." *British Journal of General Practice* 46:433–36).

3. Bronwyn Veale used four research methods: epidemiological surveys, interviews, focus groups, and health diaries kept by patients, combined with monthly interviews. The latter method enabled utilization by each patient to be studied along a trajectory.

4. Brown and her colleagues formed five focus groups from patients who had been with the practice for over 15 years ($n = 55$). The average age of participants was 55 and the average time as a patient of the practice was 21 years. About half the patients had made visits to both staff physicians and trainees, the remainder receiving care primarily from either staff physician or a succession of trainees.

3

Illness in the Community

Studies of illness in the community have revealed that physicians see only a small fraction of the health problems experienced by the population at large. Green et al. (2001) recently brought up to date a summary of the data from a number of community surveys in a diagram reproduced in Figure 3.1. Of a thousand people in the general population over the age of 16, in a typical month, 800 will report having some sort of symptom and 327 will consider seeking medical care. One hundred and thirteen will attend the office of a primary care physician, 65 will visit a complementary or alternative care provider, 21 will go to an outpatient clinic at a hospital, and 14 will receive home care. Only 13 will go to an emergency department and 8 will be hospitalized. Fewer than 1 will be admitted to an academic health science center.

In retrospective population surveys, about 90 percent of adults report a symptom during the previous two weeks. Only one in every four or five of these have consulted a physician in that period (Wadsworth, Butterfield, Blaney, 1971; Dunnell and Cartright, 1972).

In an interview survey in Glasgow, Hannay (1979) found that 86% of adults and children reported at least one physical symptom in a 2-week period. The most common symptoms were respiratory, with tiredness being second and headaches being third in order of frequency. The predominance of respiratory symptoms was similar to that in surveys in Australia and the United States. Respiratory illness is also the most common diagnosis in general practice. Fifty-one percent of adults had one or more mental symptoms in the 2-week period (e.g., anxiety, depression, insomnia, obsessional thoughts, paranoid ideas). Twenty-four percent of the children were reported by parents to have behavioral problems (e.g., developmental problems, enuresis, school problems, discipline problems). Almost a quarter of the adults had at least one social problem (e.g., unemployment, financial difficulties).

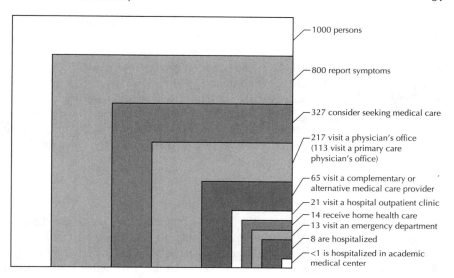

1000 persons

800 report symptoms

327 consider seeking medical care

217 visit a physician's office
(113 visit a primary care
physician's office)

65 visit a complementary or
alternative medical care provider

21 visit a hospital outpatient clinic

14 receive home health care

13 visit an emergency department

8 are hospitalized

<1 is hospitalized in academic
medical center

Figure 3.1 Monthly prevalence of illness in the community and the roles of various sources of health care. (From Green et al., 2001.)

Analysis of simple correlations in the Glasgow survey showed that a high prevalence of symptoms was associated with increasing age, female sex, unemployment due to illness, marital separation or divorce, passive as opposed to active religious affiliation, living on or above the fifth floor in high-rise flats, and a high number of moves of domicile (mobility). The neuroticism score increased with all the adult symptom frequencies. Subjects with low extroversion scores had significantly more mental and social symptoms. On regression analysis, the neuroticism score, age and sex, living in high-rise flats, passive religious affiliation, and mobility all remained significant variables.

Health diary studies have provided useful insights into the symptom burden that exists in the population. In a prospective study using the health diary method, adults recorded at least one complaint on 21.8% of days and only on 6% of these days was a doctor consulted (Roghmann and Haggerty, 1972). In a study of 107 participants extending over a 3-week period, 3.25 problems were recorded, but less than 6% of these resulted in professional care being sought (Demers, Altamore Mustin, Kleinman, Leonardi, 1980). In a group of elderly people self-treatment was found to be common, with prescription and over-the-counter medications being the most frequent interventions. The decision to seek professional help among this group of people had more to do with the level of pain or discomfort, interference with daily activities, or whether they thought it was something serious, rather than with familiarity with the symptom or causal explanations (Stoller, Forster, Portugal, 1993). In another prospective study of women using health diaries, symptoms were recorded on 10 days out of 28 on the average. The yearly average of symptom episodes was 81. A doctor was consulted for 1 out of every 37 symptom episodes (Banks, Beresford, Morrell, Waller, Watkins, 1975). Women consistently report more physical symptoms than men and in a study comparing health diary entries of a group of women and men over a 4-week period; it was found that negative mood was the strongest predictor of physical symptoms which were, in turn, the strongest predictors of illness behavior. Differences in mood states seems to mediate gender differences in symptom reporting (Gijsbers van Wijk, Huisman, Kolk, 1999). It is clear that the occurrence of symptoms is the norm rather than the exception. The important questions, therefore, are not whether symptoms are present, but how serious or frequent they are, and how they are acted on.

The Sick Role and Illness Behavior

Two concepts are helpful in analyzing the decision to consult a physician: the sick role and illness behavior. The concept of the sick role was introduced by Sigerist (1960) and Parsons (1951). According to Parsons, when a person has consulted a physician and been defined as sick, he or she occupies a special role in society. Entering the sick role has certain obligations and privileges. The individual is exempted from normal social obligations and is not held responsible for his or her incapacity. On the other hand, the sick person is expected to seek professional help and to make every effort toward recovery. Whether a person decides to enter the sick role when he or she becomes ill is dependent on many individual and group factors that are independent of the severity of the illness.

Illness behavior is defined by Mechanic (1962) as "the ways in which given symptoms may be differentially perceived, evaluated, and acted (or not acted) upon by different kinds of persons." The illness behavior exhibited by an individual determines whether or not he or she will enter the sick role and consult a physician. Lamberts (1984) has introduced the concept of problem behavior: the actions of a patient with a problem of living as distinct from an illness.

The importance of distinguishing between illness and illness behavior is illustrated by the irritable bowel syndrome. People with functional gastrointestinal disorders (FGD), including irritable bowel syndrome, were compared to the general population with respect to psychological traits, recent life events, social support, self-rated health, and frequency of physician consultation. The FGD group had significantly worse scores than the general population for depression, emotionality, and physical symptoms. They worried more about their health and their quality of life was lower, they had more negative life events in the previous 12 months, their rating of overall health was lower, and they had fewer social supports. However, when the FGD group were divided into those who consulted a physician and those who did not, the nonconsulters differed from the general population in fewer variables (somatization, emotionality, quality of life, health rating, and social support). Visits to physicians were highly correlated with depression, subjective health rating, and duration of periods with symptoms. Also important was the opinion of the health-care system. It would seem that in people with functional gastrointestinal disorders, there are two kinds of psychological conditions—those related to the illness itself and those related to the decision to seek medical care. Importantly, in this study, life events, whether perceived as positive or negative, correlated with consultation behavior (Herschbach, Henrich, von Rad, 1999).

An understanding of illness behavior can change the perspective of the physician. The key question may be "why did the patient come?" The aim of therapy may be not to remove the symptoms but to help the patient to live with them, as many others in the population have learned to do.

Underreporting of Serious Symptoms and Consultation for Minor Symptoms

Variations in illness behavior are responsible for two phenomena of interest to family physicians: failure to consult with serious symptoms and attendance with minor symptoms.

In the Glasgow survey, Hannay estimated the degree of incongruous referral, defined as either failure to consult with symptoms being assessed by the patient himself or herself as serious, or consulting for symptoms assessed by the patient as minor. Physical, mental, and behavioral symptoms were graded for pain, disability, seriousness, and duration, using the patient's own (or for children's behavioral symptoms, the parents' own) assessment. A mean severity score was then calculated for each subject. Social symptoms were graded separately for worry or inconvenience. The extent of incongruous referral of both kinds is shown in Figure 3.2. Twenty-six percent of people with physical, mental, or behavioral symptoms did not seek professional help for serious symptoms. Eleven percent sought professional help for minor symptoms. For social symptoms, the figures were 16% and 12%, respectively. Of the medical symptoms, behavioral symptoms in children were most likely to be referred for professional help, followed by physical symptoms in all subjects, mental symptoms in adults being the least likely to be referred.

In the Glasgow survey, failure to consult for serious symptoms was associated with unemployment due to illness, passive religious allegiance, lower social class, living alone, and higher neuroticism scores. On regression analysis, neuroticism, poor past and present health, increasing age, female sex, and mobility were significant associated variables.

Consultation for minor symptoms was associated on regression analysis with greater number of present illnesses, separation or divorce, increasing age, female sex, few years in present residence, poor experience with doctors or hospitals, difficulty in contacting doctor, and number of hospital stays.

Other investigators have described factors affecting illness behavior. In his book *The Health of Regionville*, Koos (1954) noted that upper-class persons more often reported themselves ill than did lower-class persons, and were more likely to seek treatment when ill. Lower-class persons had more symptoms, but reported themselves to be less often ill and were less likely to visit a physician. Some of these differences in relation to specific symptoms are illustrated in Table 3.1.

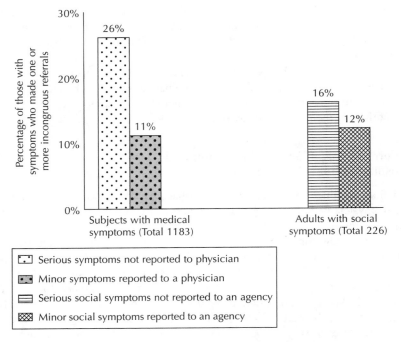

Figure 3.2 Incidence of incongruous referral in the Glasgow survey. (Hannay, Routledge and Kegan Paul 1979. Reprinted with permission.)

In a study of women aged 20 to 44, Banks et. al. (1975) found that those with a high level of free-floating anxiety were more likely to consult their general practitioners about their symptoms. The nature of the symptoms had a strong correlation with the decision to seek care. Table 3.2 illustrates the wide variation in response to different symptoms.

Mechanic (1962) found that persons reporting high stress levels, especially interpersonal difficulties, showed a high inclination to use medical services.

Zola (1966) interviewed Italian-American and Irish-American patients before they saw the physician on new visits to hospital clinics. Information on the primary diagnosis, secondary diagnosis, potential seriousness, and degree of urgency was obtained from the physician. Besides comparisons between the two groups, comparisons were also made between matched pairs of one Irish and one Italian patient of the same sex who had the same primary diagnosis, the same duration of illness, and the same degree of seriousness.

Major differences emerged. The Irish denied that pain was a feature of their illness more often than did the Italians. More Irish described their chief problem in terms of specific dysfunction; more Italians described it in terms of a diffuse difficulty. The Irish tended to limit and understate their difficulties, whereas the Italians tended to spread and generalize theirs. In the matched pairs, the Italians complained of more symptoms, more bodily areas affected, and more kinds of

Table 3.1 Percentage of respondents in each social class recognizing specified symptoms as needing medical attention

Symptom	Class I (N = 51) (%)	Class II (N = 335) (%)	Class III (N = 128) (%)
Loss of appetite	57	50	20
Persistent backache	53	44	19
Continued coughing	77	78	23
Persistent joint and muscle pains	80	47	19
Blood in stools	98	89	60
Blood in urine	100	93	69
Excessive vaginal bleeding	92	83	54
Swelling of ankles	77	76	23
Loss of weight	80	51	21
Bleeding gums	79	51	20
Chronic fatigue	80	53	19
Shortness of breath	77	55	21
Persistent headaches	80	56	22
Fainting spells	80	51	33
Pain in chest	80	51	31
Lump in breast	94	71	44
Lump in abdomen	92	65	34

From Koos, 1954.

Table 3.2 The likelihood of symptom episodes leading to consultation with physician

Symptom	Ratio of Symptom Episodes to Consultations
Changes in energy	456:1
Headache	184:1
Disturbance of gastric function	109:1
Backache	52:1
Pain in lower limb	49:1
Emotional/psychological	46:1
Abdominal pain	29:1
Disturbance of menstruation	20:1
Sore throat	18:1
Pain in chest	14:1

Adapted from Banks et al., 1975.

dysfunction than did the Irish, and more often felt that their symptoms affected their interpersonal behavior.

Zborowski (1951) studied reactions to pain in patients of Jewish, Italian, and "Old American" stock. Data was collected from interviews with patients, from observation of their behavior when in pain, and from discussion with doctors and nurses involved in the care of the individual.

Jews and Italians were described as being very emotional in their responses to pain. Italians, however, were mainly concerned with the immediacy of the pain, whereas Jews focused their concern on the meaning of the pain and its long-term implications. The two groups also differed in their attitudes to analgesic drugs. The Italians called for pain relief and soon forgot their sufferings when this occurred. The Jews were reluctant to accept drugs, were concerned about their side effects, and regarded them as giving only temporary relief.

The "Old American" patients tended to have a detached and unemotional attitude to their pain. Like the Jewish patients, "Old Americans" were concerned about the meaning and future implications of their pain; but, whereas the anxieties of Jews were tinged with pessimism about the outcome, "Old Americans" tended to retain an attitude of optimism born of their confidence in the skill of the expert.

In summary, illness behavior is related to ethnic origin, social class, age, sex, nature of illness, religious affiliation, personality, and environmental factors. Hannay's findings challenge the widely held belief that neuroticism is strongly related to high utilization of services and to consultation about trivia. In the Glasgow study, it was the less neurotic who were more likely to seek professional advice both in general and for "trivia." It was the more neurotic who were most likely to be part of the symptom "iceberg."

Self-Care and Other Alternatives to Medical Care

It will be clear from the studies mentioned that the majority of symptom episodes are managed by the sufferers themselves without recourse to medical advice. Self-care refers to all the actions taken by a sufferer on his or her own behalf. These actions may replace medical advice or they may precede consultation with a physician. Self-care can take a number of forms:

1. Studies in Britain and the United States (Freer, 1978) have shown high rates of self-medication (between 50% and 80% of adults reported taking an over-the-counter medication in a 2- to 4-week period). The great majority of these are analgesics, cold remedies, and antacids. The pharmacist is often a source of advice on over-the-counter medication. In a study of primary care given by pharmacists in London, Ontario, Bass (1975) found that in neighborhood pharmacies, for every 100 prescriptions issued, about 19 other people asked for advice on health problems. The most common of these were upper respiratory infections, stomach and bowel complaints, pain, and inquiries about vitamins.

2. Although most attention has been focused on medication, a large number of other remedial actions may be taken. In a study using the health diary method, Freer (1978) found that a large number of nonmedical actions were reported. Some of these were social actions, like talking to friends or relatives, attending a club, or going out for a meal; others were individual actions, like doing housework, going out shopping, or gardening. All these actions were recorded because they were viewed as being therapeutic.

3. There may be lay referral, or consultation with family members, friends, neighbors, and other nonprofessional people whose advice may be sought. Certain individuals in a neighborhood may have a reputation for being knowledgeable in health matters. Others may be valued for their advice on personal problems. All societies have resources of this kind, quite independent of the health care system. It is likely, however, that in highly mobile societies there is less opportunity for such informal aid systems to develop. This may help explain the large number of personal problems that are presented to family physicians in industrialized societies.

4. Folk healers and practitioners of alternative medicine are widely available in most societies. They may be used as the initial source of care, or as an additional resource when the health-care system has not met the patient's expectations. Alternative medicine is widely used in Western countries (see Chapter 21).

References

Banks MH, Beresford SAA, Morrell DC, Waller JJ, Watkins CJ. 1975. Factors influencing demand for primary medical care in women aged 20–44 years: A preliminary report. *International Journal of Epidemiology* 4:189.

Bass M. 1975. The pharmacist as a provider of primary care. *Canadian Medical Association Journal* 112:60.

Demers RY, Altamore R, Mustin H, Kleinman A, Leonardi D. 1980. An exploration of the dimensions of illness behavior. *The Journal of Family Practice* 11(7):1085–92.

Dunnell K, Cartwright A. 1972 *Medicine Takers, Prescribers and Hoarders*. London: Routledge and Kegan Paul.

Freer CB. 1978. Self care: A health diary study. Master of Clinical Science thesis, University of Western Ontario.

Gijsbers van Wijk CM, Huisman H, Kolk AM. 1999. Gender differences in physical symptoms and illness behavior. *Social Science & Medicine* 49(8):1061–74.

Green L, Fryer GE, Yawn, BP, Lanier D, Dovey SM. 2001. The ecology of medical care revisited. *The New England Journal of Medicine* 344;26:2021–2025.

Hannay DR. 1979. *The Symptom Iceberg: A Study in Community Health*. London: Routledge and Kegan Paul.

Herschbach P, Henrich G, von Rad M. 1999. Psychological factors in functional gastrointestinal disorders: Characteristics of the disorder or of the illness behavior? *Psychosomatic Medicine* 61:148–153.

Koos EL. 1954. *The Health of Regionville: What the People Thought and Did about It*. New York: Columbia University Press.

Lamberts H. 1984. *Morbidity in General Practice: Diagnosis Related Information from the Monitoring Project*. Utrecht: Huisartsenpers.

Mechanic D. 1962. The concept of illness behaviour. *Journal of Chronic Disease 15:189*.

Parsons T. 1951. *The Social System*. Glencoe, IL.: Free Press.

Roghmann KJ, Haggerty RJ. 1972. The diary as a research instrument in the study of health and illness behaviour. *Medical Care* 10:143.

Sigerist HE. 1960. The special position of the sick. In: Roemer MI, ed., *The Sociology of Medicine*. New York: M.D. Publications.

Stoller EP, Forster LE, Portugal S. 1993. Self-care responses to symptoms by older people. A health diary study of illness behavior. *Medical Care* 31(1):24–42.

Wadsworth MEJ, Butterfield WJH, Blaney MEJ, Butterfield WJH, Blaney R. 1971. *Health and Sickness: the Choice of Treatment*. London: Tavistock.

Zborowski M. 1951. Cultural components in responses to pain. *Journal of Social Issues* 8:16.

Zola IK. 1966. Culture and symptoms: An analysis of patients' presenting complaints. *American Sociological Review* 31:614.

4

A Profile of Family Practice

It is difficult to convey in statistical terms a true picture of the content of family practice. One approach is to record the diagnosis made at each patient–doctor encounter. By this means, it is possible to obtain an accurate picture of the family physician's experience with well-defined diseases such as diabetes. Many illness episodes seen by family physicians, however, are much more difficult to define and label. The reader will obtain some idea of the difficulty by reading Case 8.1 in Chapter 8. This patient's problems cannot be expressed by simple disease labels. There is no diagnosis in the usual sense of the term. Another approach is to record the patient's main symptom or complaint. Here again, however, the result may be a very partial picture of the illness because a statement of the symptoms says little or nothing about its origins. If we were classifying Case 8.1 by disease labels, we could call the illness anxiety state or insomnia. If we were classifying the case by symptoms, we could call it insomnia or gastrointestinal symptoms. Whichever route we take, we provide only a partial picture, because we are doing something equivalent to taking a two-dimensional slice through a three-dimensional object. Another difficulty is that we have no assurance that any two physicians will classify the same illness in the same way. If one physician classifies the illness as anxiety state, it will appear in the statistics under the rubric of mental illness. If another classifies it as gastrointestinal symptoms (not yet diagnosed), it will appear under the rubric gastrointestinal diseases. Given these difficulties of nomenclature and standardization, it is small wonder that there are wide variations in such estimates as the amount of psychiatric illness in family practice.

Despite this, however, there are some important areas of agreement regarding the content of family practice in countries with high general standards of living. The collection of reliable data has been enhanced by development of standardized coding systems for primary care (e.g., ICHPPC-2, and ICPC-2-R) by the training of recorders, and by the validation of data. Morbidity studies, some of them national in scope, have been carried out in the United States, Britain, the Netherlands, Australia, Norway, West Germany, Austria, and Barbados. In this chapter we have used several of these studies to give a profile of the work of the family physician, emphasizing especially those features common to all these parts of the world.

Classification of Primary Care

Difficult as it may be, some way of classifying and recording the experience of family practice is necessary if we are to make comparisons between practices or countries, to relate process of care to outcome, or follow trends in illness over time. It is also necessary if we are to learn from our experience by retrospectively reviewing our cases in different disease categories. Accurate classification is required for studies of the natural history of disease and for clinical trials.

Before the development of the International Classification of Primary Care (ICPC), only the ICD (International Classification of Disease) was available. The ICD was based on well-defined disease categories and therefore more suitable for classifying hospital discharges and causes of death than for the earlier manifestations of illness seen in primary care. The ICD classified illness at a high level of abstraction; family physicians operate for much of the time at lower levels of abstraction. Moreover, the ICD, lacking organizing principles, had "become an unstructured amalgam of chapters based variously on anatomy, clinical manifestations, changing views of 'causation,' clinical specialities, and age groups" (White, 1985). ICPC was first published in 1987 by the World Organization of National Colleges, Academies, and Academic Associations of General Practitioners/Family Physicians (WONCA). Since publication, it has received widespread acceptance and use especially in Europe and Australia. Originally designed for paper records, ICPC-2-R was released in 2005 for use in electronic databases.

ICPC breaks new ground by classifying three elements of an encounter between patient and doctor: the reason for encounter (RFE), the diagnosis or problem, and the process of care. Rather than being organized around end points of illness (definitive diagnoses or causes of death), the ICPC is based on episodes of care defined as "a problem or illness in a patient over the entire period of time from its onset to its resolution" (Lamberts and Wood, 1987). One episode therefore, may last over many encounters, and a single encounter often includes several different illness episodes in various states of evolution. An episode of care is different from an episode of illness, which is the period during which a patient has symptoms, and from an episode of disease, which is a health problem from onset to resolution or death. A person may have an illness or disease without coming under care, and may have care (e.g., prenatal) without having an illness or disease. The duration of care for a disease may be different from the duration of the disease.

Classifying the RFE is especially important in family practice where it has much stronger influence in determining costs than it has in specialty care where diagnostic labels tend to drive investigations (Bernstein, Hollingworth, and Viner, 1994).

The structure of ICPC is biaxial, with 17 chapters on the horizontal axis and 7 components on the vertical (Figure 4.1). In the chapters, body systems take precedence over etiology. The patient's reason for encounter is the patient's given reason as interpreted by the doctor. Most are symptoms and complaints, which are recorded under the appropriate chapter heading. Each chapter has rubrics for fear or disability associated with a symptom. If the RFE is a preventive procedure, prescription, test result, or medical certificate, this is recorded under the appropriate chapter heading under components 2, 3, 4, or 5. The process of care and the diagnosis are encoded and recorded under the appropriate chapter heading.

With this structure, ICPC can provide a profile of family practice that represents its complexity (see Figure 4.1).

As in all classification systems, the accuracy of ICPC depends on the skill of the recording physician. The RFE is not necessarily the same as the presenting complaint, and underlying reasons may not emerge at the first encounter. Much depends on the physician's knowledge of the patient and consulting skills. Consistency in assigning diagnostic labels is difficult to attain in the many illnesses that cannot be differentiated to more than low levels of abstraction. All

COMPONENTS \ CHAPTERS	A—General	B—Blood, blood forming	D—Digestive	F—Eye	H—Ear	K—Circulatory	L—Musculoskeletal	N—Neurological	P—Psychological	R—Respiratory	S—Skin	T—Metabolic, Endocrine, Nutr.	U—Urinary	W—Pregnancy, Child bearing, Family planning	X—Female genital	Y—Male genital	Z—Social
1. Symptoms and complaints																	
2. Diagnostic, screening, prevention																	
3. Treatment, procedures, medication																	
4. Test results																	
5. Administrative																	
6. Other																	
7. Diagnoses, disease																	

Figure 4.1 The biaxial structure of ICPC. (From Lamberts H, Wood M, eds. 1987. Copyright 1987 World Organization of National Colleges and Academies of General Practice/Family Medicine. Reproduced with permission.)

classification systems are simplifications of complex processes. We cannot expect them to fully represent the complexity of family practice.

Case 4.1 An episode of care

First visit: Mrs. C is an 80-year-old woman who lives alone since her husband died 8 years ago. She is active in her local church and is locally well known for continuing to regularly attend classes at a local fitness club. She has been diagnosed with diabetes for the past 10 years and takes an active interest in the management of it. Her glycosylated hemoglobin has consistently indicated good control. She attends her physician's office today, however, outside of her usual time for checkup. She relates that she has now come up with the courage to tell her physician that she had an episode of vaginal bleeding 3 months ago. This settled down over two days but then recurred only three days ago and that prompted her to make this appointment. She freely admits that she is afraid of cancer. "I have a lot more things that I want to do." Her physician arranges for a repeat appointment to undertake an endometrial biopsy.

RFE × 12 (postmenopausal bleeding), × 25 (fear of cancer); diagnosis × 12 × 25

Second visit: the bleeding has settled down and no new symptoms are elicited. An endometrial biopsy is completed in the office without problems.

RFE × 37 (diagnostic procedure, histological)

Third visit: the results of the biopsy confirm endometrial carcinoma. When this information is conveyed to her she became understandably upset and had many questions about what treatments were available. She can't understand how she could have cancer when she feels so well. Her physician spends time discussing next steps and arrangements are made for her to see a gynecologist.

RFE × 60 (attending to receive test results), × 45 (health advice/information)

Diagnosis × 77 (malignant neoplasm genital female other) × 60 (test results), × 67 (referral to specialist)

Fourth visit: after seeing the gynecologist and being told that she would have surgery "as soon as possible," she wishes to discuss her concerns with her family physician. Will she need to have chemotherapy? She feels well now, should she go through with treatment that she feels will make her feel sick?

RFE × 45 (health advice/information) Diagnosis × 77 (malignant neoplasm genital female other), × 58 (therapeutic counseling)

Fifth visit: six weeks after complete hysterectomy, she is feeling reasonably well though still a bit weak. She has been told by the gynecologist that they were able to "get everything" and there appears to be no cancer remaining. Nevertheless, she is to see an oncologist in the next week for consultation. Her blood sugars indicate that control has not been as good as in the past even though she has lost some weight after the surgery. Her family physician reviews the need for more regularity in her diet and adjusts her medication. Her daughters have become more solicitous and interfering (in her opinion) and she expresses discomfort about this.

RFE × 45 (health advice re: test results), Z20 (relationship problem parent/children), Diagnoses × 77 (malignant neoplasm genital female other), T90 (diabetes non insulin dependent), T45 (health counseling/advice)

Sixth visit: she returns to see her family physician after seeing the oncologist who has not recommended any further treatment at this time, but will see her regularly in follow up. She asks if her family physician can do the follow up. "that cancer clinic makes me nervous." Her blood sugars are once again in good control and she is feeling generally better. She wants to discuss living wills with her family physician. RFE × 45 (health advice), P01 (feeling anxious/nervous), Diagnosis × 77 (malignant neoplasm genital female other), T90 (diabetes non insulin dependent), P74 (anxiety state).

This case outlines a case consisting of two episodes of care: cancer of the uterus an intercurrent illness and diabetes a chronic one.

Symptoms

Table 4.1 gives the ranking order of the 30 most common problems,complaints, or symptoms presented to family physicians in the Netherlands, Japan, Poland, and the United States (Okkes et al., 2002).

Only 35 groups of symptoms/complaints covered the top 30 in all databases and this list represented 45% to 60 % of all reasons for encounter. Further, the top 30 represented 70% to 75% of all encounters per 1,000 patients per year. Limitations to this study are that the data are derived from research practices and may not be representative of all family practices in the represented countries, and that the US data did not include reasons for encounter. Differences exist between the countries in the degree to which family practice contributes to psychological and gynecological care.

These may be compared with the 10 most common presenting complaints in one Canadian and one British study (Tables 4.2 and 4.3). When comparing these figures, allowance must be made for the different ways in which symptoms were classified. Even so, there is substantial agreement between the two lists, both for males and females.

Diagnoses

Table 4.4 lists the 30 most common diagnosis clusters recorded on ambulatory patients by office-based physicians in the National Ambulatory Care Survey (NACS). Table 4.5 shows the ranking order of the ICD-9 chapters in the Fourth National Morbidity Study, England and Wales 1991–1992 (McCormick, Fleming, and Charleton, 1995). The diagnoses were recorded by general practitioners in a representative sample of practices in England and Wales. The table also shows the percentage of patients from the defined practice populations consulting in each category. Table 4.6 shows the number and proportion of visits to primary care physicians in the U.S. National Ambulatory Care Survey (Cherry, Woodwell, and Rechsteiner, 2007). Note that the denominator in this table is the number of patients visiting, not the practice populations as in Table 4.5. In spite of wide variation in time and place, these lists exhibit a broad consistency. The Direct Observation in Primary Care (DOPC) study provides important insight into the content of the practices of 138 family physicians in the state of Ohio. In this multimethod study 4,454 patient visits were observed by trained research nurses.

Table 4.1 Most frequent (groups of) reasons for encounter in the form of a symptom/complaint per 1,000 patients per year, standardized for the 1996 sex/age distribution of the US population

ICPC Codes	Symptom/Complaint	Netherlands	Japan	Poland	United States (% family physician)
R05/R07	Cough/sneezing/nasal congestion	163	292	684	295 (41)
R21/R22/R23	Throat/voice/tonsil symptom/complaint	66	81	250	102 (33)
A02/A03	Fever/chills	71	158	155	99 (29)
L02/L03/L05	Low back/back/flank symptom/complaint	88	28	64	135 (51)
D01/D06	Abdominal pain	77	34	76	42 (34)
A04	Tiredness	76	21	35	60 (26)
R02/R03	Shortness of breath/wheezing	73	9	14	59 (27)
S06/S07	Redness of skin	72	52	42	64 (31)
N01	Headache	48	49	39	68 (40)
H01	Earache	47	12	24	59 (33)
L15	Knee symptom/complaint	45	20	28	55 (12)
P03	Feeling depressed	16	—	8	53 (16)
S04	Localized swelling skin	53	14	19	28 (56)
L14	Leg/thigh symptom/complaint	38	11	14	51 (25)
K01/K02/L04	Heart/chest pain/tightness	48	15	49	42 (34)
D09/D10	Nausea/vomiting	34	49	24	42 (37)
F05/F07	Vision problems	8	2	38	48 (8)
P01	Feeling anxious/nervous/tense	26	1	14	47 (17)

Code	Symptom/complaint					
U01/U02/U03	Urination symptom/complaint	22	3	47	37	(25)
L01	Neck symptom/complaint	36	16	18	44	(48)
L08	Shoulder symptom/complaint	42	12	16	40	(52)
S03	Warts	40	1	4	12	(27)
D11	Diarrhea	20	38	21	28	(36)
S02	Pruritis	37	19	25	25	(29)
L12	Hand/finger symptom/complaint	27	12	14	36	(21)
D02/03	Stomach pain/heartburn	28	25	33	34	(33)
L17	Foot/toe symptom/complaint	34	10	19	22	(17)
N17	Vertigo	29	14	17	32	(34)
H02	Hearing complaint	29	2	15	12	(15)
R09	Sinus symptom/complaint	24	2	14	29	(37)
H13	Plugged feeling in ear	22	1	10	12	(36)
P06	Sleeping disturbance	18	6	9	20	(25)
S18	Laceration	18	17	14	10	(46)
D19/D20	Mouth/tongue/teeth symptom/complaint	15	15	12	2	(51)
S12	Insect bite	3	11	2	3	(42)
	Total top 30s	1491	1052	1867	1747	
	All symptoms/complaint reasons for encounter per 1,000 patients per year	3362	1923	3375	2598	(31)

Source: Based on top 30 of the reasons from the Netherlands, Japan, Poland, and United States (from NAMCS data) (Okkes et al., 2002).

Table 4.2 The 10 most common presenting symptoms in males from Canadian and British group practice

Canadian Practice	British Practice
Cough	Cough
Sore throat	Rash
Colds	Sore throat
Abdominal/pelvic pain	Abdominal pain
Rash	Bowel symptoms
Fever/chills	Chest pain
Earache	Back pain
Back problems	Spots, sores, ulcers
Skin inflammation	Headache
Chest pain	Joint pain

Source: From Bass, 1977; and Morrell, 1972.

Table 4.3 The 10 most common presenting symptoms in females from a Canadian and British group practice

Canada	Britain
Abdominal/pelvic pain	Cough
Cough	Rash
Sore throat	Sore throat
Menstrual disorders	Spots, sores, ulcers
Colds	Abdominal pain
Rash	Bowel symptoms
Depression	Back pain
Vaginal discharge	Chest pain
Anxiety	Gastric symptoms
Headache	Headache

Source: From Bass, 1977; and Morrell, 1972.

The nurses gathered information on the content of each visit using validated instruments (Davis Observation Code), direct observation of services offered, a patient exit questionnaire, medical record review, a practice environment checklist, billing data and ICD-9-CM diagnoses, a physician questionnaire, and field notes. The most common diagnostic clusters were hypertension, upper respiratory infection, and general medical examination. The top 25 diagnoses represented 61% of visits. The fact that nearly 40% of visits were not classifiable in one of these clusters, again emphasizes the great variety of problems addressed in family practice (Stange, Zyzanski, Jaén, Callahan, Kelly, and Gillanders, 1998). These tables illustrate some of the key features of morbidity in family practice: the great variety of problems encountered; the high incidence of infectious disease, especially of the respiratory tract; the high prevalence of chronic disease, especially hypertension, diabetes, ischemic heart disease, and arthritis; the high frequency

Table 4.4 Number and percent distribution of office visits with corresponding standard errors, by the 20 leading primary diagnosis groups according to patient's sex: United States, 2005

Primary Diagnosis Group and ICD–9–CM Code(s)[1]	Number of Visits in Thousands	Standard Error in Thousands	Percent Distribution	Standard Error of Percent	Female[2] Percent Distribution	Female Standard Error of Percent	Male[3] Percent Distribution	Male Standard Error of Percent
All visits	0	963,617	40,611	100.0	...	100.0	...	100.0	...
Essential hypertension	401	44,670	4,318	4.6	0.4	4.4	0.4	5.0	0.5
Routine infant or child health check	V20.2	41,816	4,044	4.3	0.4	3.3	0.3	5.7	0.6
Acute upper respiratory infections, excluding pharyngitis	460–461, 463–466	36,372	2,875	3.8	0.3	3.3	0.3	4.5	0.4
Arthropathies and related disorders	710–719	34,299	4,200	3.6	0.4	4.2	0.6	2.7	0.3
Malignant neoplasms	140–208, 230–234	28,709	5,644	3.0	0.6	3.0	0.7	3.0	0.4
Diabetes mellitus	250	25,451	2,730	2.6	0.3	2.5	0.3	2.9	0.3
Spinal disorders	720–724	22,732	2,523	2.4	0.2	2.4	0.2	2.3	0.3
Rheumatism, excluding back	725–729	18,580	1,580	1.9	0.1	1.9	0.2	1.9	0.2
General medical examination	V70	17,007	2,377	1.8	0.2	1.5	0.2	2.2	0.3
Follow-up examination	V67	16,249	2,573	1.7	0.2	1.7	0.3	1.6	0.3
Specific procedures and aftercare	V50–59.9	15,662	2,000	1.6	0.2	1.7	0.2	1.5	0.3
Normal pregnancy	V22	15,509	2,534	1.6	0.3	2.8	0.5	...	...

(continued)

Table 4.4 Continued

Primary Diagnosis Group and ICD-9-CM Code(s)[1]		Number of Visits in Thousands	Standard Error in Thousands	Percent Distribution	Standard Error of Percent	Female[2]		Male[3]	
						Percent Distribution	Standard Error of Percent	Percent Distribution	Standard Error of Percent
Gynecological examination	V72.3	15,067	2,378	1.6	0.2	2.7	0.4	...	...
Otitis media and eustachian tube disorders	381–382	14,399	1,517	1.5	0.1	1.2	0.1	1.9	0.2
Asthma	493	12,823	2,102	1.3	0.2	1.1	0.2	1.6	0.4
Disorders of lipoid metabolism	272	12,650	1,416	1.3	0.1	1.1	0.2	1.6	0.2
Chronic sinusitis	473	12,621	1,302	1.3	0.1	1.2	0.1	1.4	0.2
Heart disease, excluding ischemic	391–392.0, 393–398, 402,404, 415–416, 420–429	11,473	1,490	1.2	0.1	1.0	0.1	1.5	0.2
Acute pharyngitis	462	11,064	1,941	1.1	0.2	1.1	0.2	1.3	0.3
Allergic rhinitis	477	11,028	2,099	1.1	0.2	1.1	0.2	1.2	0.3
All other diagnoses		545,437	23,756	56.6	0.8	56.8	1.0	56.4	1.0

Note: Numbers may not add to totals because of rounding.

... Category not applicable.

[1] Based on the Informational Classification of Diseases, Ninth Revision, Clinical Modification (ICD-9-CM) (23). However, certain codes have been combined in this table to form larger categories that better describe the utilization of ambulatory care service.

[2] Based on 560,355,000 visits made by females.

[3] Based on 403,262,000 visits made by males.

Source: Cherry, Woodwell, and Rechtsteiner, 2007.

Table 4.5 Ranking order of diagnostic chapters (ICD-9) in fourth national morbidity study (England and Wales, 1991–1992)

ICD-9 Chapters	Percentage of Patients Consulting at Least Once
Preventive and administrative (supplementary classification)	33
Respiratory	30
Nervous system and sense organs (includes ear and eye infections)	17
Symptoms, signs, and ill-defined disorders	15
Musculoskeletal	15
Skin	15
Genitourinary	15
Infectious and parasitic	14
Injuries and poisoning	14
Circulatory	9
Digestive	9
Mental	7
Endocrine	4
Neoplasms (all)	2.4
Neoplasms (malignant)	1
Blood and blood-forming organs	1

Source: From *Morbidity Statistics from General Practice* 1991–1992 (1995) Crown Copyright 1995. Reproduced by permission of the Controller of HMSO and of the Office for National Statistics.

of depression and anxiety; and the low frequency of diseases such as cancer, which are so common in hospital practice.

One characteristic of family practice that is not captured in tables of this kind is multimorbidity which is defined as the simultaneous occurrence of several medical conditions in the same person. Because family physicians explicitly take responsibility for a comprehensive approach to their patients, multimorbidity represents a greater proportion of the workload in this discipline than in specialties. Starfield, Lemke, Bernhardt, Foldes, Forrest, and Weiner (2003) found that, for both index conditions and their comorbidities, visits to primary care physicians greatly exceeded visits to specialists, the only exception being some uncommon chronic conditions. Prevalence estimates of multimorbidity vary depending on the source of the data (administrative data sets, population surveys, family practice registers), age, and whether the data were restricted to chronic conditions. Chronic conditions vary in severity and the clinical burden that they represent. Fortin, Bravo, Hudon, Vanasse, and Lapointe (2005) used the Cumulative Illness Rating Scale (CIRS) to measure the impact of multimorbidity in family practices in the Saguenay district of the Province of Quebec. Recruiting 980 patients from the waiting rooms of 21 family practices, charts were reviewed by trained nurses and information extracted on the number and severity of chronic medical

Table 4.6 Number and percent distribution of office visits with corresponding standard errors, by physician's primary diagnosis: United States, 2005

Major Disease Category ICD-9-CM Code Range[1]		Number of Visits in Thousands	Standard Error in Thousands	Percent Distribution	Standard Error Percent
All visits	......	963,617	40,611	100.0	......
Infections and parasitic diseases	001–139	26,720	2,062	2.8	0.2
Neoplasms	140–239	39,200	5,285	4.1	0.5
Endocrine, nutritional and metabolic diseases, and immunity disorders	240–279	56,408	4,655	5.9	0.4
Mental disorders	290–319	47,094	3,777	4.9	0.4
Diseases of the nervous system and sense organs	320–389	86,128	6,644	8.9	0.5
Diseases of the circulatory system	390–459	81,836	6,683	8.5	0.6
Diseases of the respiratory system	460–519	110,999	7,670	11.5	0.7
Diseases of the digestive systems	520–579	28,678	2,225	3.0	0.2
Disease of the genitourinary system	580–629	42,256	3,131	4.4	0.3
Diseases of the skin and subcutaneous tissue	680–709	44,443	3,189	4.6	0.3
Diseases of the musculoskeletal system and connective tissue	710–739	80,601	6,320	8.4	0.5
Symptoms, signs, and ill-defined conditions	780–799	60,536	3,916	6.3	0.3
Injury and poisoning	800–999	45,137	3,087	4.7	0.3
Supplementary classification	V01–V82	179,276	11,124	18.6	0.9
All other diagnoses[2]	......	25,609	3,533	2.7	0.3
Unknown[3]	......	8,697	1,645	0.9	0.2

Note:... Category not applicable

[1]Based on the *International Classification of Diseases, Ninth Revision, Clinical Modification* (IDC-9-CM) (23).

[2]Includes diseases of the blood and blood-forming organs (280–289); complications of pregnancy, childbirth, and the puerperium (630–677); congenital anomalies (740–759); certain conditions originating in the perinatal period (760–779); and entries not codable to the ICD-9-CM (e.g., illegible entries, left against medical advice, transferred, entries of "none" or "no diagnoses").

[3]Includes blank diagnosis.

Source: Cherry, Woodwell, and Rechtsteiner, 2007.

conditions. Nine out of 10 of these individuals had more than one chronic condition and approximately 50% had five or more. The most common diagnoses were hypertension, hyperlipidemia, and rheumatologic diseases. The number of chronic conditions and the CIRS score was higher in women than men and in both genders increased with age. However, the three most common diagnoses did not differ in frequency between men and women.

Multimorbidity impacts family practice in a number of ways: (1) healthcare delivery is complicated and individual patient encounters more complex. Family physicians address more than three problems more than one-third of the time. (Beasley et al., 2004); (2) clinical practice guidelines (CPGs) generally focus on one disease at a time and do not take into consideration that most patients that are meant to be targeted by them have more diseases than the one covered by them; randomized control trials (many of which underpin the CPGs) usually exclude participants with multimorbidity casting doubt on their applicability or transferability to family practice (Fortin et al., 2006); (3) there is a major impact on time management (Ostbye et al., 2005), and (4) multimorbidity affects the cognitive strategies of family physicians (Christensen, Fetters, and Green, 2005).

A study at the University of Southern California (USC) (Meldenhall, Girard, and Abrahamson, 1978) showed major differences in practice patterns in different regions of the United States. It also showed, however, that there was very little tendency by family physicians to restrict their practices by age or sex. Whatever the age or sex of the physicians, they saw patients of all ages and both sexes. Family practice appeared, therefore, to have maintained its character as a generalist discipline.

Some other features of general practice seem to be universal. Studies in several parts of the world have shown that women consult family physicians more often than males, even after allowing for attendances during pregnancy. The reasons for this difference are not known. Between 70% and 80% of members of a practice consult at least once a year. The average number of visits per member is between three and five.

Sources of Variation in Family Practice

Although the average morbidity and utilization patterns in family practice are remarkably similar in all parts of the world with a similar standard of living, there are some major differences between practices. The following are the main sources of variation:

1. *Local conditions.* The strongest influence on family practice is the local context, including the population structure, economic conditions, the physician–population ratio, availability of other primary care services, and administrative constraints. In poor communities with a low doctor–population ratio, family physicians see more patients per hour. When the ratio becomes extremely low, physicians have to delegate much of the patient care to other personnel and act

as resources, teachers, and administrators for a primary care organization. The use of diagnostic tests is related to local resources.

The services provided by family physicians are influenced by the availability of other primary-care services in the area. Where there are specialized emergency services, family physicians are less involved with trauma. The same applies with such services as family-planning clinics, sexually transmitted disease clinics, well-baby clinics, and so on. The availability of other physicians providing primary care (pediatricians, obstetricians, internists) has a strong influence on the content of family practice. Because alternative primary-care services are more readily available in urban areas, rural family physicians usually provide a wider range of services.

2. *The age of the physician.* As doctors grow older, so do their patients. In the USC study, there was a linear relationship between the age of the doctor and the mean age of his patients. A family practice is like an organism, developing, changing, and adapting over the years as the physician also grows older and changes. Demographic differences between practices result in differences in morbidity patterns and therefore in utilization. For these reasons, older doctors see more chronic illness and do less obstetrics.

3. *The gender of the physician.* Female physicians see a higher proportion of female patients than male physicians. In the USC and NAMCS studies, 75% of the patients seen by women physicians were female, compared with 58% seen by male physicians. This appears to be a common finding in countries where women have only recently begun to enter family practice in large numbers. Whether it will change as the number of women family physicians begins to equal or exceed the number of male family physicians remains to be seen.

4. *Distribution of diagnoses.* Some diagnoses are associated with high- or low- utilization patterns (Lamberts, 1984). Chronic disease, for example, is associated with a high encounter rate, but few new episodes of illness or new problems, and few out-of-hours calls. Childhood illness is associated with many new problems, many out-of-hours calls, and a low encounter rate per episode. Psychological and social problems (problem behavior) are associated with both a large number of episodes of illness and a large number of encounters per episode.

5. *Vocational training.* Family physicians who are graduates of vocational training programs show differences from those who did not receive vocational training. In the USC study, residency trained physicians did more tests, prescribed fewer drugs, gave fewer injections, spent more time with patients, and did more counseling. These differences were not all explained by the fact that residency-trained physicians were younger. Another study showed that residency-trained physicians were more likely to have practices organized for prevention with such tools as age–sex registers, prevention flowcharts, and recall systems (Audunsson, 1986). In a Canadian study, Borgiel et al. (1989) found that vocational training in family medicine was significantly and positively related to criteria for quality in charting, periodic health maintenance, medical care, and use of indicator drugs.

In some jurisdictions there is a separation between general practice and hospital inpatient care. If this applies to obstetrics, then obstetrics may be completely excluded from general practice, or the general practitioner's role may be limited to antenatal and postnatal care.

The service profile of general practitioners in Europe was found to vary with whether or not they performed a gatekeeping role in the health-care system as well as remuneration methods "the concept of comprehensive and family care is included in the usual definitions of general practice, but, in some countries, separate provision is made for gynecology and pediatrics" (Boerma, Van Der Zee, and Fleming, 1997).

In economically advanced countries, family physicians can usually take it for granted that basic public health services like clean water, sanitation, and food inspection are provided. In other countries this is not so, and family practice will be correspondingly different. Even in developed countries, there are often communities where standards of public health are poor enough to make an impact on the content of practice. Because these are unusual, family physicians in developed countries are not usually well trained in the environmental aspects of family practice.

References

Audunsson GG. 1986. Preventive infrastructure in family practice. Master of Clinical Science thesis, University of Western Ontario.

Bass MJ. 1977. Symptoms in primary care. *Medifacts* 7(5): Tables 4.2 and 4.3.

Beasley JW, Hankey TH, Erickson R, Stange KC, Mundt M, Elliott M. et al. 2004. How many problems do family physicians manage at each encounter? A WReN Study. *Annals of Family Medicine* 2(5):405–410.

Bernstein RM, Hollingworth GR, Viner GS. 1994. Something Old, Something New, Something Borrowed: A Review of Standardized Data Collection in Primary Care. Journal of the American Informatics Association: Proceedings from the 18th Annual Symposium on Computer Applications in Medical Care.

Boerma WGW, Van Der Zee J, Fleming DM. 1997. Service profiles of general practitioners in Europe. *British Journal of General Practice* 47:481–486.

Borgiel AEM, Williams JI, Bass MJ, Dunn EV, Evensen MK, Lamont CT. et al. 1989. Quality of care in family practice: Does residency training make a difference? *Canadian Medical Association Journal* 40:1035.

Cherry DK, Woodwell DA, Rechtsteiner EA. 2007. National Ambulatory Medical Care Survey: 2005 Summary, Advance Data, from Vital and Health Statistics, U.S. Department of Health and Human Services, 387(June 29).

Christensen RE, Fetters MD, Green LA. 2005. Opening the black box: Cognitive strategies in family practice. *Annals of Family Medicine* 3:144–150.

Fortin M, Bravo G, Hudon C, Vanasse A, Lapointe L. 2005. Prevalence of multimorbidity among adults seen in family practice. *Annals of Family Medicine* 3(3):223–228.

Fortin M, Dionne J, Pinho G, Gignac J, Almirall J, Lopinte L. 2006. Randomized controlled trials: Do they have external validity for patients with mulitple comorbidities. *Annals of Family Medicine* 4(2):104–108.

Lamberts H. 1984. *Morbidity in General Practice: Diagnosis Related Information from the Monitoring Project*. Utrecht: Huisartsenpers.

Lamberts H, Wood M, eds. 1987. *ICPC: International Classification of Primary Care.* Oxford/New York: Oxford University Press.

McCormick A, Fleming D, Charleton J. 1995. *Morbidity Statistics from General Practice, Second National Study 1991–1992.* London: Her Majesty's Stationery Office.

Meldenhall RC, Girard RA, Abrahamson S. 1978. A national study of medical and surgical specialties: I. Background, purpose and methodology. *Journal of the American Medical Association* 240:848.

Morrell DC. 1972. Symptom interpretation in general practice. *Journal of the Royal College of General Practitioners* 22:297 (see Tables 4.2 and 4.3).

Okkes IM, Polderman GO, Fryer GE, Yamada T, Bujak M, Oskam SK et al. 2002. The role of family practice in different health care systems: A comparison of reasons for encounter, diagnoses, and interventions in primary care populations in the Netherlands, Japan, Poland, and the United States. *Journal of Family Practice* 51(1):72.

Ostbye T, Yarnall YSH, Krause KM, Pollak KI, Gradison M, Michener JL. 2005. Is there time for management of patients with chronic diseases in primary care? *Annals of Family Medicine* 3:209–214.

Stange KC, Zyzanski SJ, Jaén CR, Callahan EJ, Kelly RB, Gillanders WR et al. 1998. Illuminating the 'black box'. A description of 4454 patient visits to 138 family physicians. *Journal of Family Practice* 46(5):377.

Starfield B, Lemke KW, Bernhardt T, Foldes SS, Forrest CB, Weiner JP. 2003. Comorbidity: Implications for the importance of primary care in "case" management. *Annals of Family Medicine* 1(1):8–14.

U.S. Department of Health, Education and Welfare. National Ambulatory Care Survey. 1977–78. Public Health Service, National Center for Health Statistics.

White KL 1985. Restructuring the International Classification of Diseases: Need for a new paradigm. *Journal of Family Practice* 21(1):17–18, 20.

5

Philosophical and Scientific Foundations of Family Medicine

Like any other branch of science or technology, medicine is based on theory. It is, of course, quite possible to practice for a whole lifetime without being aware of the theory, let alone questioning it. Remarkable as it may seem, the curriculum in most medical schools devotes very little time to examining the ideas on which medicine is based. Small wonder, then, that for many physicians the ideas are a given and discussions about them are considered unprofitable. For some periods of medical history, this does not matter very much: physicians can practice quite confidently and successfully without examining their assumptions, even if it means ignoring for the time being some problems that do not seem to fit. There are other times, however, when problems we have conveniently set aside become more difficult to ignore. At these times, medicine is driven back to an examination of its fundamentals.

Academic family medicine has emerged during one of these periods of reassessment: in a sense, it is itself the product of a ferment of ideas. To understand family medicine, therefore, it is necessary to have a grasp of the ideas on which medicine is based. Moreover, it is important for a newly emergent discipline to be based on firm theoretical foundations. Thomas Kuhn's theory of paradigm change provides a useful frame of reference for a discussion of medical theory.

Paradigm Change in Science

In his influential book, *The Structure of Scientific Revolutions*, Thomas Kuhn (1967) has challenged the conventional view of how science progresses. Kuhn begins by challenging the view that science develops by the accumulation of individual discoveries and inventions. It is true, he says, that for certain periods of time science may appear to develop cumulatively, but this can be misleading. Such a progression only takes place after a scientific community has agreed on a set of shared assumptions about the phenomena that form the subject matter of the science. Once the assumptions have been made, they are no longer questioned. They become embedded in the education of scientists in such a way that they exert a deep hold on the scientific mind, all the deeper for the fact that they are not made explicit. Kuhn refers to this set of received beliefs in a science as a paradigm.[1] He calls the cumulative research that follows the acceptance of a paradigm normal science. He describes research in normal science as "a strenuous and devoted attempt to force nature into the conceptual boxes supplied by professional education."

To take an example from medicine, we might say that one of the assumptions of the existing medical paradigm is that there are such entities as diseases. Once this assumption was made, it became the agenda of normal medical science to describe and establish causes for these entities. But the justification for the assumption was not discussed in the education of physicians. The entities became our conceptual boxes, into which we attempted to force the natural phenomena of illness.

The formation of a scientific discipline begins with the acceptance of its first paradigm. The earlier stages in the history of a science are marked by many competing schools of thought. During this phase, observations are made and facts are gathered, but in the absence of a paradigm there is no organizing principle to indicate to the observer how the facts relate to each other. Kuhn calls this the preparadigm phase. Although this early fact-gathering has been essential to the origin of many sciences, the result is usually, in Kuhn's words, "a morass." "No natural history," says Kuhn, "can be interpreted in the absence of at least some implicit body of intertwined theoretical and methodological belief that permits selection, evaluations, and criticism."

The preparadigm phase is succeeded by a phase in which one of the competing schools of thought is accepted as a paradigm. To be accepted, a theory must seem better than its competitors in tying together and explaining the facts, but it need not, and never does, explain all the facts. The acceptance of a paradigm is the occasion for the formation of a professional discipline, with its own journals, scientific societies, and textbooks. Once a paradigm is accepted, the individual scientist can take it for granted. He need no longer "attempt to build his field anew, starting from first principles and justifying the use of each concept introduced." The process of normal science is referred to by Kuhn as "mopping up." The acceptance of a paradigm provides a research agenda that can keep workers in the field busy for generations.

The process of change begins when normal science encounters anomalies. Because no paradigm is a complete fit with nature, anomalies are always present. At first, however, these may be ignored, or not even perceived, for perceptions are influenced by expectations. Eventually, the anomalies are increasingly recognized. They attain both observational and conceptual recognition, and then, often after a period of resistance, are accommodated within a new paradigm. Sometimes, the anomalies are related to the use of a scientific instrument. Scientists' expectations are influenced not only by their theories but by their instruments. Instruments are designed with particular observations and results in mind. When the observations are different from those expected, the anomaly puts a whole new perspective on the instrumental procedure. The discovery of X-rays by Roentgen, for example, violated deeply entrenched expectations. At the time of the discovery, cathode-ray equipment of the kind used by Roentgen was in use in many laboratories. Other workers must have produced X-rays without observing them. The anomaly was presumably blocked out of their awareness because to have acknowledged it would have been tantamount to rethinking all the previous work done in this field.

In some cases the emergence of anomalies leads to a state of crisis. Failure of normal science to solve the problems created by the anomalies produces a sense of insecurity. From this state of crisis a new paradigm emerges, claimed by its proponents to be more successful in accounting for the anomalies. A period of conflict ensues, with one of three outcomes: success of the old paradigm in handling the crisis; failure of either paradigm to deal with it; or the triumph of the new paradigm.

The change from an old to a new paradigm is revolutionary rather than cumulative. It has been likened to a change of visual Gestalt: a fundamental shift in worldview. In Kuhn's words it is "a reconstruction of the field from new fundamentals, a reconstruction that changes some of the field's most elementary theoretical generalizations." The change, however, does not necessarily add any new facts. Just as in a change of visual Gestalt the picture itself does not change, the paradigm shift is an altered perception of how the facts are related. The fundamental nature of paradigm shift explains some of the features of the conflict. Because it is ultimately about matters that have never been made explicit, it may become extremely bitter and irrational. Adherents of the old paradigm may be incapable of understanding the new one. Proponents of a new paradigm often arise from the periphery of the discipline or from outside it altogether, or they may be young members of the discipline who are able to see it with fresh eyes.

If anomalies are always present, what produces the heightened awareness of them that leads to a state of crisis? There appears to be no single answer. Sometimes, the anomaly calls into question a fundamental generalization of the paradigm; or the anomaly may have practical implications; or a minor anomaly may become a major one when a new experimental technique is developed. Kuhn also mentions social influences in the precipitation of a crisis. At the time of the Copernican revolution there were strong social pressures for change. The Ptolemaic system developed between 200 bc and ad 200 was very successful in predicting the changing positions of both stars and planets. Ptolemaic astronomy is still in use today as a practical approximation. The minor anomalies in the Ptolemaic system became the subject of normal astronomical science in the succeeding centuries. Discrepancies were eliminated by making minor adjustments to the theory, but the cumulative effect was a theory of enormous complexity which, by the sixteenth century, was widely recognized as having failed to solve the traditional problems. In addition to this, there was social pressure for calendar reform, making a solution to the problem of precession of the equinoxes particularly urgent.

Kuhn has not been alone in questioning our assumptions about scientific progress.[2] In *Science and the Modern World*, Whitehead (1926) wrote, "When you are criticizing the philosophy of an epoch, do not chiefly direct your attention to those intellectual positions which its exponents feel it necessary explicitly to defend. There will be some fundamental assumptions which adherents of all the variant systems within the epoch unconsciously presuppose. Such assumptions appear so obvious that people do not know what they are assuming because no other way of putting things has ever occurred to them." In her book *Philosophy in a New Key*, Susanne Langer (1979) observes that when an epoch changes it is not the answers to questions that change, it is the questions themselves. The way a question is framed limits the possible answers. When an epoch changes, questions asked in the previous epoch are not answered differently: the questions themselves are rejected, along with the assumptions behind them. For example, we might respond to the question "Is disease X organic or psychogenic?" by saying "Diseases aren't organic or psychogenic."

The unquestioned assumptions behind a paradigm become embodied in language. The very words we use express our assumptions as if they were given, so when a paradigm changes, it is often necessary to find new words to replace the old. Only in this way can we break free from the shackles that words impose on us. For example, the conventional language of medicine expresses our culture's assumptions about the separation of mind and body in words like psychosomatic and somatization.[3]

Paradigm Change in Medicine

Opinion is divided on whether or not Kuhn's theory applies to medicine. Kuhn himself maintains that paradigm change occurs in applied disciplines, and even in subdisciplines. Our own view is that the theory fits well with the changes occurring in medicine. The old paradigm, also known as the biomedical model, can be described as follows. Patients suffer from diseases that can be categorized in the same way as other natural phenomena. A disease can be viewed independently from the person who is suffering from it and from his social context. Mental and physical diseases can be considered separately, with provision for a group of psychosomatic diseases in which the mind appears to act on the body. Each disease has a specific causal agent, and it is a major objective of research to discover them. Given a certain level of host resistance, the occurrence of disease can be explained as a result of exposure to a pathogenic agent. The physician's main task is to diagnose the patient's disease and to prescribe a specific remedy aimed at removing the cause or relieving the symptoms. To achieve this, the clinician is provided with an intellectual tool, the clinical method known as differential diagnosis. The physician is usually a detached observer and the patient a passive recipient in this process.

This paradigm provides a good fit with certain categories of illness, especially those that dominated medical practice in the nineteenth century. With the major exogenous infections such as cholera and typhoid, and with diseases resulting from nutritional deficiencies, the idea of specific causal agents is a useful one. Under certain conditions, the paradigm is still successful today. In other settings, notably in family practice, it is encountering anomalies that are increasingly difficult to ignore. Because family physicians are among the first to encounter changes in morbidity, they have also been among the first to encounter the anomalies in the old paradigm. In fact they have been encountering them for many years. The old paradigm has never had a very good fit with family practice, and we believe it probable that many family physicians have only partially accepted it.

Anomalies Encountered by the Old Paradigm

The Illness/Disease Anomaly

A large proportion of ill people seen in family practice cannot be assigned to a disease category based on a physiological or anatomical abnormality. Some examples are given in Table 5.1. In the first, Blacklock (1977) examined the records of successive patients presenting with chest pain in a general practice. Only half received a specific diagnosis based on pathology. In the second, the Headache Study Group (1986) followed up 265 patients for a year after they presented in general practice with new headaches. Only 27% received a diagnosis based on demonstrable physical changes such as classical migraine or sinusitis. In the third, Wasson and his colleagues (1981) followed up adult males for three months after they presented with abdominal pain to primary care clinics at veterans' hospitals. Only 30% received pathology-based diagnoses. Of course, the remaining patients in all these examples could be given labels such as intercostal myalgia, tension headache, or irritable colon, but these categories are devoid of predictive or inferential power.

The Specific Etiology Anomaly

If the occurrence of disease depended mainly on the presence of specific causal agents, we would expect that, in a homogeneous population sharing the same environment, different diseases would be distributed evenly across the population. Hinkle and his colleagues (1974) showed that this is not the case. In a 20-year

Table 5.1 Percentage of symptoms presented to primary physicians receiving a specific diagnosis

	Symptom	Study Method	Percentage Receiving Specific Diagnosis
Blacklock, 1977	Chest pain	Chart review	50
Wasson et al., 1981	Abdominal pain in adult males	Chart review Questionnaire	21
Headache Study Group, 1986	Headache	Physician questionnaire Patient interview	27

study of a group of women, similar in age, occupation, background, and environment, they found that 25% had 52% of the illness, and another quartile had only 6% of the illness. They conjectured that the women with high illness rates were susceptible to particular recurring complaints such as headaches, or had a defect in one organ system. This proved not to be the case. The more illnesses a woman had, the more different types of illness she had, and the more organ systems were involved. They then conjectured that these women were susceptible to diseases of a particular etiology, some to infections, some to allergies, and so on. Again, they found this not to be so. Those with the greatest number of illnesses had illnesses of many different causes, more major illness, and more disturbances of mood, thought, and behavior. The main determinant of health and disease in this population was not the presence of specific agents, but the general susceptibility of the individual women.

Even with infectious diseases the doctrine of specific etiology is not very useful in technologically advanced societies, where the citizens are protected against most highly virulent agents. As Dubos (1965) has observed, most of the agents associated with current diseases are ubiquitous in the environment, exist in the body without causing harm under ordinary circumstances, and have pathological effects only when the infected person is under physiological stress. An understanding of health and disease, therefore, requires not only a knowledge of disease agents, but of those factors that protect the host from these agents, or make them more vulnerable to them. Even *Streptococcus and Helicobacter pylori* can be present in the throats and stomachs of healthy people without causing harm.

The Mind–Body Anomaly
Under the old paradigm, mind and body were separated except in certain "psychosomatic" diseases in which psychological factors were thought to be causal. The concept of causation was strongly influenced by the prevailing doctrine of specific etiology. Psychological and social factors were thought to act directly to produce pathological change. Different factors, moreover, were thought to be specific for each psychosomatic disease. This view has now become untenable in the light of recent discoveries. Factors such as social isolation and stressful life events are associated with higher mortality from all causes, not only from certain psychosomatic diseases. Eight prospective, population-based studies have now shown an association between social integration and mortality rates from all causes (Berkman, 1995). In the Alameda County Study, men and women with the fewest social ties were 1.9 to 3.1 times more likely to die in the nine-year follow-up period than those with the most social ties. This was after correcting for other determinants of health (Berkman and Breslow, 1983). Five studies have shown that patients who lack support, live alone, or have not been married have an increased risk of death after a myocardial infarction (Berkman, 1995). In one study, men who were socially isolated were twice as likely to die over a 3-year period after the infarct as those who were not isolated. When this was combined with a general measure of life stressors, the risk increased to four to five times that of men in the low-risk categories (Ruberman et al., 1984).

Studies of different populations have shown consistently that recent stressful life events are associated with an increased risk of illness of many kinds. People who have experienced recent stressful life events, or who are psychologically vulnerable, have greater deterioration of overall health, more diseases of the upper respiratory tract, more allergies, more hypertension, and a greater risk of coronary disease and sudden death (Dohrenwend and Dohrenwend, 1974; Jemmott and Locke, 1984). Coker, Tyrell, and Smith (1991) inoculated healthy volunteers aged between 20 and 55 with either a cold virus or placebo. The rates of respiratory infection and colds increased with the level of psychological stress in a dose–response manner.

Short-term stressors such as student exam stress can delay wound repair and modulate the immune response to a vaccine (Kiecolt-Glaser, McGuire, Robles, and Glaser 2002a). Chronic stress, such as caring for a spouse or parent with dementia has been associated with prolonged endocrine and immune dysregulation as well as changes in health, vaccine response, and wound healing. Burnout, imprisonment, job stress, and unemployment have also been associated with immune modulations (Kiecolt-Glaser, McGuire, Robles, and Glaser, 2002b).

Kiecolt-Glaser, McGuire, Robles, and Glaser (2002c) regard the link between personal relationships and immune function as one of the most robust findings in psychoneuroimmunology: for example, higher NK cell activity was associated with higher level of support in women whose husbands were being treated for cancer. A low sense of coherence in healthy adults was associated with the poorest level of NK cell lysis (sense of coherence is a construct formulated by Antonovsky, 1979). High hostility individuals exhibited greater increases in NK cell cytotoxicity following self-disclosure than those with low hostility (Kiecolt-Glaser, McGuire, Robles, and Glaser, 2002c).

Events involving a loss of important personal relationships appear to have the greatest potential for harm (Kiecolt-Glaser and Glaser, 1995). This emerges strongly in studies of the mortality of bereavement. One prospective study of conjugal bereavement, for example, found increased mortality among widowers, especially between the ages of 55 and 74, for 10 years after the deaths of their wives (Helsing, Szklo, and Comstock, 1981). Divorce and marital separation are also associated with increased risks of illness that are even greater, on an actuarial basis, than those associated with bereavement (Kiecolt-Glaser and Glaser, 1995). Disruption of relationships is a possible explanation for the association between unemployment and an increase in rates of illness and death (Jin, Shah, and Svoboda, 1995).

In addition to the evidence on the effects of social integration and stress, a large body of research supports the influence of personality traits and emotions on the outcome of some disease states. The strongest associations are those between anger, hostility, and depression and poor outcomes in coronary heart disease (CHD). There is some evidence linking emotional suppression with breast cancer incidence and the occurrence of CHD. Emerging evidence is beginning to suggest that pessimism and fatalism may be associated with poorer outcomes in AIDS, cancer, and CHD (Scheier and Bridges, 1995).

Scheier and Bridges (1995) contend that age and stage of disease seem to modulate the strength of the relationship between emotional variables and health. These variables appear to have a stronger effect in younger than in older people and in the earlier rather than the later stages of disease.

The lack of specificity of illness after stressful life events has focused attention on the neuroendocrine and immune systems as the possible pathways through which the emotions can alter susceptibility to illness. Depression of immune function has been found in widowers and widows, divorced men and women, family caregivers of patients with Alzheimer's disease, and students under academic stress (Kiecolt-Glaser and Glaser, 1995). Discussing psychological factors on immune function, Kiecolt-Glaser, Dura, Speicher, Trask, and Glaser (1991) write "However, only a few studies have so far shown a correlation between stressors, immunodepression, and illnesses. We do not know how far immune function must be suppressed to make a person more vulnerable to disease. Studies now in progress may answer this question. Kiecolt-Glaser and Glaser (1995) suggest that stress-related immunosuppression may have its most serious consequences in people whose immune function is already impaired, such as the aged. As noted above, however, a number of studies have shown stronger relationships between emotional factors and health status in younger than in older people, and no studies have reported the opposite (Scheier and Bridges, 1995). The answers to these questions have therapeutic implications, for the same questions could be asked about the therapeutic effect of supportive therapies.

Therapeutic Implications of the Mind–Body Connection

Because of the strong evidence for the health consequences of emotions, relationships, and social integration, we must ask whether supportive therapies can affect the duration or outcome of illness. Several studies have shown that assurance given to patients prior to surgery can reduce the length of postoperative recovery. Patients who reported that doctors who ascertained the patient's meaning of the illness recovered more quickly from a variety of minor illnesses than patients whose doctors did not ascertain the meaning (Bass, Buck, Turner, Dickie, Pratt, and Robinson, 1986).

Several randomized controlled trials have compared groups of cancer patients receiving psychosocial supportive treatment with groups of cancer patients receiving no supportive therapies. No significant difference in life span was found (Goodwin, Leszcz, Ennis, Koopmans, Vincent, Guther et al., 2001; Kissane, Love, Hatton, Bloch, Smith, and Clarke, 2004).

It seems clear, therefore, that supportive group therapy does not prolong the life span in breast cancer patients under the conditions tested. However, this does not prove that the mind has no effect on survival in cancer. Cunningham makes it clear that these studies show "that certain types of short-term group psychological interventions fail to prolong the *mean* or *median* life span of *groups* of cancer patients...What should not be dismissed, however, is the possibility that some therapies may have the potential to extend life in certain patients under some conditions.To rule this out risks making a type II error that could inhibit further research on an issue that is of great importance to many cancer patients" (Cunningham and Edmonds, 2005).

Cunningham cites evidence from his own studies that patients who have gone through a significant life change after psychotherapy, which includes spiritual aspects of healing, survive much longer than their expected prognosis (according to a panel of oncologists). Patients in the same study, who did not go through a life change, did not have prolonged survival.

A randomized controlled trial cannot resolve this question. Research on the effects of psychotherapy is not the same as research on a new drug. There are ways of assessing whether a patient has responded to the drug. The only way of knowing whether a patient has gone through a life change is to examine patients one by one.

In addition to the evidence for the therapeutic benefits of social support, many studies have shown that adults and children can learn to voluntarily control autonomic physiological responses and to alter their cellular and humoral immune responses, by relaxation/imagery, self-hypnosis, and/or biofeedback (Hall, Minnes, and Olness, 1993). Children can reduce the frequency of migraine headaches by self-hypnosis (Olness, MacDonald, and Uden, 1987). Studies in cancer patients suggest that self-hypnosis can lessen pain in patients with breast cancer, and that relaxation and imagery can reduce the nausea and vomiting associated with chemotherapy. Other studies suggest that both individual and group therapies enhance coping skills and reduce anxiety and depression in cancer patients (Classen, Hermanson, and Spiegel, 1994).

There are important implications for family physicians. The support provided by the family doctor, like other supportive therapies, can help improve patients' health and enhance their general resistance; it can combine cognitive approaches with emotional expression and support, and the family doctor is well placed to mobilize support from the patient's family. Other members of the primary care team are also important sources of support. All these therapeutic interventions act not on specific disease states, or on causal agents, but on the patient's resistance, helping patients to become agents of their own healing.

Reviewing the subject of social environment and host resistance Cassel (1976) made three postulates:

1. Social factors enhance or lower susceptibility to disease generally, not to specific diseases.
2. The mechanisms involved are general in nature.
3. Social supports act by buffering the effects of environmental stressors.

The experimental evidence accumulated has supported these postulates.

Much of the discussion of the role of the social environment in disease has been concerned with the concept of stress, a term that is often used rather loosely. In his pioneering work on stress, Selye (1956) used the term to indicate a bodily state resulting from the interaction of the organism with noxious stimuli. The stress state described included adrenal hypertrophy and elevated corticosteroid levels. Since this time, the term stress has been used to denote both the stimulus and the response. Confusion can be avoided by using stressor for the former and stress state for the latter. With social stressors, the issue is complicated by the fact that there is no constant relationship between stressor and stress state. Whether or not a social stimulus is stressful depends very much on its meaning for the individual and on his psychological vulnerability. Hinkle and his colleagues, for example, observed that women with high illness rates were of a different personality type from the women with low illness rates.

The relationship of stressors to mental health has been controversial. Recently, the prevailing view has been that stress is of little significance in accounting for variations in mental health. Using a new method of assessing traumatic events, however, Turner, Wheaton, and Lloyd (1995) reported significant associations between traumatic events in childhood and adult life, and subsequent mental illnesses such as major depression and substance abuse. The lifetime risk of illness increased with the number of traumas prior to the age of 18, and the risk of a recurrence of the illness was strongly associated with the number of additional traumas experienced since the first episode. The childhood traumas included physical abuse, separation from home, substance abuse in a parent, parental unemployment or divorce, serious injury, and sexual abuse (in females). Adult traumas included divorce, substance abuse in spouse, physical abuse by spouse, and infidelity by spouse. The authors noted that the average age at the first episode of illness was 21 and suggested that preventive efforts should be targeted to children and adolescents. Although many of these traumas are unavoidable, their effects on the young can be mitigated.

Because social stimuli act by virtue of their symbolic meaning for the individual, their pathogenicity is of a different order from that of physicochemical stimuli. The latter tend to damage the organism directly; the former act indirectly by modifying the host's response to disease agents.

As family physicians, interested in health as well as disease, we should also think in terms of factors that increase host resistance and strengthen resistance against noxious stimuli. Psychological factors such as coping ability may increase resistance. Social factors can be not only stressful, but supportive. Antonovsky (1979) has called these factors general resistance resources (GRR). There is evidence that social supports can modify the harmful effects of stressful life events. In a prospective study of pregnant women, Nuckolls, Cassel, and Kaplan (1972) studied the relationship of life events and social supports to complications of pregnancy. Life changes were recorded at the 32nd week of pregnancy, using Holmes and Rahe's cumulative life change index (1967). At the same time, social supports were measured by an instrument designed to record the woman's feelings about her pregnancy, her relationship with her husband, and her perception of support from her family and community. After delivery, the records were reviewed blindly for complications of pregnancy or delivery. Ninety percent of women with high life change scores and low social supports had one or more complications. Among women with equally high life change scores, but high social supports, only 33% had one or more complications. In a large prospective study in Israel, Medalie and Goldbourt (1976) found that men with severe family problems were three times more likely to develop angina than those with few family problems. In men with high anxiety levels, the risk of developing angina was significantly lower in those who received much support and love from their wives than in those who did not. Social support protects men from the health consequences of loss of employment, including the physical indicators of arthritis (Cobb and Kasl, 1977; Gore, 1978). A number of studies also indicate that social support influences the course and outcome of illness and injury (Turner, 1983).

There is evidence for the influence of social support on mental health, especially on depression (Turner, 1983). Much of this evidence points to the protective or buffering effects of social supports in individuals experiencing stressful events. Other studies, however, have suggested that social support has a main and independent relationship with mental health, as well as moderating the effect of stressful life events. Education of families in coping and providing support reduces the relapse rate in patients with schizophrenia (McFarlane, 1992). After an extensive review of the evidence, Turner (1983) draws three tentative conclusions:

1. Social support tends to matter for psychological well-being independent of stressor level.
2. Support tends to matter more where stressor level is relatively high.
3. The extent to which conclusions 1 and 2 are true varies across subgroups of the population (e.g., by social class).

Another issue raised by social support research is the one of causal inference. It is well recognized that social support is not simply a matter of a network of relationships. What matters to a person is his subjective feeling of being "loved, wanted, valued, esteemed, and able to count on others should the need arise" (Cobb, 1976). The perception of being loved and esteemed may be strongly influenced by the person's own self-esteem: his social supports may be as much a reflection of his mental health as the cause of it. How then can we be sure that the association between low social support and poor mental health is causal in one direction? In human behavior, cause and effect rarely act in a linear unidirectional manner. Causation in complex systems is circular or spiral, each effect having reciprocal effects on the cause by feedback loop, as well as more distant effects on other parts of the system. A person's early life experience may make him or her vulnerable to depression. Frequent depressions may lead to a withdrawal from social contacts. The lack of social contacts may then act to reinforce the depression and delay recovery. Given the complexity of causation in human affairs, we cannot assume that cause and effect are all in one direction. Nevertheless, after an extensive review of the evidence, Turner (1983) concludes that an important part of the causation goes from support to psychological distress. Because we cannot isolate simple causal chains does not mean that we cannot act on our knowledge about the importance of life experience and social supports. We know enough to give close attention to a patient's supporting relationships in all types of illness, and especially to the support we ourselves can provide.

The evidence reviewed here makes untenable the separation of mind from body in the old paradigm and the notion that there is a group of psychosomatic diseases. Social and psychological factors may be influential in any disease state, either as a cause of the disease itself or as a factor determining its severity and course.

The Placebo Effect as a Mind–Body Anomaly

In some respects, *placebo effect* is an unfortunate name for the phenomenon, because it focuses attention on the placebo as a substance administered to the patient. In fact, the placebo effect does not depend on the administration of a substance. It may follow any therapeutic modality, including those where no physical treatment of any kind is given. The placebo effect occurs when a patient responds to the form but not the content of therapy. The patient exhibits a biological response to the symbolic significance of the treatment. Moerman (1983) prefers to call this "general medical effectiveness" rather than placebo effectiveness.

The placebo effect occurs if a patient in a healing context is administered an intervention as part of that context, if the patient's condition is changed, and if the change is attributable to the intervention, but not to any specific therapeutic effect or to any known pharmacologic or physiologic property of the intervention (Brody, 1980). By using the term *changed* rather than *improved*, this definition allows for the fact that the placebo effect can be harmful as well as therapeutic. It also excludes general effects of the intervention that are not symbolically mediated, such as diet and exercise.

A recent experiment exemplifies the power of the placebo effect in patients with severe coronary disease. Patients with end stage coronary disease had long-term beneficial effects of placebo therapy in a study of angiogenesis and laser myocardial revascularization trials. Patients were randomly assigned to therapy or placebo. Improvements in mean angina class, exercise treadmill time, and quality of life were mostly maintained at 90 days from baseline. The benefits of placebo therapy were maintained at 2-year follow-up (Rana et al., 2005).

It is important to correct some misconceptions about the placebo effect. Some of these are not so much misconceptions as attempts to explain it away as a matter of little significance. The first is that placebo effectiveness is only found in subjective conditions such as pain and anxiety. In fact, placebos affect objectively measurable processes as well as subjective reports. The second is that placebos are harmless. In fact, placebos can produce undesirable effects and addiction like pharmacologically active drugs. The third is that only highly suggestible or neurotic personality types respond to placebos. People responding to placebos are of very varied personality types (Brody, 1980). The fourth is that the placebo effect is constant at about 35% of patients. Placebo effectiveness has been found to vary between 10% and 90% (Moerman, 1983), 35% being the generally accepted mean figure.

The explanation of the placebo effect that fits best with the evidence is provided by the meaning model (Brody, 1980). This may be stated as follows. The placebo effect is most likely to occur when the following conditions are met:

1. The patient is provided with an explanation of his or her illness that is consistent with his or her worldview.
2. Individuals in socially sanctioned caring roles provide support for the patient.
3. The healing intervention leads to the patient acquiring a sense of mastery and control over the illness.

The placebo response can be learned by association, as in classical conditioning. Pavlov was the first to report a conditioned placebo effect in dogs who showed morphine-like effects, whenever they were placed in the experimental chamber where they had previously received morphine. Several studies have shown that the placebo response can be conditioned in humans (Peck and Coleman, 1991). Olness and Ader (1992) have reported on the case of a child with lupus erythematosus who needed only half the usual dose of cyclophosphamide after conditioning with cod liver oil. Because classical conditioning depends on a response to something that symbolizes the unconditioned stimulus, the symbolism of our therapeutic acts assumes practical importance. The continuing doctor–patient relationship and the familiar surroundings of the practice are fertile ground for symbols of healing. Conditioning is maintained and enhanced by every new experience of effective treatment. On the other hand, the effect can be reduced or extinguished by negative experiences. The familiar doctor's face, in a familiar place, associated with healing on many past occasions, is a strong foundation for the working of the placebo effect.

Little progress has been made in our understanding of the placebo effect in recent years. However a meeting at the National Institute of Health promises to give more attention to research on the placebo effect (*The Science of the Placebo: Towards an Interdisciplinary Research Agenda*: BMJ books, 2002). There is much still to be learned about the patient–doctor relationship in family medicine.

Physiological Pathways

Research points to the nervous, endocrine, and immune systems as the main pathway by which nonmaterial phenomena influence bodily health. The cardinal manifestations of the general adaptation syndrome (GAS) described by Selye (1956) are adrenal hypertrophy, thymic involution, and elevated corticosteroid levels. High levels of corticosteroids are immunosuppressive, and high physiological levels are required for several normal immune functions. In the GAS, noxious stimuli cause the hypothalamus to release a corticotropin-releasing factor, which in turn causes the pituitary to release adrenocorticotropic hormone (ACTH). This stimulates the adrenal cortex to secrete corticosteroids. Thyroid, growth and sex hormones, and insulin are also required for the normal development and function of the immune system.

Walter Cannon (1932), the American physiologist who gave us the concept of homeostasis, also described the fight or flight response—a sympathetic outflow leading to the secretion of norepinephrine in target organs and epinephrine in the adrenal medulla. Lymphocytes have receptors for catecholamines, and stimulation of the beta-adrenergic (epinephrine) fibers decreases cellular immune response. Beta-adrenergic drugs have been shown to be immunosuppressive. Studies in animals have shown relationships between social environment, changes in the endocrine system, and morbidity and mortality. Abrupt change in the social environment in mice, either from isolation to group or vice versa, results in adrenal hypertrophy and increased growth of an implanted tumor. Male mice housed one or two per cage had a lesser ability to reject lymphosarcoma than those in larger groups. Anxiety stress in mice increases the risk of malignancy, and this increased risk is associated with elevated plasma corticosterone. Benign virus infections can also produce an elevated corticosterone level and increase the risk of malignancy. Some of the evidence from animal experiments is conflicting. Stressful stimuli have been found in some experiments to reduce the risk of malignancy. The contradictions may be explained by the finding that chronic stress can produce immunosuppression followed by immunoenhancement (Riley, Fitzmaurice, and Spackman, 1981). Activation of T lymphocytes releases lymphokines that control lymphoid cell activation, transformation, and clonal expansion. The experimental evidence suggests two regulatory mechanisms for the immune system: homeostatic autoregulation depending on internal immunologic signals and an external system mediated by the central nervous and endocrine systems (Besedovsky and Sorkin, 1981). The way in which these control systems interact is extremely complex, making inferences about cause and effect very uncertain.

New Knowledge of the Immune System

Until recent years, the immune system was regarded as isolated from other body systems. Research has now shown close reciprocal relationships between the immune and neuroendocrine systems. The autonomic nervous system, through its innervation of lymphoid organs, provides a pathway for communication between both systems. Cells of the immune system have receptors for neuropeptides and the latter have been shown to modulate immune response. Every hormone secreted or regulated by the pituitary gland has some effect on the immune system (Bellinger, Madden, Felten, and Felten, 1994). The cells of the immune system can produce substances previously identified as neurotransmitters, suggesting that there is a commonality of signal molecules that can act on the nervous system, the immune system, or both.

Felten and Felten (1991) describe the implications of recent research in these terms:

The unequivocal demonstration of direct neural innervation between the nervous and immune system and the demonstration of functional consequences of signaling in both directions suggest that these two great memory and communication systems, poised to respond to internal and external challenges for the protection and preservation of the organism, are interdependent. No longer can we think of the immune system as autonomous, and no longer can we think of behavior and neural responsiveness as unaffected by the immune status of the organism.

One of the most striking examples of the relationships between behavior and the immune system is the fact that the immune response can be altered by conditioning. In other words, the immune system can learn from experience. In the same way as Pavlov's dogs learned to salivate at the sound of a bell, animals learn to alter their immune response when given an inert substance previously paired with a suppressor or enhancer of immune response. In a key experiment by Ader and Cohen (1991), saccharin paired with the immunosuppressant cyclophosphamide was administered to rats, which were immunized 3 days later with sheep red blood cells (SRBC). On the day of immunization, the animals were divided into three groups. One group received a second dose of saccharin; one received a second dose of cyclophosphamide; and the third were not reexposed to either substance. Antibodies to SRBC were measured 6 days later. The animals given a second dose of saccharin and those given a second dose of cyclophosphamide showed reduced anti-SRBC response compared with those who did not receive a second dose, and with unconditioned animals injected with SRBC. As already indicated, we also know that humans can be conditioned in the same way to respond to an inert substance (placebo).

The significance of this finding is the response of the immune system to a symbol of the active agent. The organism responded to the stimulus because it had meaning for it. This process is difficult to describe in the ordinary mechanistic language of medical science. To capture it, we have to use words like meaning, message, and symbol. If we insist on eschewing such terms, we miss the point that organisms in health and disease respond at multiple levels, and that each level poses its own questions for us, as well as its own therapeutic possibilities. As well as asking the lower level question, "What are the neuronal and chemical pathways?" we should ask the upper level questions, "Can humans help to heal themselves by altering their immune response by their own volition?"

A New Paradigm

In spite of its many critics, the biomedical model reigned supreme for most of the twentieth century; the model is exemplified by the clinicopathological conference, a procedure that has shown generations of students how to approach a patient's clinical problem. An invited clinician would be presented with a patient's history, physical signs, and test results, after which he or she would present a differential diagnosis and a probable diagnosis, giving his or her reasons. The pathologist would then present the definitive diagnosis. Within its limits, it was an excellent teaching tool, but patients' personal aspects were rarely mentioned and the patient's own story was not included.

The biomedical model was very successful and continued to be so within the walls of the teaching hospital. Outside the walls, however, it was very different.

Until very recently, general practitioners were trained in teaching hospitals according to the biomedical model. In practice, they found that many of their patients had illnesses that did not fit with any diagnosis, or had problems that were a complex of illness, problems of living, and emotional turmoil.

It is not surprising, therefore, that one of the earliest attempts to change the medical model came from a group of general practitioners working with Michael Balint, a psychoanalyst and physician, who sat with the group while they discussed patients who troubled them. The result was Balint's book: *The Doctor, His Patient, and the Illness.* The book and the seminars that followed had a profound effect on general practice and "marked the beginning of a shift away from the purely biomedical model of medical practice which was the prevailing one at the time" (Gillies, 2005). Although influential in general practice Balints' teaching made no impact on the medical schools.

Twenty years later, another psychoanalyst, George Engel, published a seminal paper on the shortcomings of the biomedical model, advocating a Biopsychosocial model based on general system theory. Engel, himself, was not satisfied with the name Biopsychosocial and welcomed the term Infomedical coined by Foss and Rothenberg whose book had a Foreword by Engel (Foss and Rothenberg, 1987). A term for a new paradigm should convey its essence and while "infomedical" made a step forward by focusing on the crucial role of information at all levels of the human body it fails to include a holistic approach which is so central to family medicine.

We have called this the Goldstein Paradigm in honor of Kurt Goldstein (1878–1965) (Goldstein, 1995) scientist, neurologist, psychologist, and above all a pioneer of the holistic approach to medicine. Although his major work was in neurology, we in family medicine share with him the conviction that it is impossible to consider any illness without reference to the patient's self. The essence of the Goldstein paradigm is to see the patient as a whole, an integrated being with a history, a present, and a future that is ensconced in a myriad psychological realities, social relationships, and environmental challenges against a background of genetic propensities. Within this ontological framework, symptoms are seen as a manifestation of the organism attempting to achieve a new adaptation to circumstances brought about by an illness or accident. At times, these adaptations can be more far reaching than the original deficit or illness. To fully understand a symptom complex, therefore, you must take a holistic view. Meticulous observation and understanding of the patient's self is necessary for the physician to assist the patient through a period of chaos to a new equilibrium.

The new paradigm is especially applicable to family medicine. We define ourselves in terms of relationships, not by diseases or technologies. We form relationships with patients before we know what their illnesses will be. Our commitment to them, therefore, is unconditional. We are available to them for any problem they bring to us. Our special skill is the assessment of undifferentiated clinical problems. Our long-term relationships with patients and their families give us privileged knowledge about their lives, gathered often by listening to their stories. We tend, therefore, to think in terms of individuals: of patients, rather than abstractions. General practice is the only major field of medicine that transcends the dualistic division between mind and body. Note, however, that this does not mean bringing mind and body together: a much more difficult task. In a relation-based discipline, says Gillies (2005), decision making must include both emotional and intellectual aspects.

To bring about paradigm change in medical practice, however, it is necessary to describe in detail a new clinical method as done in Chapter 8.

As the consultation begins, the patient is seen as a whole, before any attention to detail. The encounter is an emotional engagement between doctor and patient. The doctor's attention should be outward toward the patient, and his feeling with, or his compassion for, the patient should be an imaginative grasp of the patient's whole situation (Macnaughton, 2002). The capacity of bodily empathy is central to the general clinical competence of the family practitioner. Bodily empathy is a route to the understanding of the emotions and bodily experience (Rudebeck, 1992).

Whatever the outcome of the consultation, the doctor may reflect on the knowledge he or she has gathered of the patient's life history and family relationships—knowledge that may have relevance for the present illness, being careful not to make unfounded assumptions.

Almost any illness has reverberations among the patient's relationships. A new illness may have reverberations on existing chronic illnesses or disabilities. The patient's reason for coming may be a problem of living, or a problem of living affecting a chronic illness.

Medicine is, at the very deepest level concerned with loss, or the possibility of loss. In many illnesses and consultations, general practitioners deal with patients who are afraid of loss: loss of function due to illnesses or ageing, loss associated with the stigma of a disease, loss of employment, friends or family, or even their own lives...a consultation that seems to be about a minor symptom may have been interpreted by the patient as an indicator of serious, perhaps fatal disease. At the very heart of meaning, is this knowledge of the possibility, and in the end, the inevitability of loss. (Gillies M.A. Occasional Paper 86, p. 23, Royal College of General Practitioners)

Facing this suffering, week in, week out, makes great demands on us. Avoidance is a great temptation. Yet it is so important that we give ourselves to these suffering patients. At the same time we must be quite clear that what we are doing is not self-serving. This is why self-knowledge, and an understanding of our own countertransference, is so important for physicians, and especially for general practitioners.

The patient-centered clinical method is described in detail in Chapter 8. Its essence is to ascertain the meaning of the illness to the patient. A proper use of the method requires that we carefully listen to the patient's needs, be sensitive to their cues and body language, and explore the circumstances surrounding the onset of their symptoms. The patient's illness is not separate from the patient's life. That ideas and events in the patient's life can trigger or cause the illness is one of differences between the Goldstein and the biomedical paradigms. It follows, also, that bringing this knowledge to the patient can be therapeutic (Broom, 2007).

According to the emerging paradigm—designed to take into account the anomalies referred to earlier—disease is not separated conceptually from the person, nor is the person from his or her environment. Conventional disease categories are still used as a frame of reference, but always in context. All illnesses affect the patient at multiple levels. All have multiple causes, although it may be useful to focus therapy on a single causal chain. Causation acts not only in a linear, but also in a reciprocal fashion. The relationship between doctor and patient has a profound effect on the illness and its course. The task of the physician is to understand the nature of the illness on all its levels. For practical purposes, attention may be focused on only one level, at least for a time. In all serious illness, however, attention should be paid at multiple levels. Our clinical method should be adequate to this task. To understand the illness at the higher psychological and social levels, the physician has to identify with the patient and loved ones through qualities of empathy and compassion. This is necessary both for humanitarian reasons and for the scientific practice of medicine. It is through these couplings that new qualities emerge in all the participants.

The new paradigm has important implications for clinical method and for how the physician treats the patient. The contrast between the old and the new paradigms is illustrated very vividly by the clinicopathological conference (*Clinicopathological Conference*, 1968).

The subject of the conference was a 50-year-old man with adult celiac disease, resistant to treatment. Initially, the patient had responded well to a gluten-free diet, but he had later gone downhill very rapidly and died. In opening the discussion, the professor of medicine asked, "Why did this patient's intestine suddenly become wrecked and remain so wrecked that he died from his disease?"

After a discussion about the pathology of the patient's intestine, the professor commented:

So it appears that we are completely at sea over the cause of the gut lesion in this man. This is not like the ordinary coeliac disease with a response to a gluten-free diet. This is an exception which in Dr._____'s experience affects about 30% of the patients he sees.... But of some 30% of adult patients who will not respond to a gluten-free diet only a few will be like this, running almost a malignant course resulting in death; and the question we have to ask is what would cause it. Dr._____ 'you were this patient's family physician, would you like to comment...?'

To this, the patient's family physician replied:

I would like to suggest that the main reason for this [failure to account for the course of the illness] is the inadequacy of the concepts which they [the discussants] are using in their attempted explanations. If we treat the patient as a biochemical machine and exclude any concepts which refer to him as a person, then it seems to me that explanations of his illness must be extremely limited. If we turn our attention to this man's life pattern and what little we know of his inner feelings, this illness becomes much more understandable. Perhaps we should be using more relevant concepts as the basis for our explanations.

In this case, I know there were major emotional conflicts in all the main areas of his life.

The onset of the illness followed the death of his father, an event with which a lot of family feeling was associated. The exacerbation of his illness coincided with rising tension between himself and his adopted daughter within the context of a sterile marriage. The final stage of his illness coincided with the collapse of his work relationship after a long period of devoted service...I feel that he died because all that he had lived for had somehow come to nothing.

To this the professor of medicine responded

Thank you very much. The possibility of a psychogenic influence in coeliac disease has been suggested by Pauley, and clearly if the basic abnormality of coeliac disease is due to a genetically determined enzyme defect, I would find it difficult to believe that psychogenic influences could play much part. It is more likely to be a sensitivity. Do you think that the mucosal lesion was due to an enzyme factor, Dr.——?

This encounter between a professor of medicine and a family physician is full of interest, for it brings into sharp focus the two contrasting views of disease we have been discussing. Note that the family physician answered the professor's question very precisely. He had not asked "Why did the patient get celiac disease?" but "Why did the patient die?" The family physician shifted the focus of the discussion from the organ and the disease to the whole person and his response to his environment. In his reply, however, the professor showed himself to be the prisoner of his concepts. First, he was unable to transcend disease categories and think in terms of the patient as an organism rather than a case of celiac disease. Second, he was unable to think about cause in any other way than as a specific etiology. The likelihood of a genetically determined enzyme deficiency was thought to rule out any possibility of environmental factors acting concurrently.

This exchange took place in 1968, before the scientific evidence for the influence of relationships and emotions on health had begun to accumulate. The professor's reluctance to discuss this aspect of the case is therefore understandable. He was also constrained by a model of disease that is unable to account for it. This has not changed.

Although we have been thinking of recent changes in medical thought in terms of old and new paradigms, a more historical perspective indicates that the new paradigm is not without precedent. Crookshank (1926) has traced two theories of medicine back to the schools of Cos and Cnidus in ancient Greece. To the school of Cos, understanding a disease included understanding the patient in his or her environment. Therapy consisted of prescribing a regimen that would help the patient to overcome his or her disease. To the Cnidians, diseases were entities in their own right. The task of the physician was to categorize the disease and to prescribe the specific remedy. For a more extensive discussion of the Coan and Cnidian schools, see Chapter 8.

These two philosophies have vied with each other over the centuries, one or other being dominant at different times. The wisest physicians have been those who have taken something from each. What I have described as the new paradigm is the heir of the Hippocratic tradition. Of course, historical events and movements never recur in exactly the same way. The new paradigm is new in the sense that although it has roots in tradition, it also embodies all that we have learned from the experience of the past 100 years. The patient-centered clinical method is a way of implementing these principles in current practice (see Chapter 8).

The Biological Basis of Family Medicine

Medical science is based on a mechanistic metaphor of biology. Its ideal goal, as expressed by the geneticist Arthur Zucker (1981), is "diagnostics accomplished by a biochemical–biophysical survey of the body. Ideally, psychological problems could be captured by this technique. It is part of the assumption of reductionist medicine that, at the very least, mental states have clinically useful physical correlates."

Reduction undoubtedly confers benefits by reducing the number of explanatory principles for otherwise disparate phenomena (Foss, 1994). As Foss points out, however, reduction can become generalized into reductionism: "a belief in the universal applicability of *upward* causation: the universe is composed of fundamental entities—organs, cells, organelles, genes, ultimately perhaps elementary particles—whose intricate interactions account for complex behaviour" (Foss, 1994). The difference between reduction and reductionism is illustrated by the development of sumatriptan for migraine. Reducing migraine to its biochemical correlate produced a clinically useful drug. But to suggest that the syndrome is now fully explained, or that pharmacotherapy is a complete solution to the problem of migraine, is reductionism.

The biologist F.E. Yates (1993) writes:

...biological sciences now suffer from permeation by a mechanistic reductionism in the guise of two limiting and inappropriate metaphors: (1) the dynamic metaphor of organisms as machines, and (2) the information metaphor, of life as a text written in DNA...both metaphors are false and destructive of conceptual advances in the fundamental understanding of complex living systems that self-organize, grow, develop, adapt, reproduce, repair, and maintain form and function, age and die. The rise of the sciences of complexity offers a fresh, non-reductionist avenue toward the nature, origin, and fabrication of life.

Even though the body has machine-like features, everything we do for the health of the body depends on the healing powers of nature. At its most successful, medicine works in supporting these natural processes. Surgeons drain abscesses, set fractures, repair wounds, and relieve obstructions. Immunization strengthens the organism's defenses. The most effective drugs are those that support natural defenses and maintain balance in the milieu interieur. The traditional regimens of balanced nutrition, rest, sound sleep, exercise, relief of pain and anxiety, and personal support are all measures that support the organism's healing powers.

Family medicine is based on an organismic metaphor of biology. It is natural for family physicians to think organismically. "In contrast with physics, biology presents diversity and specialness of form and function, and sometimes a striking localness of distribution of its objects. Biological systems are complex by any definition of the term" (Yates, 1993).

What does it mean to think organismically? An organism is a particular, that is, "it occupies a region of space, persists through time, has boundaries, and has an environment" (Gorovitz and MacIntyre, 1976). The point about particulars is that their behavior cannot be explained or predicted solely by applying the general laws of science. The degree to which a law will apply to a particular organism will depend on its history and its context or environment. There is an inherent uncertainty about all particular applications of general scientific principles. The more complex the particular organism, the greater the uncertainty, and a sick patient is a very complex organism. Family medicine operates at a high level of complexity.

Organismic thinking is multilevel and nonlinear. Organisms maintain themselves in a state of dynamic equilibrium by a reciprocal or circular flow of information at all levels, and between organism and environment. Through these multilevel channels, change in any part can reverberate through the whole organism and to its surroundings. The necessity of constant information flow can be seen in the destabilizing effects on humans of sensory deprivation. Information is carried in the form of symbols conveying messages that are decoded at the appropriate level of the organism. At lower levels information is carried by hormones and neurotransmitters. At the level of the whole organism it is carried by stimuli reaching the special senses, such as the words and other symbols by which meaning is expressed in human relationships. This provides the background for our accumulating knowledge of the effect of relationships on health and disease.

The transition from mechanistic to organismic thinking requires a radical change in our notion of disease causation. We have learned to think of a causal agent as a force acting in linear fashion on a passive object, as when a moving billiard ball hits a stationary one. In self-organizing systems such as living organisms, causation is nonlinear. The multiple feedback loops between organism and environment, and between all levels of the organism, require us to think in causal networks, not straight lines. The organism, moreover, is not a passive object. The "specific cause" of an illness may only be the trigger that releases a process that is already a potential of the organism. The causes that maintain an illness and inhibit healing may be different from the causes that initiated it, and they may include the organism's own maladaptive behavior. Therapeutic measures may act not on a causal agent but on the body's defenses, as appears to be the case with the therapeutic benefits of human relationships. In a complex system, cause and effect are not usually close to each other in time and space (Briggs and Peat, 1989); and because organic processes are maintained or changed by multiple influences, it is difficult to predict the consequences of an intervention. It is true that we can still isolate one link in the causal network as our point of intervention, as when we prescribe an antibiotic, but even in these instances we should be aware of the whole context in which we are operating, and of the reciprocal effects of our intervention. The complexity of the illnesses we encounter in family medicine makes it natural for us to think in this way. Does isolation from social supports cause depression, or does depression cause the isolation? Did this life event cause the depression or was it only the trigger, releasing a depression in a susceptible individual? In human science we can establish relationships between events, but it is often difficult to establish cause. Does this imply therapeutic impotence? No, but it does require a change from simplistic causal thinking to thinking about how change can be facilitated in complex systems.

Self-Organizing Systems

General system theory is a response to the limitations of nineteenth-century science. The mechanistic worldview and reductive methods of nineteenth-century science were not able to deal adequately with organic phenomena such as organization and growth. The reductive method dealt with problems by cutting them down to size, separating them from their surroundings and reducing them as far as possible to simple, linear, causal chains. System theory seeks to do the opposite: to approach problems by including all their significant relationships. A system is defined by Von Bertallanfy (1968) as "a dynamic order of parts and processes standing in mutual interaction with each other." Some of the basic concepts of system theory are as follows.

Nature is ordered as a hierarchy of systems, both living and nonliving. Living systems go from organelle to cell, to tissue, to organ, to organism, to family, to community, to society. Each level in the hierarchy is both a whole in itself and part of a greater whole: in Koestler's (1979) words, it is Janus-faced, having one face toward a higher order system and another toward a lower order subsystem (see Figure 5.1). Systems are related to each other, not only hierarchically and vertically, but also horizontally. The immune system "talks" to the nervous system

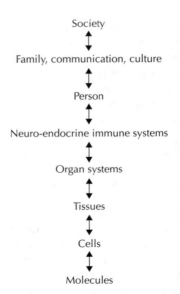

Figure 5.1   Systems hierarchy (level of organization). (After Engel, 1980.)

on the same level of the vertical hierarchy. Social systems—family, community, culture—relate to each other on the same level, and a person can be a component of all three.

If we think in terms of human systems, a person is at the highest level of the organismic hierarchy and at the lowest level of the social hierarchy. Each system has features that are unique to that level and can only be explained by criteria that are appropriate to that level. A social system like the family, for example, cannot be explained in biological terms, and a living system cannot be explained in terms of physics and chemistry. Nor can a system be understood by studying each part individually. Understanding the whole requires a knowledge of the purpose of the system and how its parts interact to attain that purpose. This feature of systems is known as emergence. A system has properties that are not present in the individual parts: they arise from the relationship between the parts—the organization. When a system is broken down into its component parts, the emergent properties are lost.

All living systems are open systems, in that they exchange both energy and information across the system interfaces or boundaries. Each system exists in a state of dynamic internal equilibrium between its parts and in a state of external equilibrium with the systems that form its environment. If the equilibrium is disturbed by changes inside or outside a system, corrective forces come into play, which may restore the equilibrium or return the system to a new steady state. Mutual interdependence of a system's parts is a basic concept of systems theory. Any change in a part produces changes in the whole and, because nature is a continuum, the change reverberates up and down the system hierarchy.

These changes cannot be broken down into simple causal chains without grossly oversimplifying the process. To do so is to think in the closed-system way typical of nineteenth-century science. The limitations of this mode of thought have been illustrated by the effects on whole ecosystems of technological innovations like pesticides. In a complex system, cause does not operate in a linear fashion. A chronic illness may cause depression, which may in turn lead to neglect of treatment, resulting in a worsening of the illness, which then exacerbates the depression, and so on.

Living systems have regulatory mechanisms to maintain their equilibrium. One of these is cybernetic regulation, which involves three steps: the return of information by feedback loop from the system's output; matching of this information to the system's rules; and adjusting the output to correct any mismatch. In systems theory, the terms positive and negative feedback are used in a different sense from the one we are accustomed to in education. In teaching, negative feedback implies criticism of a student's performance, positive implies praise. In systems language, negative feedback stabilizes a system by reducing deviation from its normal range, as when a thermostat adjusts a heating or cooling system. Positive feedback amplifies a deviation and drives the system into excess. If a doctor confronted by an angry patient responds with anger (positive feedback), the patient is likely to become more angry, then the doctor more angry still, in an escalation of emotion that threatens the relationship. If the doctor makes a conciliatory response (negative feedback), the patient's anger is likely to be reduced, with a stabilizing effect on the relationship.

A living system is constantly adjusting itself to feedback from its own body—engaging in a monologue with itself. In proprioception, for example, the motor impulses of muscles are fed back to the central nervous system through a sensory loop via receptors in tendons and joints. The term *umwelt* was introduced by the ethologist von Uexküll to express the idea that an organism's environment is not simply a neutral piece of space "out there," but rather a subjective universe constructed of features that have a meaning for it (von Uexküll, Geigges, and Herrmann, 1993). The *umwelt* of a bat is a subjective world of sonar impulses; a dog inhabits a world of smells. A blind person, deprived of one mode of perception, has to construct a new *umwelt* based on the remaining senses. The blind person's stick becomes a probe, transmitting vibrations from the environment. As Kay Toombs (1995) has observed, serious disabilities, whether motor or sensory, always require a change in our subjective universe—a reconstruction of our world in synchrony with our altered activities and perceptions. Because our sense of self comes from the sense of coherence generated by the internal monologue, and by the interaction with our environment, any serious disturbance of the interactions is a crisis for our "self."

This can be seen in the effects of sensory deprivation and social ostracism, as well as in the onset of blindness, deafness, and other disabilities.

Living systems also experience growth, development and adaptation, all of which require change in response to new conditions. A family changes as its children grow through adolescence to adulthood. The health-care system changes in response to new health problems. If a system cannot adapt to a changing environment, it may disintegrate and collapse.

One of the most important contributions of system theory has been the conceptual separation of the regulating from the dynamic processes of systems. Because information is the key to regulation, this is equivalent to the separation of information from energy. This distinction between information and energy helps us to see how very large dynamic effects can be set in motion or released by the very small amounts of energy required to process information. An electronic signal can explode a bomb. Breaking an electric circuit can open a large metal door. The ingestion of a minute amount of antigen can lead to fatal anaphylaxis in a sensitized individual. A minor annoyance may trigger a depression in a person predisposed by heredity and life experience. In all these cases the information acts by releasing energy that is already present in the system. The distinction between the regulating and dynamic processes of systems has implications for our thinking about the causes of events. The cause of anaphylactic shock is both the hypersensitivity of the individual and the antigen that releases the anaphylactic response.

The flow of information is essential to the function of medical systems: the doctor–patient system, the doctor–family system, and the different teams that make up the health-care system. Failure of communication is the most common reason for medical error. Yet we still pay much more attention to technical aspects of care than to communication.

The Question of Medical Knowledge

This brings us to a discussion of the knowledge required of the physician working in the new paradigm—the question of the epistemology of medicine. Epistemology (from the Greek *episteme*, "knowledge") is the theory of knowledge. The epistemology of medicine is concerned with questions such as "what is medical knowledge, what should we know about our patients, and how can this knowledge be acquired?"

Since the nineteenth century, medicine has been dominated by the positivist view of knowledge—the belief that the only valid knowledge is that obtained by the empirical method: the verification of hypotheses by recourse to data accessible to our five senses. In the English-speaking tradition, empiricism is indissolubly associated with the experimental method. In the Continental tradition, other rigorous routes to scientific knowledge are recognized: in German, *natur wissenschaften* and *geistenwissenschaften*; in French, *la science de la nature* and *la science de l'humanite*. In medicine, we have recognized only one of these routes to valid knowledge, and this route has to us become synonymous with science. Medical scientists sometimes make a distinction between hard and soft data, usually implying a judgment about their relative value. To do this is to compare two categories of data that are not comparable. Data from natural science is about the world of the senses; data from human science is about meaning. Both types of data can be verified, but the means of verification are different.

The physical phenomena of the illness of the patient discussed earlier were all empirically verifiable: the wasting of her muscles, her loss of weight, her sweating and flushing. The mental phenomena, however—her thoughts and feelings, her own perceptions of the injury and illness—required a different form of inquiry. In European philosophy this is known as hermeneutic (*hermeneutike*, the art of interpretation) or phenomenological inquiry. In empirical inquiry, as it is commonly understood, the observer collects data with his five senses from an object, in this case a patient. Hermeneutic inquiry is intersubjective. One person, in this case a physician, reaches an understanding of another's thoughts, feelings, and sensations by entering into a dialogue in which the meaning of words and other symbols is progressively clarified. In an intersubjective inquiry, neither party is unchanged by the process. In this case, the patient may gain a deeper level of self-knowledge as well as a resolution of her existential crisis; the physician also may learn something about the human condition, and perhaps about himself.

Knowledge attained by hermeneutics is intersubjective and is, therefore, not scientific in the conventional sense of the term. Yet it has its own canons of verification. In this case, verification depended on intersubjective agreement between doctor and patient. In other cases, verification may include more than two people. Another physician, for example, may verify a colleague's understanding of a patient's pain. The whole process of taking a history is hermeneutic, in that it seeks to understand a patient's sensations, perceptions, and feelings. Although in medicine we have followed the trend toward positivism, we have all the time, without acknowledging the fact, been relying on knowledge that can be obtained only by intersubjective agreement.

In the historical perspective, positivism can be viewed as a modern heresy. All the great religions and schools of philosophy are remarkably consistent about many things, including their teaching about levels of being. This distilled wisdom of the ages, called by Liebnitz the perennial philosophy, recognizes a hierarchy of levels of existence. The simplest has three levels: the transcendental, the mental, and the physical. Whitehead (1926) maintained that if we wish to know the general principles of existence, we must start at the top and work down. Each higher level has capacities not found at lower levels. The higher cannot be derived from the lower. Biology cannot be fully explained in terms of physics, or psychology in terms of biology. Each higher level includes the lower levels, but transcends them.

Each level of being has its own level of knowing. To have knowledge at any of the levels, the understanding must be adequate to the thing known. "When the level of the knower is not adequate to the level of the object of knowledge," wrote Schumacher (1977), "the result is not a factual error, but something much more serious: an inadequate and impoverished view of reality."

For the physical level, the way of knowing is sensory. As we well know, the simple use of the senses is not usually enough. Our perceptions have to be trained. In this way, the radiologist "sees" more in an X-ray film than a clinician; an ophthalmologist "sees" more in a retina than an internist. For the mental level, the way of knowing is symbolic. We understand another person's thoughts and feelings by interpreting symbols: words, gestures, movements, and expressions. Again, simple listening is not enough. Our inward ear has to be trained so that we can listen in the way described below. And even this is not enough. How can we understand the inner life of another person? The perennial philosophy is clear on this: we can understand others only to the extent that we know ourselves. How could we understand what a patient means by pain unless we had experienced pain ourselves? Schumacher wrote:

A person who had never consciously experienced bodily pain, could not possibly know anything about the pain suffered by others. The outward signs of pain—sounds, movements, a flow of tears—would of course be noticed by him, but he would be totally inadequate to the task of understanding them correctly. No doubt he would attempt some kind of interpretation; he might find them funny or menacing or simply incomprehensible. The invisibilia of the other being—in this case his experience of pain—would remain invisible to him. ... The example of bodily pain is instructive precisely because there is no subtlety about it. ... Few people doubt the reality of pain, and the realization that here is a thing we all recognize as real, true, one of the great "stubborn facts" of our human existence, which nonetheless is unobservable by our outer senses, may come as a shock. If only that which can be observed by our outer senses is deemed to be real, "objective," scientifically respectable, pain must be dismissed as unreal, "subjective," unscientific. And the same applies to everything else which moves us internally: love and hatred, joy and sorrow, hope, fear, anguish and so on.

It is at the mental level that we understand the meaning of a person's experience and the values he lives by. It is at this level that we encounter the spiritual aspects of medicine, the things that give significance to a person's life.

For the transcendental, the way of knowing is contemplative and intuitive. Knowledge at this level is difficult to express in words and cannot be attained by the intellect alone. We know a person has attained it because it transforms the whole personality. This level of knowing also requires an understanding adequate to the level of being.

The kind of preparation that can give us both self-awareness and an insight into the inner lives of others cannot be a matter for the intellect alone. This kind of understanding comes from the heart. The first prerequisite is faith that there is a level of meaning beyond the reach of our senses. Without such faith we are not likely to have the commitment to undertake the search for this understanding. The intellect and the heart are not—or should not be—in conflict. The understanding that comes from the heart can enrich the intellect, and the intellect can act on the heart's insights. Each form of understanding reflects a different kind of truth. For the intellect, truth is the truth of a proposition, to be established by logical argument. For the heart, truth is something that penetrates one's whole being and transforms one's life. The truth of a proposition can be accepted without having the slightest impact on the way we live. Limiting our understanding to the intellect alone gives us a shallow and impoverished vision of reality. Samuel T. Coleridge saw this happening even in his own day: "I have known some men who have been rationally educated as it is styled. They were marked by a microscopic acuteness, but when they looked at great things, all became blank and they saw nothing." Coleridge (1853).

It follows, then, that medicine should include both knowledge derived from empirical science and knowledge derived from hermeneutics. Using Dr. Stetten's case as an example (see Chapter 6), it should include both a knowledge of vision and a knowledge of the experience of blindness. These two fields of knowledge are of a very different order. One is a knowledge of abstractions; the other is a knowledge of concrete experience as it is lived through. Whitehead (1926) criticized professional education for its concentration on abstractions, the result of which is people with minds in a groove: "to be mentally in a groove is to live in contemplating a given set of abstractions. The groove prevents straying across country and the abstraction, abstracts from something to which no further attention is paid. But there is no groove of abstraction which is adequate for the comprehension of human life. Thus, in the modern world, the celibacy of the medieval learned class has been replaced by a celibacy of the intellect, which is divorced from the concrete contemplation of complete facts."

The Place of the Observer

One of the assumptions of positivism has been the separation of the observer from the observed and the subjective from the objective. Medicine has followed science in its view of the physician as a detached and uninvolved observer. In our clinical records, the history is often written under the heading of subjective and the physical examination under objective. What this implies is that the knowledge gained from these two modes of enquiry is of a different order: in the physical examination, knowledge of the bodily state comes from the physician's five senses without interpretation by the patient; in the history, knowledge comes from the patient's interpretation of his or her bodily sensations and feelings. These differences dissolve on analysis. The physical signs are not raw data; they are the physician's interpretations of his or her own sensations. Physicians do not feel the liver or hear pleural friction: they feel a resistance as they palpate the abdominal wall, or hear a sound in the chest that they interpret as pleural friction. Clinicians often disagree about physical signs, and postmortem findings often contradict the physical examination. The examination is also not without the patient's interpretation. The decision to remove the appendix may depend on the patient's "Yes, that hurts." The knowledge gained from the history is interpreted not only by the patient, but by the physician. The result is some sense of order that the clinician has given to the patient's story, an order that has a meaning in the context of a disease taxonomy.

The distinction between subjective and objective data is artificial because perception and interpretation always go together. Learning to be a skilled observer is a training in interpretation. Well-trained and experienced clinicians can achieve close agreements on their observations, so we call their findings objective. But the criterion of objectivity is intersubjective agreement by different observers: reproducible findings require observers who are skilled in the use of their senses and their instruments.

The separation of observation from interpretation was expressed by Newton's dictum: "hypotheses non fingo." Phenomena, he believed, should be described without prior hypotheses, by an observer who is neutral and detached. Newton's viewpoint has dominated Western thought, with a few dissenting voices, notably that of Johann Wolfgang von Goethe, who maintained that the observer, as part of nature, stood within the phenomena observed. Not until our own century, however, has there been a revolutionary change of view. The change has come in physics: according to quantum theory, the consciousness of the observer is essential to the observation; moreover, it is the act of observation that collapses the probability functions of quantum mechanics into actualities (Harman, 1994). So far, other fields of science have not followed physics in making this change. But when we look closely at the conduct of science, or think about our own experience in research, we find the person of the observer involved at every stage.

In his searching inquiry into the nature of scientific knowledge, Michael Polanyi (1962) rejects as false the ideal of scientific detachment. Scientific knowledge comes from the exercise of the knower's intellectual powers and his passionate participation in the act of knowing. Personal Knowledge [is] manifested in the appreciation of probability and of order in the exact sciences... and in the way the descriptive sciences rely on skills and connoisseurship. At all these points, the act of knowing includes an appraisal; and this personal co-efficient, which shapes all factual knowledge, bridges in doing so the disjunction between subjectivity and objectivity. It implies the claim that man can transcend his own subjectivity by striving passionately to fulfil his personal obligations to universal standards.

Establishing contact with the reality hidden in nature involves the recognition of order. This comes, not from a study of separate parts, but from an intuition of how the parts are organized together in the whole. The observer does this by identifying with the phenomena. Piaget (1973) described this as a process by which the subject assimilates the object and accommodates to it. The higher the whole is in the systems hierarchy, and the greater its degree of complexity, the more involvement by the observer is required. It is this kind of involvement that is required by the Goldstein model. To attend to a patient's illness at all its levels, the physician must identify with the patient as a whole person with memories, emotions, interpretations, values, and intentions. To do this accurately, avoiding the many pitfalls, we have to attend to our own emotions, interpretations, and intentions. The physician is not only an observer of the patient, but a meta-observer of self and patient altogether.

The training of an observer in medicine or any other branch of science or technology is a training in the skills of attention, observation, and interpretation. What the new paradigm requires is that the physician becomes aware of himself or herself as an agent with the patient in bringing forth order and meaning from the patient's experience of illness: "…the individual in search of knowledge is locked in an embrace with the world. Out of this knowledge emerges a generated reality that bears the imprint of both natures involved in the process" (Goodwin, 1994).

Although we should be prepared by self-reflection, in actual practice the self/other distinction between doctor and patient may almost disappear. The craftsman feeling at one with his material, the surgeon absorbed in an operation, the inhabitant's sense of connectedness with her own landscape, the intimacy between doctor and patient: all are familiar to us. By "dwelling in" an experience with our whole being, we gain what Polanyi (1962) calls "tacit knowledge": the embodied knowledge that cannot be fully articulated in words and concepts. The difference between theoretical and embodied knowledge—"knowing about" and "knowing"—can be appreciated by reflecting on the experience of using a new drug. Even though we have full information about the drug—its absorption, excretion, half-life, dosage range, and so on—we feel awkward in using it at first. It is not until we have experienced it in action with many patients—learned its nuances, its different effects on different people, the variations in its actions—do we then begin to use the drug as an extension of ourselves.

Broom invokes Husserl's concept of the life-world. "If we want to see the world more the way it is we need a radical change of attitude, when we turn from the objectified meaning of the sciences to meaning as immediately experienced in the *leberswelt* or 'life-world" (Kockelmans, 1999; Broom, 2007).

The notion of the life-world is very relevant to the "seeing" of meaning-*full* disease. The life-world is the real, experienced, lived in world…a much richer world than that of mere objects, or that defined by the objective existence of things. The life-world *gives-rise* to the scientific world but it is much more than the world described by science (Broom, 2007).

The trouble is that we are so often blind to the patient's life-world: a world which, if we knew it, can explain the meaning of the disease which we have diagnosed—a meaning which perhaps reached far into the past, and which may hold the prospect of a therapy. We are blind because the paradigm which rules our medical schools does not believe such things exist.

Broom wrote:

> When I work with patients, with disease, I employ a phenomenological method continuously. Typically, I start with my attention on the 'thing' of illness, the disease manifestation, and then I slide my attention seamlessly towards, the 'meaning' of the same illness, whilst still holding them together in the same clinical time/space. Throughout the consultation I am moving seamlessly backwards and forwards, backwards and forwards, attending to the physical 'object', disease aspect in one moment, and then attending to the subjective 'meaning' aspect in another moment; in a zig zag way I am gradually building a picture of multifactorial, multidimensional emergence and perpetration of disease in this person in front of me" (Broom, 2007).

The nature of this weaving back and forth has been described as well in the patient-centered method (Stewart, Brown, Weston, McWhinney, and Freeman 2003).

Broom's method is reminiscent of Balint's teaching, especially Balint's way of listening with total attention. There is, however, one big difference. Balint makes a clear distinction between patients with clear cut diseases, and with neurotic illnesses; Broom seeks for meaning in all diseases.

Family physicians have the great advantage of knowing the life stories of many of their patients. When new illnesses make their appearance, our store of knowledge can be a starting point, with cues as to the meaning of the "new" illness. But we must not be too complacent: we may not know our patient as well as we think we do.

> *Case:* I (IRMcW) had cared for an elderly couple for a number of years. The husband was disabled by a neurological illness which had progressed until he had great difficulty in walking. Intensive investigation had not resulted in a diagnosis. Also in the home was an elderly woman who I used to see when making home visits. I understood that she was the wife's Aunt.
>
> I used to see the husband and the Aunt quite frequently, but the wife was in good health until one day she came to the surgery (office) complaining of persistent watery stools. Suspecting ulcerative colitis, I referred her to a surgeon who confirmed the diagnosis and his report came with a cryptic remark about the patient's Aunt. When the patient came back to see me she told me that she had suddenly discovered that the "Aunt" was actually her mother. I already knew that the Aunt owned the house and used this power to make their lives difficult, but of course I did not know her true relationship. Feeling somewhat humiliated, I asked her why she had told the specialist, but not me, her family doctor. "Well" she said, "when I was going to see the specialist my husband said: tell him everything." Is it not possible that the meaning of her illness was the life change she had undergone? At this stage of my career I did not give it a thought. Nor did I ask her how the news came to her, or how it had affected her.

Abstraction and Experience (Map and Territory)

The importance of abstraction in human understanding is illuminated by Alfred Korzybski's (1958) vivid metaphor of the map and the territory. We make a map by abstracting certain features from a territory and ignoring others. The features we abstract will depend on the purpose of the map: topographical, geological, ethnographic, and so on. To be useful, the map should have the same structure as the territory but, in the words of Korzybski's aphorism, "the map is not the territory." Knowing the map is not the same as knowing the territory. A native of the territory knows it by living in it and identifying with it. The native is immersed in his landscape: his experience of it is sensuous, affective. Korzybski calls this experience a "first order abstraction." It does not distinguish between body and mind: the experience is one of immediate feelings and is ultimately indescribable—in Polanyi's (1962) terms, it is tacit knowledge. A word may be found for it, but "the word is not the thing." Once we have used a word, it becomes a second-order abstraction.

The maps and schemas we have constructed have added enormously to our knowledge of the world. In medicine, we take people with similar illnesses and identify features that they have in common, while ignoring the many things they do not share. These collections of abstractions we call diseases and our classification system is a map of the territory of illness experienced by our patients. The system greatly increases our knowledge by the power of generalization. Once we have correctly classified (diagnosed) the patient's illness (found our place on the map), we can make inferences about its course and outcome, its relationship to other illnesses, its response to treatment, and so on.

The power of generalization increases with each degree of abstraction, the ultimate degree being a scientific law or mathematical formula. In medicine, some of our categories are low-level abstractions, such as the clusters of clinical observations we call syndromes. At the next level, other ways of describing the illness are added—pathological, biochemical, radiological—each one increasing the power of genealization. Names are given to each level of abstraction and the language is also a map of the territory. The words in Table 5.2 stand for increasing degrees of abstraction from patients' original experience to the highest levels arising from "translation" of the illness into the languages of physical pathology.

The power of the abstraction depends on its having the same structure as the illness it represents—a feature exemplified by the case of multiple sclerosis.

Table 5.2 Levels of abstraction in a patient with multiple, fluctuating, neurological symptoms and signs

Level 1	Level 2	Level 3	Level 4
Patient's sensation and emotions	Patient's expressed complaints, feelings, interpretations	Doctor's analysis of illness: clinical assessment	MRI scan
Preverbal	Second-order abstraction	Third-order abstraction	Fourth-order abstraction
Illness	"Illness" (doctor's understanding)	"Disease" (clinical diagnosis: multiple sclerosis)	"Disease" (definitive diagnosis: MS)

However, no abstraction is ever a complete picture of what it represents: it becomes less and less complete as the levels of abstraction and power of generalization increase. Every patient's illness is different in some way. As we increase the levels of abstraction, the differences are ironed out in the interests of increasing our power of generalization. And something very important is lost in the process. As we increase the levels of abstraction, the affective contribution to our understanding of the original experience becomes less and less. Abstraction distances us from experience. We cannot experience the beauty or the terror of a landscape by reading the map. Of course, one can get passionate about maps. There is a thrill in making a good diagnosis (finding our place on the map), and there can be beauty in a radiograph. But this is not the same as a feeling for the patient's experience of illness.

"The map is not the territory" seems like a statement of the obvious, yet we repeatedly fall into the trap of mistaking the abstraction for the experience it represents. We ask whether such and such a disease is an "entity," when what we really mean is, "does the map have the same structure as reality?" Patients may be told, "the disease you think you have doesn't exist," and, by many subtle cues, may feel that they are not believed. The doctor, perhaps unconsciously, feels that because the illness is not on his map, the patient is not ill. It is often taught that a "disease" is the cause of a "syndrome," when what they really are is different levels of abstraction.[4] Western medicine often reverses the status of abstraction and experience: a patient's illness is not considered "real" until it has been put on the map. The opposite is true; diseases, like maps, are not "real"—they are mental constructs having the same structure as reality. Sometimes we find that our maps are wrong. Mitral valve prolapse, for example, should not have been on any map; the relationship we had mapped between symptoms and valve prolapse turned out not to correspond to relationships in the real world. Sometimes the map is correct, but we misread it. A patient's backache may be called osteoarthritis on the strength of X-ray changes that are normal for his age. Such spurious diagnoses can have serious consequences in delayed recovery and inappropriate management.

One of the features of family practice is intimacy arising from long-term patient–doctor relationships, so much so that family physicians often tend to think more in terms of individual patients than in terms of abstractions. Describing a series of interviews with general practitioners, Reid (1982) noted that some "could not talk about general practice except in terms of their specific patients." Our experience does not allow us to forget the limitations of abstractions, even when we use them. Korzybski maintained that we should constantly remind ourselves of the uniqueness of each object. We need to remind ourselves that knowing the map is not the same thing as understanding the patient's illness experience—the first order, preverbal experience. Patients are very sensitive to the difference. The path to this understanding is not abstraction, but identification. This nonverbal identification with the patient may be the most important factor in healing. Identification engages all our cognitive powers, especially our feelings. Undifferentiated illness is illness that has not been through a process of abstraction by clinical assessment. The process of differentiation is one of increasing abstraction, and the level of abstraction reached depends on the extent to which the illness can be reduced to markers at the level of cells, molecules, and images. Much of the illness seen in family practice cannot be reduced in this way, and so, for much of the time, family physicians operate at lower levels of abstraction.

Because Western medicine and the modern paradigm of knowledge are heavily biased toward abstraction, we all tend to feel drawn away from the attempt to identify with the patient's experience. The biopsychosocial model is itself an abstraction; so is the system theory on which it is based. The model could be misconstrued simply as a call to interpret the patient's illness in terms of biological, psychological, and social science theory. When it comes to healing, abstractions can only get in the way. There comes a time when we have to set aside our maps and walk hand-in-hand with the patient through the territory.

References

Ader R, Cohen N. 1991. The influence of conditioning on immune responses. In: Ader R, Felton DL, Cohen N, eds., *Psychoneuroimmunology*. San Diego, CA: Academic Press, Inc.

Antonovsky A. 1979. *Health, Stress and Coping*. San Francisco, CA: Jossey-Bass.

Bass MJ, Buck C, Turner L, Dickie G, Pratt G, Robinson CH. 1986. The physician's actions and the outcome of illness in family practice. *Journal of Family Practice* 23:43–47.

Bellinger DL, Madden KS, Felten SY, Felten DL. 1994. Neural and endocrine links between the brain and the immune system. In: Lewis CE, O'Sullivan C, Barroclough J, eds., *The Psychoimmunology of Cancer: Mind and Body in the Fight for Survival*. New York: Oxford University Press.

Berkman LF, Breslow L. 1983. *Health and Ways of Living: The Alameda County Study*. New York: Oxford University Press.

Berkman LF. 1995. The role of social relations in health promotion. *Psychosomatic Medicine* 57:245.

Besedovsky HO, Sorkin E. 1981. Immunologic-neuroendocrine circuits: Physiological approaches. In: Ader R, ed., *Psychoneuroimmunology*. New York: Academic Press.

Blacklock SM. 1977. The symptom of chest pain in family practice. *Journal of Family Practice* 4:429.

Briggs J, Peat DF. 1989. *Turbulent Mirror: An Illustrated Guide to Chaos Theory and the Science of Wholeness*. New York: Harper & Row.

Brody H. 1980. *Placebos and the Philosophy of Medicine*. Chicago, IL: Chicago University Press.

Broom B. 2007. *MEANING-full DISEASE. How personal experience and meanings cause and maintain physical illness*. London: Karnac Books.

Cannon WB. 1932. *The Wisdom of the Body*. New York: W.W. Norton.

Cassel J. 1976. The contribution of the social environment to host resistance. *American Journal of Epidemiology* 104:107.

Classen C, Hermanson KS, Spiegel D. 1994. Psychotherapy, stress, and survival in breast cancer. In: Lewis CE, O'Sullivan C, Barroclough J, eds., *The Psychoimmunology of Cancer: Mind and Body in the Fight for Survival*. New York: Oxford University Press.

Clinicopathological Conference. 1968. A case of adult coeliac disease resistant to treatment. *British Medical Journal* 1:678.

Cobb S. 1976. Social support as a moderator of life stress. *Psychosomatic Medicine* 38:300.

Cobb S, Kasl SV. 1977. *Termination: The Consequence of Job Loss.* Washington, DC: US Department of Health Education and Welfare.

Coker S, Tyrell DAJ, Smith AP. 1991. Psychological stress and susceptibility to the common cold. *New England Journal of Medicine* 32:606.

Coleridge ST. 1853. *Biographia Literaria; or, Biographical Sketches of My Literary Life and Opinions.* New York: Harper, p.609.

Crookshank FG. 1926. The theory of diagnosis. *Lancet* 1:939.

Cunningham A, Edmonds C. 2005. Possible effects of psychological therapy on survival duration in cancer patients. Journal of Clinical Oncology 23(22):5263.Dohrenwend BS, Dohrenwend BP, eds. 1974. *Stressful Life Events: Their Nature and Effects.* New York: John Wiley.Downie R. 2002. *Arts and Humanities in Medical Education in GP Tomorrow, 2nd edn.* Harrison J, van Zwanenberg T (eds) Oxford: Radcliffe Medical Press.

Dubos R. 1965. *Man Adapting.* New Haven, CT: Yale University Press.

Engel CL. 1980. The clinical application of the biopsychosocial model. *American Journal of Psychiatry* 137:535.

Fawzy FI. 1994. Immune effects of short-term intervention for cancer patients. *Advances* 10:32.

Felten SY, Felten DL. 1991. Innervation of lymphoid tissue. In: Ader R, Felton DL, Cohen N, eds., *Psychoneuroimmunology.* San Diego, CA: Academic Press.

Fleck L. 1979. The Genesis and Development Of A Scientific Fact. Chicago, IL: University of Chicago Press.

Foss L, Rothenberg K. 1987. *The Second Medical Revolution: From Biomedicine to Infomedicine.* Boston, MA: New Science Library, Shambhala.

Foss L. 1994. The biomedical paradigm, psychoneuroimmunology, and the black four of hearts. *Advances* 10(1):32.

Gillies JCM 2005. Getting it right in the consultation: Hippocrates; problem; Aristotle's answer. Occasional Paper 86, Royal College of General Practitioners.

Glass RM. 1996. The patient–physician relationship: JAMA focuses on the center of medicine. *Journal of the American Medical Association* 275:147.

Goldstein K. 1995. *The Organism: A Holistic Approach to Biology Derived from Pathological Data in Man.* New York: Zone Books.

Goodwin BC. 1994. Toward a science of qualities. In: Harman W, Clark J, eds., *New Metaphysical Foundations of Modern Science.* Sausalito, CA: Institute of Noetic Sciences.

Goodwin PJ, Leszcz M, Ennis M, Koopmans J, Vincent L, Guther H, Drysdale E, Hundleby M, Chochinov HM, Navarro M, Speca M, Hunter J. 2001. The effect of group psychosocial support on survival in metastatic breast cancer. *The New England Journal of Medicine* 345(24):1719.

Gore S. 1978. The effect of social support in moderating the health consequences of unemployment. *Journal of Health and Social Behavior* 19:157.

Gorovitz S, MacIntyre A. 1976. Toward a theory of medical fallibility. *Journal of Medical Philosophy* 1:51.

Guess HA, Kleinman A, Kusek JW, Engel LW (Eds.). 2002. *The Science of the Placebo: Toward an Interdisciplinary Research Agenda.* Guess London: BMJ Books, p. 343.

Hall H, Minnes L, Olness K. 1993. The psychophysiology of voluntary immunomodulation. *International Journal of Neuroscience* 69:221.

Harman W. 1994. A re-examination of the metaphysical foundations of modern science: Why is it necessary? In: Harman W, Clark J, eds., *New Metaphysical Foundations of Modern Science*. Sausalito, CA: Institute of Noetic Sciences.

Headache Study Group of the University of Western Ontario. 1986. Predictors of outcome in headache patients presenting to family physicians: A one year prospective study. *Headache* 26:285.

Helsing KJ, Szklo M, Comstock GW. 1981. Factors associated with mortality after widowhood. *American Journal of Public Health* 71(8):802.

Hinkle LE. 1974. The effect of exposure to culture change and changes in interpersonal relationships in health. In: Dohrenwend BS, Dohrenwend BP, eds., *Stressful Life Events: Their Nature and Effects*. New York: John Wiley.

Holmes TH, Rahe RH. 1967. The social readjustment rating scale. *Journal of Psychosomatic Research* 11:213.

Jemmott JB, Locke SE. 1984. Psychological factors, immunologic mediation and human susceptibility to infectious diseases: How much do we know? *Psychological Bulletin* 95:78.

Jin RL, Shah CP, Svoboda TJ. 1995. The impact of unemployment on health: A review of the evidence. *Canadian Medical Association Journal* 153:529.

Kiecolt-Glaser JK, Dura JR, Speicher CE, Trask OJ, Glaser R. 1991. Spousal caregivers of dementia victims: Longitudinal changes in immunity and health. *Psychosomatic Medicine* 53(4):345.

Kiecolt-Glaser JK, Glaser R. 1995. Psychoneuroimmunology and health consequences: Data and shared mechanisms. *Psychosomatic Medicine* 57:269. Kiecolt-Glaser JK., McGuire L, Robles TF, Glaser R. (2002a). Psychoneuroimmunology and psychosomatic medicine: back to the future. *Psychosomatic Medicine* 64(1):15.

Kiecolt-Glaser JK, McGuire L, Robles TF, Glaser R. 2002b. Psychoneuroimmunology: Psychological Influences on Immune Function and Health. *Journal of Consulting and Clinical Psychology* 70(3):537–547.

Kiecolt-Glaser JK, McGuire L, Robles TF, Glaser R. 2002c. Emotions, morbidity, and mortality: New perspectives from psychoneuroimmunology. *Annual Review of Psychology* 53:83–107.

Kissane DW, Love A, Hatton A, Bloch S, Smith G, Clarke DM, Miach P, Ikin J, Ranieri N, Snyder RD. 2004. Effect of cognitive-existential group therapy on survival in early-stage breast cancer. *Journal of Clinical Oncology* 22(21):4255–4260.

Kockelmans JJ. 1999. *Phenomenology*. In: R. Audi, ed., *The Cambridge Dictionary of Philosophy,* 2nd edn, Cambridge University Press, p. 665.

Koestler A. 1979. *Janus: A Summing Up*. London: Picador.

Korzybski A. 1958. Science and Sanity: An Introduction to Non-Aristotelian Systems and General Semantics, 4th edn. Lake Bille, CT: International Non-Aristotelian Library Publishing Co.

Kuhn TS. 1967. *The Structure of Scientific Revolutions*. Chicago, IL: University of Chicago Press.

Langer SK. 1979. Philosophy in a New Key. Cambridge, MA: Harvard University Press.

McFarlane WR. 1992. Psychoeducation: A potential model for intervention in family practice. In: Sawa RJ, ed., Family Health Care. Newbury Park, CA: Sage.

Macnaughton J. 2002. Arts and Humanities in Medical Education. In: Harrison J and van Zwanenberg T (Eds.). GP Tomorrow. Oxford: Radcliffe Medical Press, p. 72.

Medalie JH, Goldbourt U. 1976. Some epidemiologic aspects of the high mortality rate in the young widowed group. *Journal of Chronic Disease* 10:207.

Moerman DE. 1983. General medical effectiveness and human biology: Placebo effects in the treatment of ulcer disease. *Medical Anthropology Quarterly* 14:3.

Nuckolls KB, Cassel JC, Kaplan BH. 1972. Psychosocial assets, life crisis and the prognosis of pregnancy. *American Journal of Epidemiology* 95:431.

Olness K, MacDonald JT, Uden DL. 1987. Comparison of self-hypnosis and propranolol in the treatment of juvenile classical migraine. *Pediatrics* 79:593.

Olness K, Ader R. 1992. Conditioning as an adjunct in the pharmacotherapy of lupus erythematosus. *Developmental and Behavioral Pediatrics* 13:124.

Piaget J. 1973. *The Child and Reality*. New York: Grossman.

Peck C, Coleman G. 1991. Implications of placebo theory for clinical research and practice in pain management. *Theoretical Medicine* 12:247.

Polanyi M. 1962. *Personal Knowledge: Towards a Post-critical Philosophy*. Chicago, IL: University of Chicago Press.

Rana J, Mannam A, Donnel-Fink L, Gervino EV, Sellke FW, Laham RJ. 2005. Longevity of the placebo effect in the therapeutic angiogenesis and laser myocardial revascularization trials in patients with coronary heart disease. *American Journal of Cardiology* 95:1456–1459.

Reid M. 1982. Marginal man: The identity dilemma of the academic general practitioner. *Symbolic Interaction* 5(2):325.

Riley V, Fitzmaurice MA, Spackman DA. 1981. Psychoneuroimmunologic factors in neoplasia: Studies in animals. In: Ader R, ed., *Psychoneuroimmunology*. New York: Academic Press.

Robert Wood Johnson Commission Report on Medical Education. 1992.

Ruberman W, Weinblatt E, Goldberg JD, et al. 1984. Psychological influences on mortality after myocardial infarction. *New England Journal of Medicine* 311:552.

Rudebeck CE. 1992. General practice and the dialogue of clinical practice. *Scandinavian Journal of Primary Care*. Supplement 1.

Scheier MF, Bridges MW. 1995. Person variables and health: Personality predispositions and acute psychological states as shared determinants for disease. *Psychosomatic Medicine* 57:255.

Schumacher EF. 1977. *A Guide for the Perplexed*. New York: Harper and Row.

Selye H. 1956. *The Stress of Life*. New York: McGraw-Hill.

Stewart M, Brown JB, Weston WW, McWhinney IR, Freeman TR. 2003. *Patient-Centered Medicine: Transforming the Clinical Method,* 2nd edn. Oxford, UK: Radcliffe Medical Press Ltd.

Toombs SK. 1995. *The Meaning of Illness: A Phenomenological Account of the Different Perspectives of Physician and Patient*. Dordrecht: Kluwer.

Turner RJ. 1983. Direct, indirect and moderating of social support on psychological distress and associated conditions. In: Kaplan HB, ed., *Psychological Stress*. New York: Academic Press.

Turner RJ, Wheaton B, Lloyd DA. 1995. The epidemiology of social stress. *American Sociological Review* 60:104.

Von Bertallanfy L. 1968. *General System Theory*. New York: George Braziller.

von Uexküll T, Geigges W, Herrmann JM. 1993. A fresh look at the immune system: The principle of teleological coherence and harmony of purpose exists at every level of integration in the hierarchy of living systems. *Advances* 9(3):50.

Wasson JH, Sox HC, Sox CH. 1981. The diagnosis of abdominal pain in ambulatory male patients. *Medical Decision Making* 1:215.

Whitehead AN. 1926. *Science and the Modern World*. Cambridge: Cambridge University Press.

Yates FE. 1993. Self-organizing systems. In: Boyd CAR, Noble D, eds., *The Logic of Life: The Challenge of Integrative Physiology*. New York: Oxford University Press.

Zucker A. 1981. Holism and reductionism: A view from genetics. *Journal of Medicine and Philosophy* 6:2.

Notes

1. The word "paradigm" is now commonly used in many different contexts. So much so that it has lost much of its original meaning. Both molecular medicine and evidence-based medicine have been described as new paradigms (Robert Wood Johnson Commission, 1992; Glass, 1996), when, in Kuhn's terms, they are no more than developments within an existing paradigm.

2. Kuhn had a precursor in Ludwig Fleck, a Polish physician and scientist, who, in 1935 published a book in German, later to be translated into English as *The Genesis and Development of a Scientific Fact* (1979). At the time when the book was written, the idea that facts could have a natural history, and could go through a process of social conditioning, was so unfamiliar as to pass unnoticed. Fleck's book is of particular interest to us because he uses the discovery of the Wassermann reaction to illustrate his thesis.

3. For a fuller discussion of these implications, see my article, The Importance of Being Different. *British Journal of General Practice*, 1996, 46:433–436, McWhinney IR, Epstein RM, Freeman T. 1997. Rethinking Somatization. *Annals of Internal Medicine* 126(9):747. and McWhinney IR, Epstein RM, Feeman T. 2001. Rethinking somatization. Advances in Mind-Body Medicine 17(4):232.

4. When a condition previously described as a syndrome is redefined as a disease by the inclusion of a specific pathology, the symptoms and signs that defined the syndrome become part of the new definition. The new category is symptoms and signs plus the pathology. Without the clinical features, the pathology would have no clinical significance. To say that the disease is the cause of the syndrome is tantamount to saying that the category is the cause of itself—the equivalent of saying that lions are the cause of quadripeds.

6

Illness, Suffering, and Healing

The central tasks of a physician's life are understanding illness and understanding people. Because one cannot fully understand an illness without also understanding the person who is ill, these two tasks are indivisible. "He felt that he must know the man before he could do him good," wrote Nathaniel Hawthorne of Harrison, the physician in *The Scarlet Letter*. One approach to the understanding of illness is through the application of our knowledge of science and technology. This will give us an understanding of the illness on one level, but it will not enable us to understand the patient as a person, with unique life story, feelings, values, and relationships. Nor will it help us to understand the deeper meaning the illness may have for him or her. Science, as seen in Chapter 5, gives us a knowledge of abstractions. These abstractions are very powerful. They enable us to make the precise inferences and predictions on which the technology of medicine is based. But they do so by ignoring and excluding the concrete experience of illness as lived through by the patient. In Richard Baron's words (1985), "a great gulf now exists between the way we think about disease as physicians and the way we experience it as patients."

The grip that abstraction has on modern medicine is, we believe, at the root of one of the paradoxes of the doctor–patient relationship. At a time when medicine has never been more technologically successful, physicians have never been more criticized and attacked. In the past two decades there has been a remarkable increase in the number of books and articles describing personal experiences of illness. These writings, by patients themselves or by their relatives, are often bitterly critical of physicians. They are uncomfortable for us to read, and it is tempting to become defensive or to dismiss the writers as complainers. It is important, however, that we pay attention to what they say. They tell us something about the state of medicine and, if we do not regard the criticisms as applying only to others, they can teach us something about ourselves.

Arthur Frank (1991) developed testicular cancer at the age of 40. "I always assumed," writes Frank,

that if I became seriously ill, physicians, no matter how overworked, would somehow recognize what I was living through. I did not know what form this recognition would take, but I assumed it would happen. What I experienced was the opposite. The more critical my diagnosis became, the more reluctant physicians were to talk to me. I had trouble getting them to make eye contact; most came only to see my disease. This "it" within the body was their field of investigation; "I" seemed to exist beyond the horizon of their interest.... After five years of dealing with medical professionals in the context of critical illness, as opposed to the routine problems I had had before, I have accepted their limits, even if I have never become comfortable with them. Perhaps medicine should reform itself and learn to share illness talk with patients instead of imposing disease talk on them. Or perhaps physicians and nurses should simply do what they already do well—treat the breakdowns—and not claim to do more.

The novelist Reynolds Price (1994), writing of his experience with a spinal cord tumor and subsequent paraplegia and chronic pain, has good words for his surgeon but says this about his encounters with other doctors:

...surely a doctor should be expected to share—and to offer at all appropriate hours—the skill we expect of a teacher, a fireman, a priest, a cop, the neighborhood milkman or the dog-pound manager.

These are merely the skills of human sympathy, the skills for letting another creature know that his or her concern is honored and valued and that, whether a cure is likely or not, all possible efforts will be expended to achieve that aim or to ease incurable agony toward its welcome end. Such skills are not rare in the natural world. What else but the urge to use and perfect such skills on other human beings in need could drive a man or woman into medicine? What but massive failure to recognize one's stunted emotions before they blunder against live tissue—that and an avid taste for money and power? And having blundered on other creatures, how can the blunderer not attempt to change? Is he or she legally blind as well? Maybe we have the right to demand that such a flawed practitioner display a warning on the office door or the starched lab coat, like those on other dangerous bets—*Expert technician. Expect no more. The quality of your life and death are your concern.*

When Price was referred to a pain clinic for his chronic neurologic pain, the physicians there did not even mention therapies for pain that were available on another floor of the same building. Eventually, 2 years later, Price found that two of these—biofeedback and hypnosis—helped more than anything else to make his pain tolerable.

Some of the most revealing accounts of illness have come from physicians who have become patients. Dr. DeWitt Stetten (1981) wrote of his experience with progressive loss of vision caused by macular degeneration:

Through all these years and despite many encounters with skilled and experienced professionals, no ophthalmologist has at any time suggested any devices that might be of assistance to me. No ophthalmologist has mentioned any of the many ways in which I could stem the deterioration in the quality of my life. Fortunately, I have discovered a number of means whereby I have helped myself, and the purpose of this essay is to call the attention of the ophthalmological world to some of these devices and, courteously but firmly, to complain of what appears to be the ophthalmologist's attitude: "We are interested in vision but have little interest in blindness."

What we see in Dr. Stetten's physicians, I think, is an extreme literal-mindedness: a poverty of feeling that renders them incapable of recognizing the suffering of a person going through this devastating disruption of his "lifeworld," and a lack of that imaginative power that might have given them some sense of it. To these ophthalmologists, it appears, macular degeneration is a condition of the retina, not a human experience. The fault, moreover, is not unique to ophthalmologists. We are all guilty, family physicians included. In his attempts to compensate for his disorientation in space and time, Stetten learned about a machine that projects enormously magnified printed material onto a television monitor, the Talking Books Program, the Talking Clock, and a reading machine that converts the printed word to synthesized speech. In no instance did his information come from ophthalmologists.

Modern physicians have not been trained to understand illness as a human experience. In our formal education, we live mainly in a world of abstractions. Medical knowledge is defined implicitly as a knowledge of diseases. Macular degeneration is part of medical knowledge, but not the experience of going blind. The boundaries drawn between specialties reflect this tacit definition of medical knowledge. The patient's adaptation to illness and disability may be defined as "rehabilitation," and therefore the concern of a different specialist or another profession. Patients often find such rigid boundaries difficult to understand. Even though some differentiation of function is inevitable, we need to be alive to the ways in which too rigid a drawing of boundaries can impair our capacity as healers. Because family medicine is defined in terms of relationships, we have no need to feel restricted by the way medicine is subdivided. The resources of the specialties can be used without relinquishing our healing role.

How can we teach ourselves to understand the experience of our patients? We can learn, first of all, by paying attention to their experience, by practicing the very difficult art of listening, by reading the appropriate literature, and by reflecting on our own experience.

Autobiographies and biographies that describe experiences of illness—now known as pathographies (Hawkins, 1993)—provide us with rich opportunities for deepening our knowledge and understanding. Although—like the ones I have quoted—they are sometimes critical of physicians, they are often profound meditations on illness and healing. Some are works of literature in their own right. Book-length pathographies are a recent phenomenon. Before 1950 they were rare; now there are many. Besides the books, there have also been numerous articles in magazines and medical journals. Why this abrupt appearance of a new literary genre? Hawkins (1993) sees it as a possible reaction to a medicine "so dominated by a biophysical understanding of illness that its experiential aspects are virtually ignored." She describes three groups of pathographies: testimonial, angry, and those advocating alternative therapies. Testimonial pathographies, mostly from the 1960s and 1970s, are didactic in intent, "blending a personal account of illness with practical information." In the 1980s these mainly uncritical accounts give place to those expressing anger at "a medical system seen as out of control, dehumanized, and sometimes brutalizing." According to Hawkins, two themes recur in these stories: "the tendency in contemporary medical practice to focus primarily not on the needs of the individual who is sick but on the nomothetic condition we call the disease, and the sense that our medical technology has advanced beyond our capacity to use it wisely." The third group, also a feature of the 1980s, is less critical of physicians, but treats orthodox medicine as only one of a large number of therapies available to sufferers.

To these three groups I would add another: books written by philosophers, anthropologists, physicians, and literary critics, who bring a professional interest and expertise to bear on the subject of illness narratives. Hawkins' book is one of these.

Some of these writers bring their professional expertise to bear on their own illness. Kay Toombs (1992) writes on the meaning of illness as a philosopher and sufferer from multiple sclerosis. Oliver Sacks (1984) brings his knowledge as a neurologist and medical theorist to bear on his own experience of illness.

Hawkins views pathography as "a re-formulation of the experience of illness" using formulation in Robert Lifton's (1967) sense of a restorative process. Like the authors of pathographies, Lifton is writing about a devastating experience: survival of the atomic attack on Hiroshima.

[T]he act of formulation... involves the discovery of patterns in experience, the imposition of order, the creation of meaning—all with the purpose of mastering a traumatic experience and thereby re-establishing a sense of connectedness with objective reality and with other people.

Note that what these reformulations provide—the sense of coherence, the feeling of mastery, the creation of meaning—are the elements also of a healing relationship. A pathography can be healing for its author and for its readers; it can also help physicians to be healers for their patients, to act as their guides through terrifying and devastating experiences. The message to us from many pathographies is that we have almost forgotten what it is to be a healer.

It is not easy for us to attend to our patients' experience. To do so requires us to step out of our usual way of attending to a person's illness. We are trained to see illness as a set of signs and symptoms defining a disease state as a case of diabetes or peptic ulcer or schizophrenia. The patient, on the other hand, sees illness in terms of its effects on his or her life. The physician, therefore, must learn to see illness as it is lived through, before it has been categorized and interpreted in scientific terms. Although every illness is different in some way because everybody's life story is different, there are certain common features of illness as a lived experience (Toombs, 1992).

The Patient's Experience of Illness

A healthy person takes his or her body for granted. It does, of course, impose limitations on what he or she can do, but the person does not have to bring into consciousness the everyday acts of living. As I write this, I am not conscious of the coordinated movements of my hand. The sick become very much aware of the body and the limitations it imposes. They have to think about activities that previously were carried out below the level of awareness. Will I manage this flight of stairs? Will I be able to get on the bus to do my shopping? Bodily functions, which previously formed the background to one's world, become the foreground; the rest of world recedes into the background. In health, the body and the self are one: we are *our* bodies. In sickness, the body becomes something other than the self, something alien, over which the self has limited control.

Physicians see illness in terms of a disturbance of bodily function. Patients see it as a disruption of their "being in the world."

Critical illness leaves no aspect of life untouched. The hospitals and other special places we have constructed for critically ill persons have created the illusion that by sealing off the ill person from those who are healthy, we can also seal off the illness in that ill person's life. This illusion is dangerous. Your relationships, your work, your sense of who you are and who you might become, your sense of what life is and ought to be—these all change, and the change is terrifying. (Frank, 1991)

In Kay Toombs' words, "A patient does not so much have an illness as exist an illness." She takes to the physician a problem of existence but finds the physician's attention directed to her body rather than to her problems with existence. The patient feels "reduced to a malfunctioning biological organism" (Toombs, 1992).

Chronic disease, especially if it brings successive losses of independence and control, often engenders profound sensations of grief. With grief come the feelings associated with it: sadness and anger, guilt and remorse. If the illness is one that carries a stigma—such as epilepsy, cancer, or AIDS—then feelings of rejection may add to the grief. Anger may be projected onto the physician, who may be viewed as responsible for delays in diagnosis or errors in management. Given the insidious nature of many chronic illnesses and the difficulties of early diagnosis, family physicians are especially liable to encounter this level of hostility. When the patient feels responsible for causing his or her own disease, the anger is turned inward. Those physicians who would like to convince people that they are responsible for their own healing should consider the consequences in guilt and remorse if their efforts do not improve their health or prevent deterioration.

Fear and anxiety are ever-present in illness, even in minor illness. Fears are many and varied, rational and irrational. Physicians cannot assume that they know what patients' fears are until they make an effort to discover them. A patient may have come to terms with the fact that she has progressive cancer but may still fear that her death will be painful and distressing. Or she may fear for the future of her family. Dying patients may have a fear that they will be abandoned by their doctor if they complain too much. They then become reluctant to ask for a visit when they need one, and tolerate pain that could be controlled. This is why regular, rather than "on request" visits are so important for dying patients.

A number of physicians, most recently Eric Cassell (1990), have observed that illness may impair the faculty of reason. The most rational of people may become irrational, and even superstitious. This impairment of judgment is rarely considered when we are enjoined to give patients responsibility for decisions about their treatment. As an ethical principle, this is no doubt correct. In real life the issue is rarely so clearly defined.

The threats to self that illness brings—the disruption, loss of autonomy, loss of control, and loss of confidence—make sick persons very vulnerable. They not only feel vulnerable, they are vulnerable. This vulnerability makes it impossible for the relationship between the doctor and the sick patient to be an equal one, however much we may wish it to be so. This puts a great responsibility on physicians to respect patients' vulnerability and to use their power responsibly and with compassion.

Kay Toombs has commented on the changed sense of time and space that illness induces. The natural rhythms of the body—the rhythms of eating, sleeping, working, resting—are disturbed. The patient loses the sense of the future as a time of possibilities. Simple tasks like dressing and tying shoelaces may occupy a large part of the day. Hull (1990) says of his experience as a blind person:

Sighted people can bend time. For sighted people, time is sometimes slow and sometimes rapid. They can make up for being lazy by rushing later on....For me, as a blind person, time is simply the medium of my activities. It is the inexorable context within which I do what must be done. For example, the reason why I do not seem to be in a hurry as I go around the building is not that I have less to do than my colleagues, but I am simply unable to hurry.

"Perhaps all severe disabilities," says Hull, "lead to a decrease in space and an increase in time." Toombs (1992) remarks on how illness changes the character of one's sense of space. "...[O]bjects or locations [the bathroom, for example] which were formerly regarded as 'near' are now experienced as 'far.'...Spaciality...constricts in the sense that the range of possible actions becomes severely circumscribed. Rather than representing the arena of possible action, space is encountered as the restriction of possibilities."

Toombs (1992) writes of the "profound effects of the loss of upright posture." A person in a wheelchair at a social gathering, being low on the ground, may be treated like a child, in that people talk to their spouse about them, as if they were not able to speak for themselves.

In mental illness, the threat to the self is terrifying. The experience of dementia, depression, schizophrenia, or anxiety may produce the most intense suffering. The experience is not limited to those with severe mental illness. It is often surprising to find that patients who are mildly depressed will express fears of insanity.

An account of the experience of illness would not be complete without mention of the response to illness. People do triumph over their disabilities. The body has remarkable powers of compensation and adaptation. A newly defined self can emerge from suffering. Suffering engenders the kind of introspection that can add a new depth to the personality. Although the patient may have little control over the course of the illness, he or she is free to choose how to respond to it.

So far, we have been considering the experience of illness and disability in a person who was previously healthy. The process is one of alienation of the body from the self. The situation is different in those who are born with a disability. In these, the disabled body is the lived body, from the very beginning. Rather than the body becoming alien to the self, the body, with its disabilities, is the self. With some disabilities such as deafness, the person enters a culture with a strong sense of its place in the world. A child may resist a parent's attempts to correct some disability on the grounds that if they corrected it, "it wouldn't be me." Rejection of the disability may be interpreted as rejection of the child. Harm may be done by attempts to correct "disabilities" that are themselves harmless variants. At one time, left-handed children were forced to use their right hands. When a child has severe disability that can be corrected, the process of adaptation is the reverse of that in a person with an acquired disability. The child, whose body and self have grown within their limitations, has to develop a different way of "being in the world"—a world with wider horizons.

Although all sufferers from chronic disease and disability have something in common, each patient's story is an individual one. The experience of illness also varies with the course the illness takes: a sudden or gradual onset; a one-time disability like stroke or injury, which then remains static; a progressively downhill course; or a process of remissions and relapses. Loss of vision, for example, is often a very long process ending in the state of blindness—a new way of being in the world. John Hull (1992) a university professor, describes his own experience:

First, there was a period of hope that lasted for a year or 18 months. It was brought to an end by the deterioration of sight during the summer of 1981, although even as late as the summer of 1982, when I was still seeing a few lights, colours and shapes, I could not resist occasional flickers of hope.

Secondly, there was a period of busyness in overcoming the problems. This began about the summer of 1981, when visual work became impossible, and lasted until about the summer of 1984. It was not until Easter of 1985 that I began to have a feeling that I did not need any more equipment. A main drive to create a workable office system took place during 1982 and 1983. During this time, blindness was a challenge.

The third stage began some time in 1983, possibly late in the year, and lasted for about a year. This was the time when I passed through despair. These were the years during which my sleep was punctuated by terrible dreams, and my waking life was oppressed by awareness of being carried irresistibly deeper and deeper into blindness.

The fourth and current period has begun since the autumn of 1984, i.e., since the recovery from the visit to Australia, during which time blindness had engulfed me. I began writing my book on adult religious education in October of 1984 and concluded it in March of 1985.

For most of the time now my brain no longer hurts with the pain of blindness. There has been a strange change in the state or the kind of activity in my brain. It seems to have turned in upon itself to find inner resources. Being denied the stimulus of much of the outside world, it has had to sort out its own functions and priorities. I now feel clearer, more excited and more adventurous intellectually than ever before in my life. I find myself connecting more, remembering more, making more links in my mind between various things I have read and had to learn over the years. Sometimes I come home in the evening and feel that my mind is almost bursting with new ideas and new horizons.

I continue to find deep need for that kind of sustenance. Even a single day without study, away from the possibility of learning something new, can precipitate a new sense of urgency and suffering. I still feel like a person on a kidney machine, but increasingly like a person who has managed to survive.[1]

Primacy of the person has been mentioned as one of the fundamental principles of family medicine. To give primacy to the personhood of the patient requires that we attend very carefully to the meaning the illness has for him or her, not as an "add-on" after clinical diagnosis but as a central obligation. This has implications for our clinical method, which is discussed in Chapter 8.

Suffering

Eric Cassell (1991) recognizes three aspects of suffering. First, suffering involves the whole person and "requires a rejection of the historic dualism of mind and body." Second, people suffer when threatened by distress which can cause them serious harm. Third, "suffering can occur in relation to any aspect of the person."

Arthur Kleinman (Kleinman and Kleinman, 1997) adds that a suffering person not only perceives a threat, but also must resist it. Also, that suffering has a social dimension "that undergoes great cultural elaboration in distinctive local worlds." Frank regards telling stories as a form of resistance: "people tell uniquely personal stories, but they neither make these stories by themselves, nor do they tell them only to themselves. Stories of suffering have two sides: one expresses the threat of disintegration, the other the emphasis on resistance" (1997, p.171). What Frank calls the quest narrative "recognizes that the old intactness must be stripped away to prepare for something new. Quest stories reflect a confidence in what is waiting to emerge from suffering."

The suffering of the following woman was inevitably of the first kind. There was, however, an outcome which was of very great importance to her: the continuing relationship between her daughters.

Case 6.1

A woman with widespread metastases from carcinoma of the lung asked me if I (IRMcW) could assure her that she would not suffer. I told her that nobody could give her that assurance. Almost certainly, we would be able to relieve her pain, but suffering is intensely personal and not by any means synonymous with pain. There were many reasons for this woman to suffer. What we could say to her was that we would be sensitive to her sufferings, listen to her, be with her, and support her and her family during the last stages of her illness.

This woman was a widow who had lost her husband only 1 year earlier. She had two daughters, one in her twenties, the other in her teens, and suffered many anxieties about their future. She had paraplegia caused by spinal cord compression and had decided not to have surgery for this. The thoracotomy done for her primary tumor had been followed by respiratory failure, for which she had spent several months in the hospital. The steroids given for the spinal cord compression had given her a bloated appearance that caused her intense distress. She was so heavy that three nurses were needed to lift her. If she lay down, she became breathless and felt she was going to suffocate. Metastatic deposits in the cervical epidural space caused nerve root pain in the right arm, with progressive weakness and loss of function. A month before her death, she developed a pathological fracture of the femoral neck which caused severe pain on movement, uncontrollable by morphine. Because she was deemed unfit for surgical immobilization of the fracture, it was kept immobile by other means as far as possible, and she was moved with great care by a team of nurses.

The only way we could help this woman to bear her inevitable sufferings was to identify them and help her with them one by one. Her wheelchair mobility, and therefore her feeling of independence, was maintained until her fractured femur made it impossible. Discussions were held with the daughters and relatives about their future. In the course of these, the daughters became closer to each other than they had ever been before. One thing that always made the patient's eyes light up was to be complimented on her appearance, She would spend hours before her mirror and worked very hard to repair the ravages of her treatment. Her anxieties about suffocation were confronted. She had radiotherapy for the epidural metastases and morphine and a coanalgesic for her skeletal pain.

Physicians tend to equate suffering with pain and disease. As Eric Cassell observes, suffering is a very personal matter. How much suffering is caused by a pain or disease depends on many individual factors. The suffering caused by pain is greater if pain is chronic, if the reason for the pain is not known, and if the patient feels that it cannot be controlled. It is a common experience that patients with chronic cancer pain feel a great release from suffering when it has been demonstrated to them that their pain can be controlled by narcotics. Patients suffer more if their pain has not been validated by a physical diagnosis and if, as a result, their relatives or their physician convey disbelief in its reality.

The suffering produced by disruption of the sense of self depends on how a person defines his or her sense of self. A middle-aged laborer may be devastated by a physical disability that would cause little suffering to a sedentary worker. Loss of sexual function may be devastating to one person but of little importance to another. To a young woman without children, loss of her uterus may be the loss of her hope for the future; to a middle-aged woman, loss of her uterus may be a relief.

Suffering is increased if it is associated with guilt, if the pain and disability are caused by some foolish and avoidable error—an accident or some form of self-abuse, for example. The most intense form of suffering is vicarious suffering, the anguish of a relative who sees a loved one suffering, especially if the relative feels that he or she may be to blame. Parents suffer greatly through the misfortunes of their children and usually feel that they are to blame in some way.

In his book *The Doctor and the Soul*, Victor Frankl (1973) has written of the importance of finding meaning in suffering. Frankl himself suffered greatly in a concentration camp during World War II but was able to find some meaning in his suffering. Almost any suffering can be tolerated if it can be imbued with meaning. Frankl tells the story of an elderly physician—a widower—who was very depressed by chronic illness and loneliness. Frankl asked him which he would have preferred: his present situation or for his wife to have been left alone and suffering. He began to see his suffering in a new light, as a burden he was carrying for his wife's sake after a long and happy marriage.

We cannot understand suffering until we realize that it is indivisible. Cicely Saunders (1984) uses the term "total pain" to express the fact that suffering is physical, mental, and spiritual. People suffer with their whole selves. The only way we can find out how they are suffering is to ask them. One of the most common errors we make as physicians is to treat pain but ignore other dimensions of suffering.

The Physician as Healer

All that a physician does for a sick person is dependent on the healing power of nature, expressed in the old principle of *vis medicatrix naturae*. Our therapies are designed to assist the patient's own healing powers and to remove the obstacles to healing. Lacerations heal when sutured, fractures heal when set and immobilized, and abscesses heal when drained. Before the advent of antibiotics, collapse therapy for pulmonary tuberculosis helped to remove an obstacle to healing by closing the cavities maintained by physical properties of the lungs. Antibiotics are of limited value when the immune system is impaired. General, nonspecific measures such as rest, nourishment, and relief of pain and anxiety are designed to strengthen the body's own healing powers. Our dependence on nature's healing powers becomes abundantly clear when we are dealing with a person whose immune system has failed or one who presents obstacles to healing that we cannot remove.

The healing powers of nature are not limited to physical wounds. A person is equally provided with powers to heal psychic wounds. Perhaps the most common example is the experience of bereavement. The natural response to bereavement and to other types of serious loss is a grieving process in the course of which the person experiences eventual healing, although, as with a physical wound, a scar remains. As with a physical wound or disease, healing may be inhibited. The healing of the psyche may be obstructed by various forms of self-deception, including the suppression from consciousness of painful or unwelcome feelings and experiences. In a bereaved person the grieving process may be prolonged if the emotions of grief are suppressed. Shakespeare understood this well. In *Macbeth*, when MacDuff learns that his wife and children have been murdered,

Malcolm says to him: "Give sorrow words. The grief that does not speak whispers the o'erwrought heart and bids it break."

What qualities do family physicians require as healers? First, we should be masters of those tools and techniques that fall within our own field. These are the therapeutic agents of healing at the physical level—the drugs, instruments, and manual skills. Among these are the skills of early diagnosis and rehabilitation. Much suffering can be avoided by good clinical practice. One of my general practitioner father's aphorisms was "Rehabilitation begins at the time of the injury." Sometimes, the doctor has to help the patient to identify and work through problems that are inhibiting healing (see *Case 8.6*). Sometimes the doctor himself is adding to these problems (see *Case 8.7*). For patients who are struggling with progressive and permanent disabilities, there are many aids ranging from mechanical devices to counseling services. The family doctor is unlikely to know them all, but at least he should know how a patient can gain access to them. Sometimes we deny patients access to services because in our egoism we cannot accept our own need of assistance.

Second, we should master the skills of healing at the mental level—the skills of communication: attentive listening, facilitation, and the provision of reassurance. Healing at the highest level, however, is not primarily a matter of technique. Techniques are certainly helpful, but they are not sufficient in themselves. For example, the best of listening skills will not be helpful if we do not believe that what patients are telling us is interesting and helpful. To be a healer for one's patients is to recognize and acknowledge their suffering, to understand the meaning the illness has for them, to be present for them in their times of need, and to give them hope. Ian Gawler (1995) a long-term survivor of metastatic osteogenic sarcoma, describes five kinds of hope. One is the *absence of hope*—hopelessness—the belief that recovery is impossible. Even in cases of advanced cancer, Gawler urges doctors to leave patients with a little hope. Remarkable and unexpected remissions do occur.

Hope for survival (the hope not to die) is a fragile stage and may lead to trials of alternative medicine. Patients need a lot of support at this time. In *hope for a better future*, patients are looking ahead to future plans and important events like a family anniversary or the birth of a new grandchild. This may be a time when short-term sacrifices are made in the hope of a better future: strict diets for example. *Hope for spiritual realization* is the awakening to a deeper purpose in life that serious illness may provoke. The need here is for a doctor who will take this seriously. *Hope for the present moment* is the capacity for living in the moment by developing the practice of mindfulness: an awareness of experience from moment to moment that becomes so vivid that past and future lose much of their importance.

Recognition of a person's suffering sounds like such a simple thing, yet we hear so often that it is not forthcoming from doctors. In this regard, we cannot use lack of time as our excuse, for it is a question more of manner than of time. Patients are very quick to recognize indifference to their suffering in even the briefest of encounters. They are also very quick to recognize that a doctor senses their pain.

In George Eliot's story "Janet's Repentance," Janet is in despair, abused by her husband and herself addicted to alcohol. In her despair she turns to the Reverend Tryan, a man who she senses has himself known suffering and despair:

He saw that the first thing Janet needed was to be assured of sympathy. She must be made to feel that her anguish was not strange to him; that he entered into the only half-expressed secrets, before any other message of consolation could find its way into her heart. The tale of Divine pity was never yet believed from lips that were not felt to be moved by human pity.

To understand the meaning of the illness for the patient one must listen to the story of the illness. "…illness in its immediacy is not simply an isolated physical event but rather it is an episode which is embedded in the unique life narrative of the patient. …present meaning is always constituted in terms of past meanings and future anticipations" (Toombs, 1992, p. 109). An understanding of the meaning of the illness for the patient is an integral part of the patient-centered clinical method (see pp. 136–143). The doctor's interpretation should synthesize the pathological basis of the illness with the narrative context.

Listening to the story of the illness takes time, though less time in family practice than in other fields of medicine. The long-term relationships in general practice can give the doctor a prior knowledge of the patient's life story—a context into which each new event can be fitted. Often the doctor has been a witness to, or participant in, the story. However, our knowledge is never complete, and we are often surprised by the new understanding that emerges, even in patients we have known for many years.

To be present for patients in their times of need requires commitment and involvement. The healing relationship takes its place with those other human relationships where there is both commitment and involvement: husband–wife; parent–child; teacher–learner. A sufferer is not healed by a person who keeps his distance. As Toombs (1995) puts it: "I don't want to be cared for by somebody who doesn't care about me." In the real world of conflicting obligations, one cannot always be present for those we care about. Even with our children, care must often be responsibly delegated. But there are times of great need when other obligations must be set aside. The need may only be for simple presence, as in a visit to a dying patient when everything else has been done. Some of the things I have regretted most have been those occasions when I have failed to realize the importance of presence. Sometimes one is forgiven for these failures, sometimes not.

Of course, the kind of involvement in the relationship between healer and patient is different from that in relationships where there is a kinship and emotional bond. There are both right ways and wrong ways for a healer to be involved. I will return to these presently.

As we listen to patients' stories, we are trying to form a picture of what life is like for them: of their own understanding of the illness, of their hopes and fears, of the disruptions in their social world, and of the strengths and resources they bring to bear in their struggle for wholeness. A well-timed question may help the patient to express these feelings, as well as assuring him or her of our interest.

Toombs (1992) says "... no physician has ever inquired of me what it is like to live with multiple sclerosis or to experience any of the disabilities that have accrued over the past seventeen years. Perhaps, most surprisingly, no neurologist has ever asked me if I am afraid, or, for that matter, even whether I am concerned about the future." She observes that "fears for the future are nearly always concrete. 'Will I be able to walk from my office to the classroom?' 'Will my illness be prolonged and prevent me from carrying out an important project?'" Concrete fears can always be addressed. Knowing this helps to remove our own sense of helplessness, which can make us afraid to ask the question.

Because each patient deals with an illness in his or her own way, listening to their stories is a matter of attending to particulars. This is in marked contrast to our diagnostic mode of thought in which we are trying to categorize the illness. Arthur Frank (1991) writes that: "Caring has nothing to do with categories; it shows the person that her life is valued because it recognizes what makes her experience particular;"

Care begins when difference is recognized. There is no 'right thing to say to a cancer patient,' because the 'cancer patient' as a generic entity does not exist. There are only persons who are different to start with, having different experiences according to the contingencies of their diseases. The common diagnostic categories to which medicine places its patients are relevant to disease, not to illness. They are useful for treatment, but they only get in the way of care.

To be a healer is to help patients find their own way through the ordeal of their illness to a new wholeness. John Hull (1992) writes in July 1985:

I am developing the art of gazing with my hands. I like to hold and rehold and go on holding a beautiful object, absorbing every aspect of it. In a multicultural exhibition the other day, I was allowed to handle a string of beads, smooth and polished, and a South American water jar made from earthenware. There was a lovely, scraping sound when one rotated the lid of the jar, and thousands of tiny, tinkling hollow echoes were made when the full, round belly of the jar was touched with the fingernails.

Hull has long enjoyed the beauty of the English cathedrals. While he could see, his feeling for them was predominantly visual. After he became blind, he learned how their beauty could also be sensed through hearing and touch: the changing quality of sound as one moves through the building, the feel of the stone. He has now designed, with the help of others, acoustic and tactile guides for the blind in seventeen English cathedrals, including Canterbury and York.

Suppose that we could, in a small way, help a patient in such a journey. Of course, only one in a million will take the path that Hull took. But each will have his or her own way, and perhaps it is the least articulate—those who do not write their stories—who need the most help.

Involvement

Generations of medical students have been told, "Don't get involved: keep your distance." One of the assumptions of the conventional clinical method is that the correct attitude of the physician should be that of a detached observer. In my own experience, the teachers who gave this advice did not convey the complexity of the issue. They meant to say, I think, "don't get emotionally involved." But they did not explain how to avoid this while maintaining the involvement necessary for healing. Neither did they admit that we can remain emotionally detached only by suppressing our feelings, a process that can seriously inhibit our capacity to heal. Our encounters with patients can provoke in us some very disturbing feelings, including those of fear and helplessness. One defense against these feelings is avoidance of the situations that provoke them—a common experience in the care of patients who are incurably or terminally ill. But in protecting ourselves, we deny our patients the care they have a right to expect from us. If we cannot be open to our own pain, how can we be open to the pain of others?

The question is better framed in two parts: "What is 'healing' involvement?" and "How do we avoid the pitfalls of emotional involvement?" Healing involvement can be expressed in two words: attention and presence. What it means to attend to a patient is conveyed by a story told in Jacob Needleman's book *The Way of the Physician* (1992). As a boy, he had to pay a visit to the family doctor, a longtime friend of the family who was like an uncle to him. As he was going into the waiting room, he passed the open door of an examination room where his "uncle," the doctor, was examining an obese old man. For a moment, their eyes met, but the doctor did not acknowledge him. Needleman went past the door again, hoping to get a smile from his uncle. Once again there was no hint of recognition. At first he felt hurt, but then he understood that, for that brief time, the fat old man had the doctor's undivided attention: "you cared for that old man as much as you cared for me. Yet you were a friend of my family; you tousled my hair, you gave me candy, you called me by amusing names. But then and there you cared for that old man more than you cared for me." It was, says Needleman, a manifestation of "non-egoistic impersonal love" (Needleman, 1985).

I (IRMcW) have never forgotten a brief experience I had as a medical student. When at home, I used to do rounds with the surgeon at the local hospital. After the round, he was asked to see an old vagrant from the workhouse, who was complaining of abdominal pain. The experience made a deep and lasting impression on me. The patient was exactly as one would have expected: his face red and blotchy; several days' growth of beard on his chin. For those few minutes, this old vagrant seemed to be the most important person in the world for the doctor. All his attention was focused on the old man, whom he treated with the utmost respect—a respect that showed in the way he talked and listened and the way he examined him. The word that perhaps describes it best is presence: for those few minutes, the doctor was a real presence in the patient's life.

The fact that this attention is nonegoistic and impersonal means that the doctor is at the same time involved and detached. When he has finished with one patient, he can transfer the same undivided attention to the next. It is not that feelings are absent, but that they are on a different level from egoistic emotions. It would be wrong, however, to suggest that the difference between the two ways of being involved is clear-cut. This is especially true for family doctors. The long-term relationships with patients cannot often be impersonal. Feelings of many kinds enter into these relationships, some of them helpful to healing, some of them harmful. It is when our egoistic emotions become involved that we encounter the pitfalls.

Egoistic emotions can enter into the relationship in many ways, some of them very subtle. Our helplessness in the face of suffering can make us afraid to recognize the sufferings of our patients; our openness to patients may be inhibited by our fears of what questions they will ask. We are capable of using our power to punish patients who anger us. Our therapeutic recommendations may be tinged with self-interest; our advocacy of our patients' interests may become a personal crusade in which their interests become secondary to our need to advance a cause. Work of healing with patients who have suffered childhood abuse has, in some overzealous hands, become a destructive process in which patients and their families have suffered. Sometimes, at a case conference, one becomes aware that the tone of the discussion has changed from one that is helpful to the patients in practical ways, to a dissection of the patient's soul from on high. Some of the great novelists teach us how subtle these pitfalls can be.

In *The Brothers Karamazov*, Dostoevsky describes how the young novice monk Alexey has tried to give money to a poor man who has been humiliated in public by Alexey's older brother. The man refuses the gift with indignation. Later Alexey is discussing with Lisa, an invalid girl, how he might get the man to take the money. "Listen Alexey," says Lisa, "don't you think our reasoning...shows that we regard him—that unfortunate man_with contempt? I mean that we analyze his soul like this, as though from above? I mean that we're absolutely certain that he'll accept the money. Don't you think so?" Later in their discussion Alexey says to her "...your question whether we do not despise that unhappy man by dissecting his soul was the question of a person who has suffered a lot....a person to whom such questions occur is himself capable of suffering."

In *Emma*, Jane Austen describes how, in a moment of truth, Emma Woodhouse realizes that "with insufferable vanity (she had) believed herself in the secret of everybody's feelings; with unpardonable arrogance proposed to arrange everybody's destiny." Instead of, as she thought, working for the good of her young friend Harriet Smith, she had in fact brought evil on her.

What makes the intrusion of egoistic emotions into the doctor–patient relationship difficult for us is the fact that they are so often at the unconscious level. In psychoanalysis, the process is referred to as transference and countertransference. "Transference in the clinical relationship denotes the patient's displacement and externalizing of internal issues onto the clinician; countertransference denotes the reverse" (Stein, 1985). In analysis, the therapist deliberately does not respond intuitively to transference, because he or she wants the patient to face up to the immature response that the behavior represents. The therapist must try to identify responses arising from his or her own countertransference, so that he or she can avoid the harm that may be done if these feelings are acted out. It has taken a long time for us to realize that these notions apply to all therapeutic relationships, including those in family practice. Freud (Gay, 1989) described three types of transference. Negative transference is the direction of hostile feelings onto the analyst; in erotic transference, the analyst becomes the object of erotic love. Both of these obstruct healing and must be exposed and learned from. In the third type—sensible transference—the therapist is seen as a supportive ally in the process of healing. It is, said Freud, "essentially a cure through love."

In the long-term relationships of family practice, feelings may be expressed by both doctor and patient that are simply part of the relationship and have nothing to do with transference. When transference can be identified, it may not be harmful, as when a patient becomes temporarily dependent at a time of serious illness or crisis. On the other hand, all of us, at some time or other, act out our egoistic emotions in ways that are anti-therapeutic. How can we avoid these pitfalls? Only by striving for self-knowledge—that most difficult of all fields of knowledge—most difficult because it can be attained only by facing honestly those parts of our own nature that are most painful to acknowledge. Self-knowledge comes in a number of ways: sometimes at times of crisis, through illness, failure, or suffering; sometimes in moments of truth, such as one finds in the stories of the great novelists; sometimes in old age. In day-to-day experience, however, self-knowledge comes through attention to ourselves in the same way as we attend to our patients. By attending to our thoughts and feelings as they arise in us, we can become aware of them before they do harm "... it is a matter of emotions of man: how to control them, how to evoke the non-egoistic emotions, and how to free ourselves from the emotions that make wreckage of our lives individually and collectively. The question of human relationship is synonymous with the question of human emotions" (Needleman, 1992). Studying our own emotions should be the realm of psychology, but as Needleman (1992) and Bettelheim (1984) have observed, modern psychology is predominantly concerned with the study of other people's emotions. But psychology did not begin in modern times. All the great spiritual traditions have psychological theories as well as spiritual disciplines designed to do what Needleman describes. Though the disciplines differ in details, they are remarkably consistent in using contemplative methods of "mindfulness, awareness." These methods, or modifications of them, are now being used therapeutically.[2]

Moral and Spiritual Aspects of Healing

It has become quite common to refer to the spiritual aspect of healing, sometimes in a superficial way that does not do justice to its importance. It may be seen, for example, as a category of problems—a fourth category to be added to the biomedical, psychological, and social. The spiritual then becomes another kind of problem solving: an additional responsibility for the physician. I prefer to think of spirituality in healing in a much more specific sense. Spiritual experiences are those in which persons feel the presence of powers and influences outside themselves. The feeling is accompanied by a sense of awe and of deep meaning. The experience is at the root of all religions, though religious practice can, and often does, become completely separated from spirituality. Hawkins (1993) observes that, paradoxically, the feeling that illness can be an occasion for spiritual growth is "strangely absent from religious pathographies, [but]...present...in a wide variety of pathographies that acknowledge no explicit religious referent."

The classical spiritual pathography is John Donne's *Devotions upon Emergent Occasions*, of which Hawkins (1993) writes

The organizing construct that explains the meaning both of the illness itself and of the various treatments to which Donne is subjected is religious belief. In accord with an underlying sacramentalism, all physical realities have a spiritual dimension and a spiritual analogue: illness is thus inherently meaningful and purposive. Not only is the physical dimension consistently interpreted as a metaphor for the spiritual, but physical realities are always subordinated to their spiritual counterparts.

Donne's illness teaches him that man is not separate from the cosmos: "No man is an island, entire of itself; every man is a piece of the continent, a part of the main."

In modern times this sense is less likely to be expressed in strictly religious terms than in terms of cosmic consciousness: a feeling of connectedness with cosmic forces. It may be manifested in the scientist or naturalist as a feeling of awe in the contemplation of nature. In the physician it may be a sense of awe and reverence—perhaps largely unconscious—in the presence of the healing powers of nature. In older language it is the experience of being on holy ground. In *De Profundis*—a meditation on suffering—Oscar Wilde (1905) wrote: "Where there is sorrow there is holy ground. Some day people will realise what that means. They will know nothing of life till they do." Vastyan (1981) expresses a background to this feeling:

"Healing" and "holy" have a common Old English root in our language. That common etymology well describes the older origin. From cover to cover, healing—holy healing—is the central concern of the Bible: the Jewish Bible, the Christian Bible. There we find a common insistence that healing springs from spiritual insight and spiritual action; that healing—all healing—is a holy task; that all healing has a holy source; that only the wounded can heal; that healing does not follow a path of upward mobility and autonomy and competition and minimum risk, but rather has a path of downward pilgrimage and sharing and community and maximum risk; that all who are touched in any way by the Holy are called to be healers; and that all who are healers, do the work of the Holy.

Does a physician who brings this quality to a relationship enhance it? One result is likely to be that patients feel able to be open about expressing their own spiritual experiences. Patients are very quick to sense when their experiences are being greeted by skepticism and disbelief. Perhaps also the sense of presence engendered by this quality plays some part in mobilizing the patient's own powers of healing.

Although this quality may be unusual today, there is reason to believe that it may have been present in previous generations, albeit at the subconscious and intuitive level. An account of Sir William Osler's visits to a child dying in the influenza pandemic of 1918 is an example:

He visited our little Janet twice every day and these visits she looked forward to with a pathetic eagerness and joy. There would be a little tap, low down on the door which would be pushed open and a crouching figure playing goblin would come in, and in a high-pitched voice would ask if the fairy godmother was at home and could he have a bit of tea. Instantly the sick-room was turned into a fairyland, and in fairy language he would talk about the flowers, the birds, and the dolls who sat at the foot of the bed who were always greeted with, "Well, all ye loves." In the course of this he would manage to find out all he wanted to know about the little patient.... The most exquisite moment came one cold, raw, November morning when the end was near, and he mysteriously brought out from his inside pocket a beautiful red rose carefully wrapped in paper, and told how he had watched this last rose of summer growing in his garden and how the rose had called out to him as he passed by, that she wished to go along with him to see his little lassie. That evening we all had a fairy tea party, a tiny table by the bed, Sir William talking to the rose, his "little lassie," and her mother in a most exquisite way; and presently he slipped out of the room just as mysteriously as he had entered it, all crouched down on his heels; and the little girl understood that neither fairies nor people could always have the colour of a red rose in their cheeks, or stay as long as they wanted to in one place, but that they nevertheless would be very happy in another home and must not let the people they left behind, particularly their parents, feel badly about it; and the little girl understood and was not unhappy. (Cushing, 1926)

At the time of this incident, Osler was near the end of his career. He was also deeply grieving the death of his only son in World War I. One feels Osler's total attention to the child and the sense of his presence she must have had. It seems that the healer and clinician were working together in perfect harmony, for he was at the same time absorbed in the patient and collecting the clinical information he needed. Nearly three centuries separate this account of an illness from that of John Donne and the context has changed from a religious to a secular spirituality. Yet there are deeper resemblances. Just as for Donne every feature of his illness symbolizes some aspect of his spiritual life, for the mother there is a symbolic meaning in the last rose of summer. That Osler was not only a great clinician but also a great healer is evident from the accounts of his friends and colleagues. "[He] really brought Healing and Health, Life not Death," wrote one (Cushing, 1926). Although this quality in a clinician may be intuitive rather than consciously present, Osler was quite explicit in his teaching. In one address to students, he said:

I would urge upon you...to care more for the individual patient than for the special features of the disease....Dealing as we do with poor suffering humanity, we see the man unmasked, exposed to all the frailties and weaknesses, and you have to keep your heart soft and tender lest you have too great a contempt for your fellow creatures. The best way is to keep a looking glass in your own heart, and the more carefully you scan your own frailties the more tender you are for those of your fellow creatures. (Cushing, 1926)

The Moral Dimension

In all the great spiritual traditions, true spirituality shows itself in the conduct of life—likewise false spirituality. As Dante descends through the rings of the Inferno, encountering at each level greater depths of evil, the souls he meets are consumed by anger and hatred. In his journey through Paradise he is met everywhere by the most exquisite courtesy. The moral life is a reflection of the spiritual life: the outer a reflection of the inner. The great spiritual masters have sometimes been accused of breaking the moral laws; the occasion, however, is always a call to a higher morality. The written code—the letter of the law— cannot always be applied literally; without the spirit, it becomes lifeless. The spiritual masters, however, are emphatic that true spirituality means, in the first place, living according to the law. The mistake made by some self-styled spiritual movements in the West has been to believe that spiritual growth comes from throwing off restraints and discipline. The opposite is true. The mastery of all true spiritual disciplines is a long and arduous process.

The reason for saying these things is the resemblance between religious experience and sickness. "Like the sick man, the religious man is projected on to a vital plane that shows him the fundamental data of human existence, that is, solitude, danger, hostility of the surrounding world" (Eliade, 1964, p. 27). Sacks wrote, after recovering from his illness, "I have since had a deeper sense of the horror and wonder which lurk behind life and which are concealed...behind the usual surface of health" (Sacks, 1984).

This being so, it is not surprising that serious illness should often be the occasion for what may be a painful self-examination. Paul Tournier (1983), the Swiss general practitioner and psychotherapist, tells the story of a physician who consulted him at his wife's request after failing to recover completely after septicemia. The patient was full of remorse for the way he had spent his life and for betrayals he had not confessed to his wife. This remorse haunted him throughout his time in hospital, and he would have liked to unburden himself to his doctors. In fact, he saw the illness as having deep meaning for him, as being a time for introspection and change. Although he was treated with great kindness, the talk during ward rounds was all of blood cultures and antibiotics. The doctors were surprised at how slowly he recovered from the illness. For all their kindness, they could not see the illness as having a deeper meaning for the patient. On leaving the hospital, the patient had refused convalescence and returned to his old defense mechanism of frenetic overwork. Healing did not take place until he found a physician who could reach his "moral loneliness."

The point here is not that physicians have any claim to be moral or spiritual teachers: it is simply that to be a healer one must recognize and respond to all forms of suffering, at least by listening and comforting and, if not possessing the necessary experience ourselves, calling on others who have. "It is not a question of taking the clergyman's place, of teaching, preaching, indoctrinating, admonishing or proselytizing.... It is a question of perceiving the whole of our patient's suffering and of facing up to it without cowardice, without subterfuge. And if that suffering is a feeling of guilt, it is not enough to say that it is no longer in the doctor's sphere" (Tournier, 1983). To ignore spiritual suffering is to deny the wholeness of the person, to divide a person into compartments. As Tournier tells us, suffering knows no frontier. Physical illness is associated with spiritual suffering; spiritual suffering may be manifested as physical or mental illness.

We do not have to be religious ourselves, in the world's sense of religious, and certainly not in the sectarian sense, to respond to a patient's sufferings, whatever their origin.

The Pedagogy of Suffering

The pedagogy of suffering means that one who suffers has something to teach . . . and thus something to give "What is at issue is an ethic derived from a pedagogy of suffering that [sic] was stated in 1909 by Gyorgy Lukacs as he meditated the mysterious reciprocity between creative activity and the 'the primacy of ethics in life' " (Frank, 1997). The impetus of ethics for Lukacs is loneliness . . . the pedagogy of suffering begins its teaching from a ground of loneliness seeking communion . . ."Instead of one ethical person bearing all the weight of things, the weight is shared. Instead of bearing all the weight of medical decisions, the physician shares the weight with the patients he is responsible for, or the nurses he works with. The ethics that Lukacs recommends is exemplified by Dr. Hilfiker who works, and lives with, the poorest of the poor in central Washington. Hilfiker does not work with the poor with condescension or with charity. He does it because of his brokenness. Having acknowledged his own brokenness his service to the poor is that much easier, and he can receive support from his patients in return. Hilfiker calls his book: *Not All of us are Saints.*" He works with the poor not because he is morally superior, but because he is needy. When will our medical profession have the grace to acknowledge this brokenness?

Jean Vanier (1988), the founder of *L'arche*, an organization to care for those with mental disabilities makes the same point as Hilfiker. The mentally disabled give as much to their custodians as their custodians give to them. The Swiss cultural philosopher Jean Gebser sees our epoch as one in which our present ego-consciousness will give place to an openness that is founded on the transcendence of the ego. Ego-freedom is not so much a relapse into ego-lessness as a "deep affirmation of life, its forms and beyond all forms" (Fuerstein, 1995). Hilfiker and Vanier may be leading us along this path.

Because the pedagogy of suffering is taught in the testimony of illness stories, the kind of ethics it supports is a narrative ethic. Frank regards illness narratives as a postmodern development. In modern medicine, the physician took charge of the patients' illness and expressed it in medical terms, in the postmodern world, the patient insisted in telling and re-telling their own story, even thought there might still be a modern description supplied by the physician. "My concern," says Frank: "is with people's self-stories as moral acts, and with care as the moral action of responding to these self-stories" (Frank, 1997). Narrative contributions can be made in this way to collaborative decision making.

The Authority of the Healer

From the earliest times, healing has been associated with power and authority. In traditional cultures, shamans are persons who have acquired power and knowledge by going through an intense initiatory experience. Whether selected by inheritance or personal vocation, the shaman is not recognized as such until he has received two kinds of teaching: an ecstatic experience (altered state of consciousness), through which he has learned the mysteries of human destiny; and didactic instruction in the theory and practice of healing. The ecstatic experience often followed an ordeal, such as a period of isolation or a serious illness. The ecstatic "journey" of the soul to the underworld changes the person forever, and confers on him the power of healing. "The shaman is the great specialist of the human soul" (Eliade, 1964). The shaman has experienced serious illness or existential crisis himself, looked death in the face, and recovered. Eliade suggests that the ecstasy of the shaman is an archetype of "gaining existential consciousness" (p. 394). In Greek mythology, the archetype is expressed in the stories of Chiron the wounded healer, Orpheus' journey to the underworld, and the death and resurrection of Aesculapius. In modern times any manifestation of the archetype is likely to be overlaid by layers of culture and history that separate us from the ancient world.

Modern medicine has valued and emphasized technical knowledge, almost to the exclusion of the esoteric knowledge gained by reflection on the deep experience of life and death that medicine can provide. Its muted manifestations can be seen, perhaps, at the margins: in the hospice movement, in the literature on illness and healing, or in music therapy, described by one of its practitioners as "a contemplative practice with clinical implications" (Schroeder-Sheker, 1993).

The shaman is a person set apart in his society as a manifestation of the sacred, a person who, by unusual means, has "experienced the sacred with greater intensity than the rest of the community" (Eliade, 1964). For Needleman (1992), the generation of physicians preceding our own "was one of the last surviving traces of the sacred in our world." Perhaps this is what Robert Louis Stevenson meant when he said that the physician "stands above the common herd...almost as a rule." Among the classes of humankind thus distinguished by Stevenson were also the soldier, the sailor, and the shepherd—all of whom experience life and nature in the raw (or did, until our own time). It is doubtful whether Stevenson would have said this of the modern physician. Our technologies often distance us from the realities of human experience. Needleman was astonished to find that the physicians he encountered had seldom been present at a patient's death.

Of all fields of medicine, perhaps family medicine and psychiatry can best preserve and cultivate this power of healing. Bettelheim (1984) has reminded us that the term we translate into English as psyche was the German *seele* in the writings of Freud—more accurately translated as soul. The logotherapy of Victor Frankl (1973) is a direct outcome of his experience as a prisoner in Auschwitz. However, the successes of pharmacotherapy seem to be leading psychiatry in another direction. Although affected by modern trends, family medicine retains a closeness to the realities of human life, an experience captured vividly in Berger and Mohr's book *A Fortunate Man* (1967).

To value the power of the healer may seem to be at variance with the modern reaction against the authoritarian attitudes of physicians. On closer examination, however, it is clear that we are dealing with two different kinds of authority. The modern reaction is against physicians who disempower patients by taking decisions for them. The power and authority of the healer is of an entirely different order, mobilizing the patient's will to live and releasing the powers he or she alone possesses.

References

Baron RJ. 1985. An introduction to medical phenomenology: I can't hear you while I'm listening. *Annals of Internal Medicine* 103:606.

Berger J, Mohr J. 1967. *A Fortunate Man: The Story of a Country Doctor.* London: Allen Lane.

Bettelheim. 1984. *Freud and Man's Soul.* New York: Vintage Books.

Cassell EJ. 1990. *The Healer's Art.* Philadelphia, PA: Lippincott.

Cassell EJ. 1991. *The Nature of Suffering and the Goals of Medicine.* New York, Oxford: Oxford University Press.

Cushing H. 1926. *The Life of Sir William Osler.* New York: Oxford University Press.

Eliade M. 1964. *Shamanism: Archaic Techniques of Ecstasy.* Princeton, NJ: Princeton University Press.

Frank A. 1991. *At the Will of the Body.* Boston, MA: Houghton Mifflin.

Frank A. 1997. *The Wounded Storyteller: Body, Illness and Ethics.* Chicago, IL: University of Chicago Press.

Frankl VE. 1973. *The Doctor and the Soul: From Psychotherapy to Logotherapy.* New York: Vintage Books.

Fuerstein G. 1995. *The Structures of Consciousness, the Genius of Jean Gebser.* Lower Lake, CA: Integral publishing.

Gawler I. 1995. The five stages of hope: How to develop and sustain hope—an essential pre-requisite for profound healing. In: Gawler I, ed., *Proceedings of the Mind, Immunity and Health Conference: Psychoneuroimmunology and the Mind–body Connection.* Yarra Junction, Victoria, Australia.

Gay P. 1989. *Freud: A Life for Our Time.* New York: Anchor Books.

Hawkins AH. 1993. *Reconstructing Illness. Studies in Pathography.* West Lafayette, IN: Purdue University Press.

Hilfiker D. 1994. *Not All of Us Are Saints: A Doctor's Journey With the Poor.* New York: Hill and Wang.

Hull JM. 1992. *Touching the Rock: An Experience of Blindness.* New York: Vintage Books.

Kleinman A, Kleinman J. 1997. The Appeal of Experience; the Dismay of Images: Cultural Appropriation of Suffering in Our Times in Social Suffering. In: Kleinman A, Das V, Lock M. (Eds.). University of California Press.

Lifton RJ. 1967. *Death in life: Survivors of Hiroshima.* New York: Random House.

Needleman J. 1985. *The Way of the Physician.* Arkana. London: Penguin Books.

Needleman J. 1992. *The Way of the Physician.* London: Penguin Books.

Price R. 1994. *A Whole New Life.* New York: Atheneum Macmillan.

Sacks O. 1984. *One Leg to Stand On.* London: Gerald Duckworth.

Saunders C. 1984. The philosophy of terminal care. In: Saunders C, ed., *The Management of Terminal Malignant Disease, 2nd edn.* London: Edward Arnold.

Schroeder-Sheker T. 1993. Music for the dying: A personal account of the new field of music thanatology—history, theories, and clinical narratives. *Advances* 9(1):36.

Stein HF. 1985. *The Psychodynamics of Medical Practice.* London: University of California Press.

Stetten D, Jr. 1981. Coping with blindness. *New England Journal of Medicine* 305:458.
Toombs SK. 1992. *The Meaning of Illness: A Phenomenological Account of the Different Perspectives of Physicians and Patients*. Dordrecht: Kluwer.
Toombs SK. 1995. Healing and incurable illness. *Humane Medicine* 11(3):98.
Tournier P. 1983. *Guilt and Grace*. San Francisco, CA: Harper and Row.
Vanier J. 1988. *The Broken Body: The Journey to Wholeness*. New York: Paulist Press.
Vastyan EA. 1981. *Healing and the Wounded Healer*. Philadelphia, PA: Society for Health and Human Values.
Wilde O. 1905. *De Profundis*. London: Methuen.

Notes

1. The extract is from *Touching the Rock* by John Hull, copyright ©1990 by John M. Hull. Reprinted by permission of Pantheon Books, a division of Random House.

2. One example is the work of Jon Kabat-Zinn at the University of Massachusetts Medical Center, described in his book *Full Catastrophe Living: Using the Wisdom of Your Body and Mind to Face Stress, Pain and Illness*. New York: Bantam Doubleday Dell, 1990.

7

Doctor–Patient Communication

Many of the errors in medical practice have their origins in a failure of communication. The doctor either fails to understand the patient's meaning or fails to convey his or her own meaning. These misunderstandings cause frustration for doctors and patients, with all that follows in lowered morale, patients' dissatisfaction, ineffective medicine, conflict, and litigation. Effective communication is fundamental. If we have not understood the patient's problem as the very first step, everything that follows in investigation and treatment may be wrong. Even when diagnosis and therapy are technically correct, the way they are communicated to patients has important implications for their response. Moreover, communication is the essence of a therapeutic relationship.

In family practice, communication between doctor and patient has some important special features. Most of these can be summed up in one word: context. Communication usually takes place between a doctor and patient who know each other, who have shared previous experiences, and have other relationships in common, for example with other family members. It takes place, very often, over extended periods of time, and in the different environments of office, home, and hospital. It is important, therefore, for us to understand how context influences and enhances communication.

Most consultations between doctor and patient begin with the patient's account of his or her symptoms. In many cases, these will eventually be supplemented by other data. However, as we have seen, a very high proportion of patients have symptoms without physical signs or abnormal investigations. Even when signs and abnormal tests are found, the correct diagnosis is more likely to depend on the history than on the examination and investigation. This is particularly so in general practice. An understanding of the patient's symptoms is, therefore, fundamental.

Symptoms are the patient's description of what he or she perceives to be abnormal sensations. By definition, they are subjective and not open to verification by empirical methods. There is no objective test by which we can verify that a patient is actually feeling a pain. This is not to say, however, that we cannot apply rigorous methods to understanding the meaning of a patient's symptoms. The methods are those of attentive listening, clarification of meaning through dialogue, and avoidance of selection bias.

Symptoms are a form of communication—the way in which a patient conveys feelings of illness, distress, or discomfort. Symptoms are the information on which we base our understanding of the patient's problem. The starting point is the information received by the patient in the form of messages transmitted from his or her nervous system. Information about bodily functions is constantly being transmitted via the nervous system and by chemical transmitters to the brain—information that provides the basis for the body's self-regulation. Normally, we are unaware of these messages. The signals that lead to an adjustment in heart rate, blood pressure, or posture are, under usual circumstances, received and acted on below the level of consciousness. Nor are we normally aware of bodily functions like digestion and respiration. In unusual circumstances, signals reach consciousness and have to be interpreted or decoded. How the signals are decoded depends on a number of factors, including the person's past experience and culture. These all form the context within which the messages are transmitted and interpreted.

Because the memory of a significant experience has an affective component, the interpretation is both cognitive and affective.

Let us suppose that the constancy of the background feeling is broken by a sensation of chest pain on waking one morning. At first there is a moment of anxiety; then a fall the day before, when a blow was received on that part of the chest, is remembered. This explanation is accompanied by a feeling of relief. On the other hand, no such explanation may be available. Perhaps the memory instead is of a colleague who had a severe heart attack accompanied by chest pain. The anxiety results in a visit to the doctor. The presenting complaint is probably the pain, not the anxiety. But things can be even more complicated. Even though the anxiety is not expressed in words, it may be expressed in bodily ways—facial expression, gestures, heart rate and so on. An observant physician may recognize the emotion from these signs.

To complicate things even more, the original change in body state may itself be the bodily expression of an emotion. In the case described on page 273, Chapter 12, the patient suddenly became short of breath after her father's funeral. This distress signal was interpreted as the approach of death ("I thought I was going to die"). The extreme fear would probably generate more bodily changes: tachycardia, sweating, and pallor, thus adding to her anxiety. A doctor's explanation of her symptoms as an expression of grief would have been processed both cognitively and emotionally, with increased understanding and lessening of fear. As it happened, she encountered a physician who was dismissive and provoked an angry reaction that was anti-therapeutic.

Information is provided by signals that convey differences from the usual state of affairs. The information level of a signal is directly related to its capacity to surprise the receiver. A person who usually coughs up some mucoid sputum in the morning gets no information by looking at his sputum. If one morning it is bloodstained, he does get information. A person who wakes with a headache after an excess of alcohol gets little information. A person who wakes with a headache "out of the blue" gets a lot more information, especially if he has never suffered from headaches before. The information conveyed by the bloodstained sputum will depend on the context within which the message is received. A person who believes that blood in the sputum always means cancer will decode the message differently from the person who does not connect the blood with cancer. A person who coughs up blood for the first time will decode it differently from a person who has coughed up blood before.

We know from population surveys, and from our own experience, that information arising from differences in our inner state is a daily occurrence. We all experience minor aches, pains and discomforts of various kinds: headaches, muscle pains, dyspepsia, fatigue, itching, insomnia, irregularity of bowels or menses, and so on. The fact that a person consults a physician means that he has interpreted the information as a departure from his usual pattern, or as a signal that is outside his frame of reference. This interpretation varies enormously from one person to another. There is no clear relationship between the severity of the symptoms and the decision to consult. A common defense against unwelcome information is denial. It is not uncommon for people to explain away symptoms like anterior chest pain that they know may indicate myocardial infarction. People have a great capacity for self-deception. On the other hand, there are those whose tolerance is low and who consult for very minor ailments. There may, of course, be a very good reason for consulting, as with the person who comes with vague chest pain after a friend has died of a myocardial infarction.

This initial decoding of information we will call the first gate: the gate where information from bodily feelings is interpreted and acted on in illness behavior (see Chapter 3). Symptoms admitted through this gate may be acted on in different ways. For some, self-care will be tried—at least for a time; for others, advice from family, friends, or members of the person's lay referral system. The decision to consult a physician may be an individual one or may be made with the assistance of family and friends. Sometimes it is on the insistence of family and friends.

This decision brings us to the second gate. Having decided to see a doctor, the person must then decide how to code his or her symptoms for transmission to the physician, including what language to use and which symptom or problem to mention first. The decision is influenced by many factors. Very seldom is there a single symptom or problem; more usually there are many. Often there are also emotions related to the symptoms: anxieties, fantasies, fears. How can the patient convey how he or she feels? At this gate we encounter the complexities and difficulties of doctor–patient communication. First the patient has to code the information in verbal form. How well he or she can do this depends on the availability of a language and his or her own familiarity with it. For some symptoms a well-understood language is quite readily available. The message is coded in words that have a direct causal relationship with the sensation the patient is trying to communicate. There may also be a clear and direct relationship between the symptom and a diseased state, such as the one between anginal pain and ischemic heart disease. Other sensations and feelings are much more difficult to put into words: vague illness and distress, changes of mood, unhappiness, anxiety, grief, self-doubt, guilt, and remorse. These difficulties are so great that some very sick people do not consult physicians. In his population survey in Glasgow, Hannay (1979) found severely depressed people who had never consulted a doctor. It seems that disorders that threaten the integrity of the personality are particularly difficult to find expression for.

Burack and Carpenter (1983) studied the relationship between the presenting complaint and the principal problem identified during new patient visits. The problems were classified as somatic, psychosocial, or health maintenance. The presenting complaint correctly identified the category in 76% of somatic problems, but only 6% of psychosocial problems. If, however, the presenting complaint was psychosocial, the principal problem was psychosocial in all cases. If the presenting complaint was somatic, only 53% of the identified problems were somatic.

To overcome these difficulties of expression, patients find other ways of coding their message. This means using an indirect, rather than a direct, form of communication. When patients express personal distress through bodily symptoms, they are not inventing the symptoms, or imagining the sensations. They are simply selecting the aspect of the illness experience which they can most easily put into words. A patient who cannot find words for his or her feeling of despair may express the problem in terms of a familiar symptom like headaches, which may be an effect of the problem but are not the core of it. It is much easier to talk about headaches than about despair. In indirect communication, the patient may express meaning by using metaphors or nonverbal forms. Metaphors, according to Jeremy Campbell (1982), "place the familiar in the context of the strange"—or, one might add, the strange in the context of the familiar. The message is in the context. A patient with a chronic disease, who is also in personal distress, may communicate this distress in the form of a visit for the disease.

Case 7.1
A patient with multiple sclerosis came with the usual symptoms of her disease. The distress she was trying to communicate was caused by her husband's refusal to countenance birth control. This problem was related to the disease, in that she felt unfit to manage another child, but only indirectly.

It is a universal experience that words are inadequate to express feeling: "...words, like nature half reveal and half conceal the soul within," wrote Tennyson in *In Memoriam*. In all cultures, the deepest feelings are expressed in dance, drama, poetry, and other forms of symbolism. Many patients who come to see us are in the grip of powerful emotions, so it is not surprising that indirect communication is common in family practice.

Problems that arouse shame or guilt—like family and sexual problems—are often communicated indirectly. The problem may be introduced in the context of a visit for a "checkup" or for an unrelated problem. A woman suffering from dyspareunia may say that she has come for a routine examination. If asked directly about difficulty with intercourse, she may deny problems. Then, in the course of the pelvic examination, she may ask, "Should it hurt there when I have intercourse?" Note that the problem is framed in the form of a question (a common form of indirect communication) and that the most sensitive issue is raised during the physical examination.

If the context is a visit for another problem, mention of the most sensitive problem is likely to be left to the last. This has been called the "exit problem" or "doorknob comment"—the one that is not mentioned until the patient is getting up to leave, sometimes introduced by the words "By the way, Doctor." The exit problem is usually the main reason for the patient's visit.

Indirect communication protects us against rejection or embarrassment. If a patient requests a sickness absence note for an illness he is recovering from and the request is refused, he loses face. If he first complains of symptoms and allows the doctor to assess his illness, then asks for the note as an afterthought, refusal causes much less embarrassment.

A patient may introduce an embarrassing subject by hinting. A hint is somewhat ambiguous and does not reveal the problem all at once. If the physician responds to the hint, the patient still has the choice of how much to reveal.

Case 7.2
The wife of a soldier who had been away from home was disturbed to find that he had pubic lice on his return. He attributed them to dirty blankets provided in his billet. Instead of saying what was on her mind, she asked, "Can you get crab lice from bedclothes?"

How a patient codes personal distress for transmission to the physician depends also on his or her perception of how the physician will receive the information. A doctor who is perceived by the patient as working in the context of physical pathology is likely to receive messages about personal distress coded in the language of physical symptoms. A doctor who is perceived to be patient centered, encouraging the expression of feeling, is more likely to have personal distress conveyed to him or her directly. Given the difficulty of finding words for distress, it is not surprising that patients often complain first of bodily symptoms (see *Cases 7.3, 8.1, 10.1*). This is often referred to as *somatization*. If it is persistent, it is known as *somatic fixation*. There is a category of *somatoform disorders* in the *Diagnostic* and *Statistical Manual*.

Somatization

Somatization is defined as the process by which emotions are transduced to bodily symptoms, for which medical aid is sought. In its original formulation, somatization was related to the psychoanalytic concept *conversion*: the transduction of a psychological conflict into bodily symptoms. In psychoanalytical theory, conversion was viewed as a defense mechanism by which the patient unconsciously avoided having to deal with the internal conflict and gained some protection from threatening circumstances through bodily symptoms (secondary gain). The symptoms of conversion were therefore forms of communication rather than the experience of physiological disturbances. The concept has now been expanded to embrace any bodily manifestation of distress. The classical manifestation of conversion hysteria is now uncommon, and most bodily manifestations of distress are compatible with physiological correlates of emotion. However, the implication of personal gain remains. The term somatization is unfortunate in that it suggests that the process is abnormal and that the patient is the agent of the transduction. It is therefore difficult to avoid the implication that the patient is morally responsible for his own illness, especially when there is the added suggestion that the illness enables him to avoid responsibilities. The idea of somatization, therefore, always has the potential for putting the doctor and patient in conflict.[1]

It is normal to feel emotion in the body.[2] The problem is not the bodily expression of emotion but the patient's inability to make the connection between the emotion and the bodily sensations. In many patients, the understanding lies only just below the level of consciousness, and the connection is soon made, given the right approach by the physician (e.g., the case on p. 273). Some patients, however, are resistant to any suggestion that their symptoms are the bodily expression of emotion. McDaniel, Campbell, and Seaburn (1990) describe this somatic fixation as "a process whereby a physician and/or a patient or family focuses exclusively and inappropriately on the somatic aspects of a complex problem." This formulation of McDaniel, Campbell, and Seaburn thus recognizes that the family may reinforce the patient's fixation and that the doctor's biomedical bias may result in unnecessary investigations and therapies.[3]

Context

"All communication necessitates context... without context there is no meaning," wrote Gregory Bateson (1979). One of the most difficult things for a physician is knowing what context to use in decoding the patient's message. The context we all internalize in the course of our training is the classification of diseases according to their organic pathology. If a patient is using symptoms as a form of indirect communication for a problem of living, correct decoding requires the physician to identify the context as a personal one. If the physician decodes the message using the context of physical pathology, the result may be a spurious diagnosis and all its consequences. If the patient is also misreading the context, as is sometimes the case, the possibilities of misdiagnosis are even greater.

For family physicians, it is not sufficient to have one internal context for decoding patients' messages. They need to be very receptive to those information cues that indicate what context the patient's message is encoded in. These cues are referred to by Gregory Bateson as metamessages, messages that make other messages intelligible by putting them in context. Many of the illnesses encountered in family practice can only be understood by understanding their context. As in all human communication, decoding is not a once-and-for-all process. The decoder makes hypotheses, which he or she then proceeds to check by questions and observations.

In *Much Ado About Nothing*, Shakespeare provides an amusing example of the effect of a change of context on meaning.

Beatrice and Benedict have a teasing relationship, vying as to who can be more insulting to the other. Benedict's friends deceive him into thinking that Beatrice is really in love with him. No sooner has he come to believe this than Beatrice enters and says:
Against my will I am sent to bid you come in to dinner.

Instead of the usual insulting reply, Benedict answers:

Fair Beatrice, I thank you for your pains.
Beatrice: I took no more pains for those thanks than you take pains to thank me: if it had been painful I would not have come.
Benedict (after Beatrice has left): Ha. "Against my will I am sent to bid you come in to dinner," there's a double meaning in that. [She really loves me.]

As with diagnoses, so with therapy, to be successful the physician has to work in the right context. To treat at the level of symptoms, when the problem is in the doctor–patient relationship, or the way a person's life is organized, will lead only to frustration. Shifting the attention from one context to the other may of course be a very difficult process, especially when the patient himself has decoded his illness incorrectly. Conversely, trying to shift the attention to the personal context when the problem *is* the symptom also leads to frustration. In patients with chronic headache, for example, the problem may be the symptom itself, and the attitudes and coping mechanisms developed by the patient. Even if the headaches originated in a problem of living, an attempt to shift the focus on to this context after the symptom has become autonomous is usually not helpful.

Cues to Context

The following cues should alert the physician to the possibility that he or she should be working in the personal and interpersonal rather than the clinical–pathological context:

Frequent attendances with minor illnesses
Frequent attendance with the same symptoms or with multiple complaints
First attendance with a symptom that has been present for a long time
Patient initiated attendance with a chronic disease that does not appear to have changed
Incongruity between the patient's distress and the comparatively minor nature of the symptoms
Failure to recover in the expected time from an illness, injury, or operation
Failure of reassurance to satisfy the patient for more than a short period
Frequent visits by a parent with a child with minor problems (the child as a presenting symptom of illness in the parent)
An adult patient with an accompanying relative
Inability to make sense of the presenting problem

Case 7.3

A well-dressed young man of 19 came for the third time in 1 year with intercostal pain and tenderness. His age suggested that his problems might be those common to adolescence. When encouraged to talk, he revealed such despair that he had twice called the suicide prevention service. His father had died, he was unable to communicate with his mother, and he had no siblings or close friends. He was almost totally without supporting relationships at a critical stage in his development. (See also *Case 7.1*)

Culture and Context

One of the most important determinants of a person's interpretation of his or her illness and expectations of the physician is the culture or subculture to which he or she belongs. Kleinman Eisenberg, and Good (1978) have referred to this as "the cultural construction of clinical reality." It is difficult for physicians to accept that their construction of clinical reality, based on pathology, is only one of many possible constructions. If the patient's construction is different, and no attempt is made to reconcile the difference, the probable outcome will often be a breakdown of communication and a failure of treatment.

These difficulties are at their greatest when there is a very wide cultural gap between doctor and patient, as, for example, when the doctor is from the dominant culture and the patient an immigrant from a different ethnic and language group. It is a general principle of human communication that difficulties in communication increase with the cultural distance between the participants (Bochner, 1983). The difficulties arise both in verbal and nonverbal communication. It can be difficult to "read" the behavior of a person from a very different culture. It is difficult, for example, to detect depression in a patient from a widely different culture (see p. 288). Cultural differences are not only ethnic. Subcultural groups defined by age, social class, sex, education, occupation, or region may also experience cultural distance from each other, and therefore difficulties in communication. Medicine itself is a subculture with its own set of unstated assumptions and expectations. A patient entering this subculture is therefore in the same position as a traveler visiting a strange country. This puts the patient at a social disadvantage, as well as being made vulnerable by his or her illness and lack of medical knowledge. It is therefore the doctor's responsibility to be aware of potential communication difficulties and to do everything possible to mitigate them.

Although the process is difficult, a strange culture can be learned. The main problem confronting the learner is that the rules governing behavior in a culture are not explicit. Indigenous members of a cultural group learn the rules implicitly, beneath the level of awareness. Unless they have the rare ability to view their own culture from outside, indigenous members of a culture are not even aware that their behavior is governed by rules. The same applies to the assumptions of a culture: rarely are these made explicit. In the subculture of medicine, our own assumptions about what a disease is are not made explicit, and many physicians remain unaware that they are assumptions.

An illustration of the implicit rules governing behavior is the question of when a person may be addressed by his first name or by his last name without the title "Mr." The rules for first naming are quite different between Europe and North America. Yet, for a visitor, it is not easy to discover what the rules are. They are even different between occupation and age groups within the same culture. An elderly lady in my practice was outraged at receiving a letter from the practice nurse, addressing her by her first name. To a young person in our culture, using first names is a sign of friendliness; to many older people it is an invasion of privacy. Using a person's last name alone is not an uncommon practice among European men. In North America, as far as I am aware, it would be considered impolite in most circles.

How can family physicians prevent failures of communication? They can make a practice of ascertaining patients' expectations in any clinical encounter. They can try to elicit patients' explanatory model of illness and the meaning their own illness has for them. These are important principles in the clinical method described in Chapter 8. Kleinman, Eisenberg, and Good (1978) suggest a set of questions designed to elicit the patient's explanatory model: What do you think has caused your problem? Why do you think it started when it did? What do you think your sickness does to you? How severe is it? What kind of treatment do you think you should receive? Other questions are designed to elicit the patient's therapeutic goals and the cultural meaning of the illness: What are the most important results you hope to receive from this treatment? What are the chief problems your sickness has caused you? What do you fear most about it?

These questions are designed to be tailored to the individual patient. The problem with direct questions, however, is that so often they do not elicit the information we need. We certainly need to have them available in our clinical method; even if we do not ask them of the patient, we should ask them of ourselves; but much of the information we seek will only come by attentive listening and responsiveness to the subtle cues by which patients convey their meaning.

Physicians can also try to make their own expectations and assumptions explicit. If there are conflicts between their own expectations and those of the patient, they can deal with them wherever possible by negotiation rather than by confrontation. They can also try to coach their patients in how to be more effective in the subculture of medicine. Taking this approach, Greenfield, Kaplan, and Ware (1985) coached patients to ask questions and negotiate medical decisions with their physicians. When compared with a control group receiving a standard educational session, these patients were more involved in the interaction with the physician and were twice as effective in obtaining information from him.

Family physicians as teachers of their patients will only be effective if they—model the behavior they are trying to teach. For example, telling the patient to ask questions will not help unless the physician is open to receiving the questions, listens carefully to them, and takes them seriously.

High- and Low-Context Cultures

In his book *Beyond Culture*, anthropologist Edward Hall (1977) draws a distinction between high- and low-context communication. A high-context communication is one in which most of the information is in the context. The receiver of the information must, of course, be "programmed" to receive this information from the context. Because the context is usually implicit, rather than explicit, this implies a sharing of assumptions. A low-context communication is one in which most of the information is in the explicit code. The language of science and technology is low context. A paper on mathematics, physics, engineering, or immunology can be understood by a specialist in the field from any part of the world, regardless of context. The language of diplomacy is high context: the diplomat on the spot is usually much more reliable in decoding diplomatic messages than the bureaucrat in a distant office who has no knowledge of the country from which the message comes.

Similarly, cultures can be viewed as of high, medium, or low context. In a high-context culture, much communication takes place implicitly. For this to occur, there must be a high level of mutual understanding and sharing of assumptions. High-context cultures, therefore, tend to be marked by long-term human relationships, homogeneity, and a low level of social mobility. Low-context cultures, on the other hand, tend to be complex, technologically advanced, and subject to rapid change.

Another perspective on these communication differences is provided by the Canadian scholar Harold Innis (1951), known for his theory of the bias of communication. This can be stated as follows: The things we pay attention to are strongly influenced by our technology of communication. Oral forms of communication favor continuity over time in communities bound together by custom, tradition, and kinship. Visual forms of communication favor the development of codified rules and laws, specialization, fragmentation, and bureaucracy. The act of translation from oral to written form involves abstraction. Much of the contextual richness of the original data is lost in the process.

Innis maintained that once we know the dominant communication technology of a culture, we will know the shaping force of its entire structure. The dominant technology produces a bias in the culture, of which the culture is usually not aware. The danger is that the bias may become so overwhelming as to be destructive.

If we view medicine from these perspectives, we believe that we see many of its subdivisions moving toward the low-context end of the spectrum. Attention is paid less to the patient's story than to the data abstracted from him or her: the computer printout, the biochemistry panel, the scan, the echocardiogram. There are only a limited number of things we can attend to at one time. If we have our attention fixed on a monitor, it is unlikely that we are listening with attention to the patient. Increasing specialization, in large and bureaucratic institutions, reduces the opportunities for long-term relationships to develop. A family practice that remains faithful to its origins should, on the other hand, be high-context. In a practice where the population is relatively stable, and the physician and patients are members of the same community, long-term relationships can develop, with all that this implies in shared assumptions.

Conveying and receiving information through context, Hall observes, is a way of dealing with information overload. If more information is carried in the context, less has to be carried in the coded message. It is a common experience that the better a physician knows the patient, the less need he or she feels for large quantities of data. There is no significant relationship between quantity of data and quality of care. But there are pitfalls in relying too much on the knowledge that comes from a long-term relationship. Sometimes it leads to unjustified assumptions that preempt communication. The fact that family practice is usually high-context may account for economies of time made by the family physician. In other words, time spent in building relationships may be time saved in communicating about episodic problems.

Difficult Relationships

We are indebted to Dr. W.W. Weston for many of the observations in this section. Weston defines a difficult patient as one with whom the physician has trouble forming an effective working relationship. The long-term relationships with patients in general practice make this a particular problem for family physicians. Because therapeutic success depends so much on the relationship between doctor and patient, the inability to form a therapeutic relationship is usually a source of much frustration for the doctor. Paradoxically, failure of the relationship does not necessarily lead to its termination, so that dealing with the problem is a continuing struggle.

Difficult patients fall into a number of categories:

Patients who have developed a "somatic fixation," that is, express personal distress in the form of somatic symptoms and refuse to believe that no organic disease is present. These are patients we perceive as working in the wrong context. They seek answers from the medical system and the answers they get are negative: negative tests and failed therapies. The medical system often fails them by reinforcing their context error. Negative answers usually do not deter them from seeking yet more tests and consultations with specialists. Little wonder that these patients often end up having unnecessary surgery

Patients who abuse themselves with drugs or alcohol, or who use their diseases in a self-destructive way—for example, diabetics who induce attacks of ketoacidosis

Patients who have become dependent on prescription drugs

Patients who make excessive demands on us by frequent visits, out-of-hours calls, pressure for tests, medications, or referrals

Patients who move from doctor to doctor or who go to several doctors for the same problem, perhaps playing one off against the other

Seductive patients

Angry patients

Some patients fall into more than one of the above categories.

Certain cues may alert the physician to a problem—or a potential problem—in his or her relationship with a patient. Some of these have already been described as cues to a context error (see p. 121).

A new patient who comes after leaving another physician (perhaps a whole series of them) and is extravagant in his praise for you, while expressing great hostility toward the former doctor. There may be immediate demands for action in the form of referrals or prescriptions.

Frequent visits for problems that never respond to treatment; persistent complaints of symptoms with repeatedly negative tests and unhelpful consultations with specialists. This was called by Balint (1964) "the fat envelope syndrome" after the bulging charts accumulated by these patients. These patients have also been called "heartsink patients"—identified by the feeling they evoke in the doctor (O'Dowd, 1988).

Disagreements over prescription drugs. These patients may be quite content as long as they receive their monthly prescription. Often this is requested by mail or phone, so that personal contact with the physician can be avoided. The relationship is placid on the surface but only remains so as long as the doctor confines questions to safe topics and does not try to change or discontinue the medications (Balint et al., 1970). The medication may be taken for a spurious diagnosis that goes back many years and for which no evidence can be found in the record.

Cues from our own feelings. Weston enjoins us to be curious about it when a patient becomes special to us in some way—evoking feelings of anxiety, pressure, boredom, or frustration—or when we particularly want to please and impress a patient.

Grant (1996) has observed that these relationships often become self-fulfilling prophecies. What patients fear most about the relationship is what they invite by their behavior. The doctor falls into the trap of responding automatically to the behavior rather than to the patient's needs. What the patient fears most may be rejection. But his or her behavior, paradoxically, invites rejection, and the doctor, if unreflective, responds accordingly. After describing three examples, Grant writes:

... it was almost a relief to acknowledge them as heartsink patients. It was much more of a challenge to acknowledge that I was part of the problem, part of a heartsink relationship. It was relatively easy to identify their contradictory behavior—it was much more difficult to acknowledge my destructive responses. And yet, they could not be denied. I rejected a man who feared rejection; I ignored a woman who feared not being heard; I fought for control with a man who feared losing it. Their behaviors as supplicant, martyr, and adversary, contradicted their needs. My impulsive responses, as tyrant, bored bystander and antagonist, reinforced their fears. It was only when I was able to look more critically at my own and my patients' behavior, as clinical data, without shame or blame, that I was able to formulate responses that stood a chance of breaking the heartsink cycles and of rewriting scripts that had been written many years before.

There is no easy solution to these difficulties. Physicians who can correctly identify the problem, however, and avoid the many pitfalls, may not only save themselves much frustration, but also in some cases help their patients, if in no other way than protecting them from harm.

Here are some general guidelines:

Try to avoid somatic fixation by dealing with it when it first occurs. If it is already established, try to shift the context by focusing on the patient as a person: life history, expectations, feelings, and relationships. Try to respond to the inner pain, of which the symptoms may be an expression.

Be cautious in prescribing narcotics for chronic or recurrent pain (see p. 282).

Try to protect patients from harm in a medical system that is oriented toward physical pathology; from unnecessary tests, medication, or surgery.

Be alert for countertransference reactions in yourself, for example by responding to a needy patient with excessive attempts to please and pacify.

Do not overreact if a patient tests the relationship. Patients who have difficulty forming a relationship with a doctor usually have problems with other relationships too. Sometimes they have experienced a whole series of rejections and betrayals. Their provocative behavior may be a way of testing the doctor to see if he or she will respond with a rejection, like everybody else. If the doctor can avoid this temptation, the ensuing relationship may be the patient's first experience of trust.

Be prepared to set limits—to the amount of time for visits, to the number of visits, etc.

Involve colleagues in your management plan: the practice nurse and receptionist, and colleagues who take calls for you, will need to know what you expect of them. They may also have a useful contribution to make.

If conflictual relationships become persistent and pervasive in your practice, seek consultation or supervision.

Do not make things worse by being a "difficult" doctor. Sometimes the patient seems to be difficult, but the difficulty is really with the doctor, as in the following example.

Case 7.4

A resident expressed frustration with an elderly diabetic who had persistent glycosuria but would not cooperate in attempts to monitor his blood sugar or adjust his insulin. Eventually the resident was able to see that the problem was her own inability to accept the limited goals that were quite acceptable to the patient, and quite reasonable from his point of view.

Interviewing

Interviewing[4] is a process by which one person, usually a professional, reaches an understanding of another, usually a patient or client. The same principles apply to any kind of interviewing, medical or nonmedical. Medical interviewing provides the context for history taking—the collection of information about the patient's problem. Interviewing is a process of communication, both verbal and nonverbal. It is much more than asking questions and receiving answers. "The question-and-answer technique may be of some value in determining favored detergents, toothpaste and deodorants," wrote Studs Terkel (1975), "but not in the discovery of men and women." It is this "discovery of men and women" that is the aim of interviewing. Questions must of course be asked, but what questions are asked, how they are asked, and how the answers are received will determine whether the interview achieves its aim.

Although the principles of interviewing are universal, their application in the conditions of family practice requires some comment. Even if family physicians are good managers, they cannot avoid working under pressure. In a normal working day, time for a lengthy interview is difficult to find. But there is a paradox here. If time in the short term is at a premium, in the long term it is abundant. Because of the continuing relationship, family physicians have ample opportunity to "discover" the men and women who are their patients. This has several implications. First, it means that physicians do not need to devote time to establishing rapport at every visit. Rapport has already been established and needs only to be maintained. Second, they start out with some personal knowledge of the patient. Third, the process of "discovery" does not need to be hurried.

The lack of short-term time exposes the family physician to certain pitfalls. Rather than giving the patient time to express himself, the physician may resort to the question-and-answer method from the beginning of the interview. Although this may shorten the interview, it is often false economy, for the patient may then keep returning at intervals. One longer interview that accurately identifies the problem may take up less time than the aggregate of several shorter interviews that fail to do so. In their study of doctor–patient interviews in general practice, Byrne and Long (1976) found that dysfunctional interviews were significantly shorter than satisfactory interviews, and that less time in these interviews was devoted to finding out why the patient had come.

Listening

The greatest single fault in interviewing is probably the failure to let the patient tell his or her story. So often the talk is dried up by questions that divert the flow of conversation, by changes of subject, or by behavior in the physician that expresses lack of interest (thumbing through the records or glancing at a wrist-watch). At the beginning of an interview, the physician should try, by every means possible, to encourage patients to tell their own story in their own way.

Listening to the patient with undivided attention is a very difficult discipline. It requires intense concentration on everything the patient is trying to say, both verbally and in other ways, overtly and in those very subtle cues by which patients convey meaning. It is so very easy to focus only on the content of a patient's utterance, and not on how it is said. If a patient with advanced cancer says "I seem to have needed a lot more morphine recently," the physician can reply, "Yes, your needs have increased," or he or she can say, "Does that concern you?" The second response will probably lead to an unfolding of why the patient raised the issue. Possibly the patient views increased needs as the beginning of the end.

Attentive listening requires us to empty ourselves of personal concerns and distractions, and to set aside for the moment our preconceptions and frames of reference. Carl Rogers (1980) puts it very well:

Attentive listening means giving one's total and undivided attention to the other person and tells the other that we are interested and concerned. Listening is a difficult work that we will not undertake unless we have deep respect and care for the other. As counselors, we listen not only with our ears but with our eyes, mind, heart, and imagination as well. We listen to what is going on within ourselves, as well as to what is taking place in the person we are hearing. We listen to the words of the other, but we also listen to the messages buried in the words. We listen to the voice, the appearance, and the body language of the other.

We are attentive listeners when we focus entirely upon what is said and the circumstances under which it is said. We do not use selective listening by hearing only what interests us and fits with our preconceptions. We simply try to absorb everything the speaker is saying verbally and nonverbally without adding, subtracting, or amending. Attentive listening is a demanding process to be undertaken only if we truly care for the other person.

Doctors, in general, are not good listeners. We frequently interrupt. In one study, the average interval between the patient beginning to tell his story and the doctor interrupting was 18 seconds (Beckman and Frankel, 1984). A more recent study (Marvel, Epstein, Flowers, and Beckman, 1999) suggests the situation may have slightly improved with first interruption occurring after 23.1 seconds. Pursuing our own train of thought, we may not even hear the crucial remark:

Patient: And I often feel I could cry.
Doctor: Does the pain go anywhere else?

Questions from patients are often ignored or sidetracked. Interviews tend to be dominated by questions from the physician. There is a place for serial questions in the search for information, but simply asking questions is not a way of getting to know and understand a patient. It is a common experience to find that a patient who replies "no" when asked if he or she has any worries turns out to have major personal problems. So common is it that questions like "Have you any worries?" are of little value. Michael Balint wrote: "If you ask questions, you will get answers, and nothing else." One of the most common errors in interviewing is asking a question, then providing the answer before the patient has time to respond:

Doctor: How are you sleeping? All right?
Patient: Yes.

With very sick or elderly patients, the response may be a long time in coming. The doctor may have to listen in complete silence for up to a minute. Restraining oneself from interrupting in these circumstances is extremely difficult. An elderly man was dying of prostate cancer. His pain was under good control but he seemed to be very depressed:

> Doctor: How do you feel today, Mr. ?
> Patient (pause of about a minute, then): Everything seems hopeless.
> Doctor: Is any situation completely hopeless? Is there nothing you can hope for?
> Patient: I would like to see my children settled.

Open expression by the patient can be encouraged by facilitation. This is a communication, not necessarily verbal, that encourages the patient to continue. A common example of this is repetition of the patient's last words:

> Patient: I felt so awful. (Pause)
> Doctor: You felt awful?

Gestures can have the same effect—leaning forward closer to the patient or slowly nodding the head. As in the example given above, silence can be facilitating.

If questions are needed, open-ended questions encourage expression by the patient more than closed questions. Consider the difference between "Where is your headache?" and "Could you tell me about your headache?"

There is a place for both types: closed questions are for getting very specific information about the problem, and open-ended ones for reaching an understanding of the patient.

In some cases, expression by the patient may be helped by feedback of an observation in their behavior. In this way, the physician helps the patient to face up to some aspect of his behavior, for example, "You look upset" or "You seem to be angry."

The effect of this is to bring feelings into the open, where they can be more effectively dealt with. The effect may be a flood of tears, or an outburst of anger. Whatever form it takes, emotion in the consulting room should be accepted and acknowledged without surprise or embarrassment, for it deepens insight and changes the level of the relationship. Crying can be responded to with empathetic listening and by reassurance that crying is nothing to be ashamed of. Relatives of the dying, for example, sometimes need permission to cry, especially if they are men who have been brought up to believe that men do not cry.

Anger is more difficult to deal with, especially if it is directed against the physician or one of his colleagues. Anger is natural in anybody whose life is disrupted by serious illness in themselves or their family. If the physician can acknowledge the anger, without becoming angry himself, the patient may come to an understanding of his or her feelings. If the physician has provoked in some way the patient's feelings, he or she can acknowledge the anger and explore the reasons for it. In family practice, actual or perceived delays in diagnosis may be a cause of anger. Given the insidious nature of many diseases, none of us can escape this at some time or other. Sometimes, the patient's anger is accompanied by the physician's feeling of discomfort and guilt. Often these feelings are acted out by doctor and patient avoiding each other. They are much better brought into the open and discussed.

The expression of feeling is often helped by touch. Little is said about touch in medical education. I suspect that the hidden message is that touching patients is not permissible, except in the physical examination. Yet it has often been my experience that touching has helped patients to express their feelings.

A 40-year-old woman dying of cancer seemed to be full of pent-up emotions. She complained of being "beside herself," but could not say why. She did not cry or express feeling of any kind. I (IRMcW) was sitting by her bedside encouraging her to talk without success. Then I (IRMcW) reached across and held her hand. Almost immediately she started to cry and express her feelings.

Touching, however, is not always appropriate. When and how to touch are questions requiring sensitive judgment of the patient's needs. In the following case, touch was misinterpreted by the patient and had negative results.

I was discussing the question of resuscitation and artificial life support with a woman with advanced amyotrophic lateral sclerosis. During the discussion I (IRMcW) put my hand on her hand as it lay paralyzed across her chest. After I left her room, the nurse told me that she had become upset. The nurse assumed that the cause of her distress was the subject of our discussion but found that it was my touching her hand that had upset her. She had interpreted this as an expression of sympathy and did not want people to feel sorry for her.

Connectional Moments

Sometimes the obstacle to genuine communication between doctor and patient is the doctor himself. A patient is not likely to open his heart to a doctor who is detached and objective. True reciprocity may come only when the doctor has shown that he too is human. Paul Tournier tells the story of a surgeon whose son died of a sarcoma. One day he was visiting a patient in the very room where his son had died. The patient was an old lady, inconsolable over the death of her daughter and bereft of the will to go on living. He tried to console her, to no avail. Then he said to her "Do you know, my son died in this room." The next day, the old lady dressed, put on her makeup, and walked out of the hospital.

In their book *Six Minutes for the Patient*, Michael and Enid Balint (1973) have described this sudden change in the relationship between doctor and patient as the flash. Suchman and Matthews (1988) describe these as connectional experiences: moments of closeness and intimacy. They seem to occur when we cross the professional/patient boundary and begin to relate to a patient as a fellow human being. It may not be possible to make them happen, but we can probably prepare ourselves for them by avoiding the things that inhibit them. These seem to be our preoccupation with theory or the need to be "doing" something—though not knowing what to do or say—rather than simply being with the patient.

Empathy

Empathy is the capacity to enter into another person's experience. For the physician it is the capacity to sense what it is like to be the patient: to experience illness, disability, depression, and so on. On other occasions it may be the capacity to sense what it is like to be the person caring for the patient. This may seem like an impossible task. Some experiences are so different from the common run that nothing can prepare one for them. Many people have described bereavement in these terms. William Styron (1992) said the same about severe depression.

While accepting this, Toombs (1987) maintains that the alienation from the body experienced by the sick is accessible to others through everyday experience of the body as object. We all experience bodily symptoms, discomforts, limitations, which, if reflected on, can open us to the experience of being alienated from one's own body. We can all gain some intimation of the difference between unconsciously "living" our bodies, and becoming aware of them as objects apart from ourselves. This understanding can be enriched by reading patients' narratives of illness and listening to their stories with openness to their experience.

Rudebeck (1992) regards the capacity for bodily empathy as central to the general clinical competence of the family practitioner (see p. 59). Although empathy is usually understood as the professional route for the understanding of emotions, he observes that bodily processes play a part in the transfer of emotions from person to person. "Perception and intuitive imitation of facial expression and bodily posture are supposed to lead to an 'affective resonance,' including also a neuro-hormonal state...." Thus bodily empathy is a route to the understanding of both the emotions and bodily experiences. They are indeed two sides of the same coin. As Rudebeck also observes, the physical examination is an important vehicle for the exercise of bodily empathy.

The development of a capacity for bodily empathy requires a change in our perception of the clinical task. In the conventional clinical method, symptoms are conceived as avenues to the diagnosis of a patient's disease. We need also to see the patient's bodily discomforts as experiences to be understood in their own right (Rudebeck, 1992).

Key Questions

Even after listening attentively and responding to all the cues given by the patient, we may still feel that some things have been left unsaid. We need questions that will help a patient to express himself, perhaps by clearing away some inhibition.[5] It is sometimes said that asking questions about sensitive issues is an invasion of privacy. This can only be so if the question is poorly worded and if questioning is pursued against the patient's wishes. Even if a key question produces no response, it does at least convey to the patient that the doctor is open to such issues. Sometimes, as in the following case, failure to ask a sensitive question may have unfortunate consequences. The patient was a young woman who had just been released from prison to a halfway house. She complained of sore throat and fatigue and I (IRMcW) suspected early mononucleosis. I (IRMcW) asked no questions about her experience of prison or her feelings about her situation. The same evening she attempted suicide. She had been sentenced to prison for infanticide.

Breaking Bad News

Giving patients bad news is so difficult that we are often tempted to shy away from the task. We are afraid of being too frank; we fear the questions we might be asked; and we are afraid of the emotions that may be unleashed. There are many defense mechanisms we can invoke to avoid dealing with our fears. We can disguise the truth ("I think we got it all out"). We can put off the evil hour ("Let's do some more tests"). We can fail to respond to the subtle ways in which the patient opens the subject ("I seem to be getting weaker." "How are you sleeping?"). We can avoid the patient altogether, either by not visiting or by taking care not to see him alone. Nowhere have these defense mechanisms been better described than in Tolstoy's story "The Death of Ivan Illich."

We do not believe there is a single physician who has not used one of these maneuvers at some time or other; or who has not made mistakes in breaking bad news. It is something one has to struggle with. We have found some general principles to be helpful:

Never tell the patient something that is not true. At the same time, do not tell him more than he wants to know. The truth will emerge sooner or later, and, when it does, patients who have been lied to and misled feel betrayed. Not surprisingly, the result is usually irreparable damage to the relationship between doctor and patient, and often damage to family relationships too.

Applying these principles is not easy. How do we discover what the patient wants to know? First, we can find out what the patient knows, or at least suspects, already. Patients usually know much more than we think they do. In her study of patients dying of cancer, Elizabeth Kubler-Ross (1969) found that most patients knew that they were dying and did not need to be told. What they needed was the opportunity to discuss their feelings openly and without evasion. We find that the question "What is your understanding of your illness?" usually gives us a good insight into what the patient knows.

We find it helpful to let the patient ask the questions, so that we can follow where he or she leads:

"Do you have any questions about the gland that was removed from your neck?"
"Yes, what did it show?"
"You know why it was removed?"
"Yes, it was to see if the cancer had spread from my lung."
"Yes. It did show that there is cancer there. Is there anything you wanted to ask me about that?"
"Does that mean that the cancer is all through me?"
"No. It does mean that it has spread from the lung to the lymph glands, but your bone scan was normal—no sign of spread there—and there isn't any sign of spread elsewhere. With the chemotherapy you are starting, we are hoping that you will get a remission of the disease. Do you know what I mean by a remission?"
"Yes—the disease being arrested for a time."
"That's right. Any other questions at this point?"
"Not just now; I did have some, but I've forgotten."
"All right...I'll be back to see you on Thursday, so make a note of any other questions and we can discuss them then."

In this case, the patient already knew that he had cancer. When a serious diagnosis is being conveyed for the first time, one can get a feeling for how much information the patient wants by asking, "Are you the kind of person who likes to know all the facts?" When giving bad news for the first time, sometimes when it is not expected, pain is not avoidable. What can be avoided is any unnecessary addition to the patient's burden by insensitivity. Patients sometimes complain that information is given to them in a brutal fashion, as in the following instance, recounted to me by a patient:

> "We've got the results of your tests and they show that you've got cancer of the kidney."
> "What's going to happen to me?"
> "We are going to have to remove your kidney."
> "When will that be?"
> "Tomorrow morning."

The pain of devastating news is mitigated somewhat if the doctor shows consideration for the patient's feelings, takes time to answer questions, and assures the patient of continuing support. Do not give bad news, then walk away. If possible, sit down with the patient. Take time. When you leave, try to ensure that there is somebody else with the patient. Assure the patient that you will see him or her again soon and will continue your support. Bad news should be given only in the context of a continuing, supportive relationship.

An openness to indirect communication is especially important when talking to patients with devastating illness. Rather than asking, "Am I going to die?" patients, for understandable reasons, may ask, "Is it serious?" or "Why do I feel so tired?" The temptation to evade the issue is great, for example:

> "Why do I feel so tired? I've no energy."
> "Let's do a blood test. Maybe your electrolytes are out of balance."

Instead of

> "Do you understand about your illness?"
> "Yes, I know I have cancer."
> "The disease itself will make you feel tired and lacking in energy."
> "Does that mean it is progressing?"
> "It is a progressive disease, so we must expect that. How rapidly or slowly it will progress I can't tell you. However, there are ways we can help the tiredness."
> "How?"
> "By relieving pain, by making sure you get a good night's sleep, by attending to your diet."

One of the ways people deal with devastating news is denial. Such is our capacity for denial that a person may not even remember being told that he or she has a fatal disease. Denial may precede the gradual acceptance of the facts, or it may be maintained to the end. When faced with denial, it is not our place to try to break it down. An individual's way of dealing with the crisis must be respected. There is no reason, however, why we should enter into the process of denial ourselves by reinforcing unrealistic expectations. If patients who are denying their illness ask questions, we should reply honestly.

When a patient's family learns that the prognosis is serious, they may insist that the patient not be told. This may be based on their loving understanding of the patient's wishes. On the other hand, it may be more an expression of their own fears. It places the doctor in a dilemma. How can we reconcile our second-ary responsibility to the family with our primary obligation to be truthful to the patient? Our response to this is to tell the family that we will not impose the truth on the patient, but that we will not lie if the patient asks us questions. We also try to get family members to see what a strain this deception will put on their own relationship with the patient. The patient, who will almost certainly know that he or she is dying, will feel increasingly lonely and isolated, unable to share his or her feelings with those who are close to him or her.

The words we use in talking to patients will depend on the culture we are working in. Some words, in some cultures, may be so emotive that we cannot use them. Some words have associations for a patient that are quite different from the associations they have for us. I (IRMcW) once told a patient at a postpartum visit that she had superficial phlebitis in a varicose vein. Her husband came to see me later in great distress. His wife had seen her mother die of a pulmonary embolism arising from thrombophlebitis of the leg.

In some cultures, *cancer* is such a word. Other words have to be used as substi-tutes, but we should not see this as an excuse for using words that are evasive. If the patient uses an emotive word first, then we know that we can use it ourselves, remembering to ask what the word means to them:

"Is it cancer, doctor?"
"Yes, it is cancer. What is your understanding of that?"
"Does that mean I am not going to get better?"
"No. With this type of cancer you have a good chance of getting better."

If patients ask us how long they have to live, we never give them a specific time period. We do not think we should ever do so. Prognosis is a much less precise art than diagnosis. We are almost certain to be wrong, often by weeks, sometimes by months and years. The effects on patients and their families are usually negative. Hope diminishes, and they become increasingly anxious as the stated time approaches. The last guiding principle in giving bad news is to try to find some reason for hope in every patient. Even if it is not hope for survival, it may be hope for living until a task is completed or a grandchild born, or hope for a period of remission, or for a peaceful death without pain (see p. 102).

Reassurance

As Kessel (1979) has written, "The utterance of reassurance should be as planned and deliberate as the use of any other medical skill." Although it is not possible to provide specific rules for the application of this skill, there are some principles that, if followed, will help the physician to be more effective in his reassurance and to avoid some errors and pitfalls.

1. The essential basis for effective reassurance is a trusting relationship between patient and doctor. The family physician starts out with the great advantage of having in many cases already established this relationship.
2. If reassurance is to be specific, the physician must know what the patient's anxieties are. Only then can he or she take the necessary steps to achieve reassurance. If a man with chest pain is worried about lung cancer, he will not be reassured if the physician tells him—on the basis of an ECG—that he does not have coronary heart disease. Specific reassurance requires that his anxiety be identified and the investigation directed toward it.
3. Premature reassurance is ineffective and may be interpreted by the patient as a rejection. The patient must be convinced that the physician has obtained the information necessary for reassurance. If a patient says "Do you think this pain is anything to worry about?" it may be tempting to say, "No, it's nothing to worry about." It may be better, however, to say "It doesn't sound like anything serious, but before telling you there's nothing to worry about I'd like to ask you some more questions and examine you."
4. When reassurance can be given with confidence, it should not be delayed. A patient coming to hear the results of tests has little thought for anything but the news he or she is about to hear. Questions about how the patient is feeling will attract only partial attention. Better to start straight away with "Well, Mr. Smith, your X-rays are fine."
5. The patient's complaints—and his or her perception of them—should be taken seriously. It is very disturbing for a patient to be told "There is nothing wrong with you." It suggests that he or she is malingering. Better to say, "I can assure you that your symptoms are not due to cancer or any other serious disease." If this can be followed by a description of what is producing the symptoms, so much the better.
6. Some hope should always be given. This does not have to be false hope. Patients do not always want to be reassured that they will recover from their illness. They may have accepted permanent disability and need to be assured only that they will still be able to go for a walk, do their gardening, or some other activity they enjoy. Even in terminal illness, the assurance that they will not suffer pain may be a source of comfort.
7. Emphasis should be given to the hopeful aspects of the condition. To say: "Eighty percent of patients get back to normal activity with this disease," sounds very different from, "Twenty percent of patients have some residual disability after this disease." The information is the same, but its effect on the patient can be quite different. We are sometimes so hesitant and negative in our reassurance, even with diseases carrying a good prognosis, that the patient is left in doubt and anxiety.
8. When the nature of the disease is explained, everyday language should be used, with checks to see that the patient has understood. We often forget that words

we use every day have no meaning at all for many patients. I once observed a resident explaining to a patient about the need for surgery for an aortic aneurysm. When the doctor had finished, the patient asked, "What is an aorta?"

The above principles apply to the assurance of patients with what we may call "normal" anxiety: the anxiety that a person naturally feels when faced with the threat of death or disability. With abnormal anxiety, reassurance is ineffective, for it will not relieve the anxiety. In these patients, anxiety is part of a more deep-seated disorder and must be dealt with differently.

Dependence

The long-term nature of the doctor–patient relationship in family practice means that some patients may become frequent attenders because of their dependency needs. Not all dependency is pathological. We are all dependent on others for support. At some times in our lives we have special needs, especially at times of crisis, grief, and illness. It is natural that many people turn to their family physician then. K.B. Thomas (1974) has used the term "temporarily dependent patient" for patients who come mainly to be supported during a period of stress, often only for one visit. Nigel Stott (1983) speaks of the "refuge role" of the family physician. Physicians also have their dependency needs. We have a need to be seen as a good doctor, to be sought after and liked by our patients.

It is not easy to avoid pathological dependency. When in doubt, most of us would probably risk dependency rather than fail to support a patient who really needed our help. No family physician can avoid having some patients who are chronically dependent. The most we can do is to be aware of the risk of pathological dependency in our patients and ourselves and to avoid fostering it.

References

Balint M. 1964. *The Doctor, his Patient and the Illness*. London: Pitman.

Balint M, Hunt J, Joyce R, Marinker M, Woodcock J. 1970. *Treatment or Diagnosis: A Study of Repeat Prescriptions in General Practice*. London: Tavistock Publications.

Balint M, Balint E. 1973. *Six Minutes for the Patient*. London: Tavistock Publications.

Bateson G. 1979. *Mind and Nature: A Necessary Unity*. New York: E. P. Dutton.

Beckman HB, Frankel RN. 1984. The effect of physician behaviour on the collection of data. *Annals of Internal Medicine* 101:692.

Bochner S. 1983. Doctors, patients and their cultures. In: Pendleton D, Hasler J, eds., *Doctor–Patient Communication*. London: Academic Press.

Burack RC, Carpenter RR. 1983. The predictive value of the presenting complaints. *Journal of Family Practice* 16:749.

Byrne PS, Long BEL. 1976. *Doctors Talking to Patients*. London: Her Majesty's Stationery Office.

Campbell J. 1982. *Grammatical Man: Information, Entropy, Language and Life*. New York: Simon and Schuster.

Grant N. 1996. Heartsink relationships: Self-fulfilling prophecies and how to avoid them. Unpublished manuscript.

Greenfield S, Kaplan SH, Ware JE, Jr. 1985. Expanding patient involvement in care. *Annals of Internal Medicine* 102:520.

Hall ET. 1977. *Beyond Culture*. New York: Anchor Press/Doubleday.

Hannay DR. 1979. *The Symptom Iceberg: A Study in Community Health*. London: Routledge and Kegan Paul.

Innis HA. 1951. *The Bias of Communication*. Toronto: University of Toronto Press.

Kessel M. 1979. Reassurance. *Lancet* 1:1128.

Kleinman A, Eisenberg J, Good B. 1978. Culture, illness and care: Clinical lessons from anthropologic cross-cultural research. *Annals of Internal Medicine* 88:251.

Kubler-Ross E. 1969. On Death and Dying. New York: Macmillan.

McDaniel S, Campbell TL, Seaburn DB. 1990. *Family-Oriented Primary Care: a Manual for Medical Providers*. New York: Springer Verlag.

Marvel MK, Epstein RM, Flowers K, Beckman HB. 1999. Soliciting the patient's agenda: Have we improved? *Journal of American Medical Association* 281(3): 283–287.

O'Dowd TC. 1988. Five years of heartsink patients in general practice. *British Medical Journal* 297:528.

Rogers C. 1980. *A Way of Being*. Boston, MA: Houghton-Mifflin.

Rudebeck CE. 1992. General practice and the dialogue of clinical practice. *Scandinavian Journal of Primary Health Care*. Supplement 1.

Stott NCH. 1983. *Primary Health Care*. Berlin: Springer Verlag.

Styron W. 1992. *Darkness Visible. A Memoir of Madness*. New York: Vintage Books.

Suchman A, Matthews D. 1988. What makes a doctor–patient relationship therapeutic? Exploring the connectional decisions of medical care. *Annals of Internal Medicine* 108:125.

Terkel S. 1975. *Working*. New York: Avon Books.

Thomas KB. 1974. The temporarily dependent patient. *British Medical Journal* 1:1327.

Toombs SK. 1987. The meaning of illness: A phenomenological approach to the patient–physician relationship. *Journal of Medicine and Philosophy* 12:219.

Notes

1. This issue is discussed in LJ Kirmayer's essay, Mind and body as metaphors: Hidden values in biomedicine. In: Lock M, Candon D, eds., *Biomedicine Examined*. Ondrecht: Kluwer, 1988.

2. The idea of somatization is only conceivable in a culture that views diseases as entities and assigns a different status to illnesses with no verifiable physical pathology. In medical traditions with a unitary view of illness—such as Ayurvedic and Chinese medicine—the idea of somatization would make no sense. See Horatio Fabrega's essay, Somatization in cultural and historical perspective. In Kirmayer LJ, Robbins JM, eds., *Current Concepts of Somatization*. Washington: American Psychiatric Press, 1991. For a fuller discussion of these implications, see my article, The importance of being different. *British Journal of General Practice,* 1996 46:433–436 and I R McWhinney, R M Epstein, and T Freeman. 1997. Rethinking somatization. *Annals of Internal Medicine* 126(9):747–750.

3. For a good practical approach to somatic fixation, see Integrating the mind-body split: A biopsychosocial approach to somatic fixation. In: McDaniel S, Campbell T, Seaburn D, eds., *Family Oriented Primary Care*, chapter 16. 1990. New York: Springer Verlag.

4. A number of comprehensive texts on interviewing are now available. See, for example, Lipkin M, Putnam S, Fazare A, eds. 1995. *The Medical Interview: Clinical Care, Education and Research* New York: Springer Verlag and Enelow A, Forde DL, Brummel-Smith K. 1996. *Interviewing and Patient Care*, 4th edn. New York: Oxford University Press.

5. For a strategy designed to systematically develop key questions see Malterud K. 1994. Key questions: A strategy for modifying clinical communication. *Scandinavian Journal of Primary Health Care* 12:121–127.

8

Clinical Method

This chapter describes a clinical method that we believe to be both appropriate and necessary for family practice: the patient-centered clinical method. Its essence is the physician's attempt to fulfill a twofold task: understanding the patient and understanding his or her disease. From this understanding flows the process of therapy for both patient and disease. The process of diagnosing disease has been central in medical education for many years. So prominent has it been that students could be excused for thinking that this process was synonymous with clinical method. Understanding the patient and what the illness means to the patient has tended to be an afterthought, something added on after the diagnostic task has been completed. The patient-centered clinical method provides an integrated and systematic method for bringing together the patient and the disease.

For several reasons, family medicine has been at the forefront of attempts to develop a reformed clinical method. No disease-specific diagnosis is possible in 25% to 50% of patient visits to family physicians. Only by understanding the patient and the patient–doctor relationship can we gain insight into these problems. Even when a physical diagnosis can be made, successful therapy often requires an understanding of the context of the disease. In Chapters 6 and 7 we have seen how important an understanding between doctor and patient is for healing. Other fields of medicine face these issues too, but few to the same extent as family medicine.

The conceptual distinction between illness and disease helps us to understand the nature of the task (Fabrega, 1974). Illness is the patient's personal experience of a physical or psychological disturbance. It includes patients' sensations and feelings—especially their fears—disabilities and discomforts, attitudes toward their condition and toward the physician, the effect of the condition on their activities and relationships, the reasons for coming, their expectations, and their ideas. Disease is the pathological process physicians use as an explanatory model for illness. In family practice, we often encounter illness without a discernible pathological process—illness without disease. Illness without disease may be simply the inability of our existing methods to identify pathology. Disease and illness belong to two different universes of discourse: one to the world of theory, the other to the world of experience. In the vernacular, "Illness is what you have when you go to the doctor; disease is what you have when you've seen the doctor." Illness and disease also belong to different levels of abstraction[1] and have different levels of meaning. Illness is the meaning for the patient's life; disease is the meaning in terms of pathology. All significant illness is multilevel,[2] and the patient-centered method aims to understand the illness at all its levels from pathology to thoughts and feelings.

The Consultation

The consultation or clinical encounter—whether it takes place in the consulting room, the home, or the hospital—is the context for the patient-centered clinical method. In family practice, each consultation is one episode in a continuing relationship. There is much to be learned from consultation analysis, but we must always remember that in most cases, a single consultation is not the beginning or the end of the story for patient or doctor. Each new consultation carries over memories of previous ones; many consultations have some unfinished business to be taken up in due course. Some of this common memory of previous encounters is entered in the record and is available if the patient sees another doctor. Much of it, however, is tacit information that cannot easily be expressed in words.

A consultation may take many forms in addition to the common one of presentation and assessment of a new complaint. It may be for follow-up of chronic illness, preventive procedures, counseling, the communication of test results or consultants' reports, examinations for administrative purposes, and so on. The patient may be alone or accompanied by a spouse, parent, adult child, or friend. In some cases, the consultation may take the form of a family conference. Some have more to do with the pastoral than the clinical aspect of general practice.

Some observers have classified consultations in terms of the process (Marinker, 1983; Miller, 1992). Miller describes four types: routine, drama, ceremony (transitional), and ceremony (maintenance). Routines are everyday family practice problems—acute infections, minor trauma, need for reassurance—that by mutual agreement are dealt with simply and rapidly. Dramas are encounters involving uncertainty, conflict, emotion, lack of common ground, family discord, or diagnosis of an illness with grave implications. Doctors try to recognize dramas early. Often, however, they unfold in the course of a routine visit. The doctor's aim in these cases is to allow the drama to start and "buy time." This is accomplished by following four steps: the patient must know that the doctor believes him or her; the doctor must address the patient's greatest fears; he or she should perform some physical examination; and he or she should give the patient hope and something to do before the next visit. These consultations Miller describes as transitional ceremonies, whose purpose is to provide a transitional explanation and protect the patient from harm until a longer visit can be arranged.

Maintenance ceremonies are consultations that have settled into a regular, recurring pattern. These may be dramas that have resolved into a period of adjustment, visits for control of a chronic disease, or a periodic need for support and reassurance. Others are visits that physicians find disturbing: patients with chronic symptoms that do not respond to treatment, people with self-destructive tendencies, and those whose wants cannot be satisfied. Ceremonies are so called because of their ritualized, symbolic character. The same ritualized conversation, examination, or therapy may take place at each visit. Miller suggests that the physician in these consultations is acting like a shaman (see Chapter 6).

The type of consultation is usually identified by the doctor in its early stages. Typing depends on answering a number of questions: Why did the patient come? What does he or she want? What are the doctor's intuitive feelings based on past encounters? What mode of communication is the patient using?

The History of Clinical Method

Crookshank (1926) has described the development of diagnosis in terms of a tension between two schools of thought: the natural or descriptive and the conventional or academic. The natural, concerned with the organism and disease, attempts to describe the illness in all its dimensions, including its individual and personal features. The conventional, concerned with organs and diseases, attempts to classify and name the disease as an entity independent of the patient. The tension between these two schools of thought in each era of medicine has its counterpart in the controversy between the Coans and Cnidians in ancient Greece, the Coans being the natural, the Cnidians the conventional diagnosticians. The rival schools of Cos and Cnidus were said by Boinet to stand for "the two great doctrines which recur ceaselessly across the centuries."

Each of the schools of thought is associated with a different theory of disease. The Coans saw the essential unity of all disease, with various presentations depending on personal and environmental factors; the Cnidians were concerned with the diversity of diseases and the distinctions between them. For the Coans, the purpose of diagnosis was descriptive—an assay of the patient's state. The classical account is given in the First Epidemics of Hippocrates, in which he says that he framed his judgments by paying attention to

what was common to every and particular to each case; to the patient, the prescriber, and the prescription; to the epidemic constitution generally and in its local mood: to the habits of life and occupation of each patient; to his speech, conduct, silences, thoughts, sleep, wakefulness, and dreams—their content and incidence; to his pickings and scratchings, tears, stools, urine, spit and vomit; to earlier and later forms of illness in the same prevalence; to critical or fatal determinations; to sweat, chill, rigour, hiccup, sneezing, breathing, belching; to passage of wind, silently or with noise; to bleedings; and to piles.

For the Cnidians, the purpose of diagnosis was to classify the patient's illness in accordance with a taxonomy of diseases. To them, diseases had a reality independent of the patient. The Coans, on the other hand, did not separate the disease from the person, or the person from environment. The Coans employed individual description, the Cnidians abstraction and generalization. These differences were also reflected in attitudes to therapy. The Cnidians employed the specific remedy deemed efficacious for the named disease. The Coans treated each patient individually and symptomatically, attempting to assist nature in restoring the functional unity of the organism. The Cnidians prescribed remedies, the Coans a regimen.

The differences between these two schools of thought are summarized in Table 8.1. Each has strengths and weaknesses. The strength of the conventional approach is its explanatory and predictive power in certain types of illness. Its weakness is that the schema used by physicians may so influence them that they miss individual features of the illness. There is an instructive parallel with art. In his book *Art and Illusion*, Gombrich (1960) discusses the use of formulas in the training of artists, such as the schema for drawing the human head. The problem is that the schema may so influence artists' perception that they fail to notice the particular features of the head they are drawing. Using such a schema can block the path to effective portrayal unless it is accompanied by a constant willingness to correct and revise. Artists should use a schema only as a starting point that they will then clothe with flesh and blood. Similarly in medicine, a diagnostic schema should not be an end in itself, but a starting point which the physician will then clothe with flesh and blood.

The strength of the natural approach is its concreteness—the richness of its descriptions. Its weakness is that a distrust of classification and a focus on symptoms may lead to a failure to explore the origins of illness in more depth. The natural method suffers also because it is difficult to articulate. Natural diagnosticians tend to teach by example rather than by the spoken word.

The tension between the two schools of thought can be discerned in other ages. During the Renaissance, it was reflected in the controversy between the Hippocratists and the Galenists, summed up by Crookshank (1926) as one between a system founded on experience and a system founded on reason. In the seventeenth century, conventional diagnosis was greatly advanced by the work of Sydenham, who in turn was influenced by the Swedish biologist and systematizer Linnaeus, and by the philosopher John Locke. Like the best physicians in all ages, Sydenham had in him something of the natural and something of the

Table 8.1 Differences between the Coan and Cnidian schools of thought

Cos	Cnidus
Organisms and diseases	Organisms and diseases
Individual description	Classification
Concrete	Abstract
High-context	Low-context
Holistic	Reductive
Regimen	Specific remedy

conventional diagnostician. He was critical of the theoreticians who interpreted illness by reference to a priori theories that had little relation to clinical observation. Sydenham's method was to observe and record the phenomena of illness at the bedside, and this earned him the name "The English Hippocrates." On the other hand, he believed strongly in the existence of distinct disease entities, comparing them to the botanical species described by Linnaeus. He insisted that diseases were subject to laws. The symptoms "observed in Socrates in his illness," he wrote, "may generally be applied to any other person afflicted with the same disease, in the same manner as the general marks of plants justly run through the same plants of every kind."

Using this method, Sydenham was able to separate a number of infectious diseases into distinct categories: measles, scarlet fever, smallpox, cholera, and dysentery. He distinguished gout from rheumatism and was the first to describe chorea. Sydenham followed the course of diseases over time and was therefore able to test his categories for their predictive power. This correlation of clinical categories with their course and outcome—the study of the natural history of disease—was an important innovation that was not followed by his immediate successors. Eighteenth-century physicians did continue to produce classifications of disease, but these were "uncorrelated catalogues of clinical manifestations...lacking the prognostic or anatomic significance that would make the results practical or useful" (Feinstein, 1967). English physicians, on the whole, displayed little enthusiasm for these classifications and continued to regard diagnosis as a process applicable to persons rather than to diseases.

Early in the nineteenth century, clinical method took a sharp turn toward conventional diagnosis. The impetus for this turn came from the innovations of the French school of clinician-pathologists, who began to turn their attention to the physical examination of the patient. New instruments such as the Laennec stethoscope revealed a new range of clinical information. At the same time, clinicians examined the organs after death and correlated symptoms and physical signs with postmortem appearances. The result was a radically new classification of disease based on morbid anatomy—far more powerful than the nosologies of the eighteenth century. English physicians were so impressed with the result that they were soon converted to the new system. "To interpret in terms of specific diseases [became] almost the only duty of the diagnostician" (Crookshank, 1926).

In the course of the nineteenth century, the new system led to the clinical method that has dominated medicine in our own day. The emergence of the method has been described by Tait (1979) in a study of clinical records at St Bartholomew's Hospital, London, dating back to the early nineteenth century. The modern structure first appeared about 1850 in reports of necropsies. Then the physical examination and, in the 1880s, the medical history began to be recorded in their modern form. By the end of the century the evolution of the method as we know it was complete. The record was divided into presenting complaint, history of present condition, systems inquiry, and so on. The method aimed to provide students with a conceptual structure within which they could work rationally and methodically toward their goal—the formulation of a diagnosis in terms of organic pathology. For this purpose the student doctor's clinical attention was directed and made selective in character. In particular its concentration on the special points needed to achieve a diagnosis in pathological terms did result in a relative neglect of the psychological and social aspects of illness (Tait, 1979).

In the early twentieth century, textbooks on clinical diagnosis began to appear. In 1926, Crookshank commented that these "gave excellent schemes for the physical examination of the patient, whilst strangely ignoring, almost completely, the psychical." The turn toward conventional diagnosis had gone so far that the other part of the clinician's task had been all but forgotten. Conventional diagnosis in its modern form is strictly objective. It does not aim, in any systematic way, to understand the meaning of the illness for the patient or to place it in the context of his or her life story or culture. The emotions are excluded from consideration; the physician is encouraged to be objective and detached. The objectivity of the method fits well with its nineteenth-century origins: it is, indeed, a product of the European Enlightenment.

The conventional method has been brilliantly successful in paving the way for the great therapeutic advances of the twentieth century. The application of these therapies required a diagnostic method with high predictive power. With its predictive power based on organic pathology, enhanced by new diagnostic technologies such as imaging, endoscopy, and chemistry, the new method provided that. Paradoxically, it is probably the successes of medical technology that have exposed so vividly the limitations of the modern method. Concentration on the technical aspects of care tends to divert us from the patient's inner world. The complexities and discomforts of modern therapeutics have, at the same time, made it even more important for us to understand the patient's experience.

Besides providing predictive power, the conventional method did two things that no clinical method had done before. It provided the clinician with a clear injunction: conduct the clinical inquiry in this way and you will either arrive at a physical diagnosis or exclude organic pathology. And it provided clear criteria for validation: the pathologist told the clinician whether he or she was right or wrong. The clinicopathological conference became the epitome of the process.

Attempts to Reform the Modern Method

As the limitations of the modern conventional method have become apparent, attempts have been made to develop new models.

In the 1950s, Michael Balint, a psychoanalyst, began to work with groups of general practitioners to explore the patient–doctor relationship. He was struck by the inadequacies of the conventional method for reaching any deep understanding of the patient's illness. The need was to listen, not to ask questions. Balint (1964) developed the concepts of attentive listening and responding to a patient's "offers" as means of reaching an understanding of his or her illness. He distinguished between traditional diagnosis, the search for pathology, and overall diagnosis, the attempt to understand the patient and the patient–doctor relationship. Balint also spoke of physicians themselves as powerful diagnostic and therapeutic tools and of the need to understand how to use them—hence the importance of self-knowledge in physicians.

In the 1970s and 1980s, George Engel (1980), from his experience as both internist and psychiatrist, developed the influential biopsychosocial model described in Chapter 5. This model requires the physician to consider and integrate information from several levels of the hierarchy of systems: from the milieu interieur, from the person, and from the interpersonal level.

Kleinman and his colleagues (1978) have drawn attention to the frequency with which patients have explanatory models of illness that are discordant with the biomedical model. If the physician fails to explore the patient's understanding of illness, and to negotiate some rapprochement between the two models, the outcome is likely to be unsatisfactory. Although illustrated most vividly when the physician and patient come from different cultures, discordance can occur even within the same culture. Kleinman and his colleagues recommend a series of questions designed to attain this level of understanding, followed by an explanation of the doctor's interpretation of the illness, and, if necessary, a negotiation between the two views of clinical reality.

All these models have been attempts to develop a framework for a more patient-centered clinical method. So far, they seem to have had limited impact on clinical method as taught in the medical schools. One reason, we believe, is that they do not fulfill the requirements so successfully met by the conventional method. They do not provide a clear and relatively simple injunction to the physician, and they do not provide criteria for validation.

The method described here uses insights provided by Balint, Engel, and Kleinman, but goes further. It specifies the clinical task in simple terms and establishes criteria for validation. It was formulated as a clinical method and evaluated by Joseph Levenstein and a group of colleagues at The University of Western Ontario (Brown et al., 1986; Levenstein et al., 1986). The team has more than two decades of experience in developing, researching, and teaching the method (Stewart et al., 2003). The method has six integrated components:

1. Exploring and interpreting both the disease and the illness experience
2. Understanding the whole person
3. Finding common ground with the patient about the problem and its management
4. Incorporating prevention and health promotion
5. Enhancing the patient–doctor relationship
6. Being realistic about time, resources, and teamwork

It is important not to think of the patient-centered method as a strictly defined process, with sequential stages and standardized procedures and interviewing styles. If the flow of the consultation is to follow the cues given by the patient, its course will depend on how and when these cues are given, and will vary from patient to patient. As with the conventional method, the main criterion of success is the outcome. Did the doctor reach an understanding of the patient's expectations and feelings and the social context of the illness? Was the clinical diagnosis correct? Was there an attempt to reach common ground? Did the therapeutic plan follow logically from the process? If the answer to any of these questions is no, then one can look at the process to identify errors. If the answer to all of them is yes, one may still examine the process for what may be learned from it, but whether certain items are right or wrong is unlikely to be a profitable discussion. Attempts to evaluate the consultation process in terms of right and wrong, without regard for the outcome, are liable to end in controversy; experts can often be found to differ. As with any practical art, there may be wrong ways of making a diagnosis or understanding a patient's illness, but there is no single right way.

The Patient-Centered Clinical Method

Every patient who seeks help has expectations, based on his or her understanding of the illness. All patients have some feelings about their problem. Some fear is nearly always present in the medical encounter, even when the illness may seem to be minor: fear of the unknown, fear of death, fear of insanity, fear of disability, fear of rejection.

Understanding the patient's feelings, fears, ideas, expectations, and the impact of the illness on their daily functioning is specific for each patient. The meaning of the illness for the patient reflects his or her own unique world. Frames of reference from biological or behavioral science come from the doctor's world, not the patient's. They may help the physician to explain the problem, but they are not a substitute for understanding each patient as a unique individual.

The patient-centered clinical method, like the conventional method, gives the clinician a number of injunctions. "Ascertain the patient's expectations" recognizes the importance of knowing why the patient has come. "Understand and respond to the patient's feelings" acknowledges the crucial importance of the emotions. "Make or exclude a clinical diagnosis" recognizes the continuing power of correct classification. "Listen to the patient's story" recognizes the importance of narrative and context. "Seek common ground" enjoins us to mobilize the patient's own powers of healing. To these, we would add two others: "Monitor your own feelings." They may give you some vital cues; on the other hand, they may be anti-therapeutic (see Figure 8.1), and "pay attention to the patient–doctor relationship."

The key to the patient-centered method is to allow as much as possible to flow from the patient, including the expression of feeling. The consultation on page 283 is a good example. The crucial skills, described in Chapter 7, are those of attentive listening and responsiveness to those verbal and nonverbal cues by which patients express themselves. Failure to take up the patient's cues is a missed opportunity to gain insight into the illness. If cues do not provide the necessary lead, a question may help the patient to express feelings: "What is your understanding of your illness?"; "What is it like for you to ... ?"; or "Are you frightened ... ?" "What was going on when the symptoms started ... ?"

The following reconstructed example contrasts a visit which was not patient-centered with one that was patient-centered, for the same problem.[3] A 55-year-old

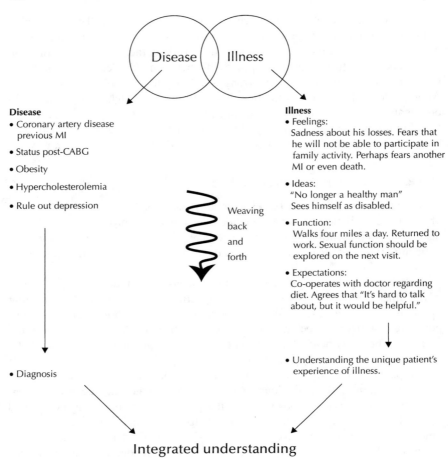

Disease
- Coronary artery disease previous MI
- Status post-CABG
- Obesity
- Hypercholesterolemia
- Rule out depression

Weaving
back
and
forth

Illness
- Feelings:
  Sadness about his losses. Fears that he will not be able to participate in family activity. Perhaps fears another MI or even death.
- Ideas:
  "No longer a healthy man" Sees himself as disabled.
- Function:
  Walks four miles a day. Returned to work. Sexual function should be explored on the next visit.
- Expectations:
  Co-operates with doctor regarding diet. Agrees that "It's hard to talk about, but it would be helpful."

- Diagnosis

- Understanding the unique patient's experience of illness.

Integrated understanding

Figure 8.1 The patient-centered method applied. (Stewart M, Brown JB, Weston WW, McWhinney IR, McWilliam CL, Freeman TR. 2003. *Patient-Centered Medicine: Transforming the Clinical Method.* 2e Oxford UK, Radcliffe Medical Press Ltd.)

female patient has been told, 1 week ago by a replacement doctor, that her breast cancer has recurred. She returns to her family doctor for the initiation of her next phase of care.

Approach That Is Not Patient-Centered

Doctor: Um, Mrs. Collins, I believe we were to talk about, about ahem, your biopsy, is that right?

Patient: Yes, I came in to see earlier Dr. Armstrong in an appointment and he gave me my results a week ago.

Doctor: Um. Yeah, I remember that now...

Patient: Um, before we begin. It's just um, I've been on the internet a lot this week, and talking to a few people and they made some suggestions about alternative procedures or treatments that might exist and...

Doctor: Excuse me.

Patient: Suggesting about fat and

Doctor: ...Let's find out exactly what's going on before you start thinking about all sorts of alternatives...Um, I think the important thing now is to go over these plans. Are you clear on exactly what this means?

Patient: Um. I think I am, but I'd appreciate it if you could reiterate it to me.

Doctor: Basically, it means the cancer has recurred on the area of your chest wall and the biopsy was taken. Um, and what we have to determine now is whether that's the only recurrence or whether it has spread elsewhere in your body.

Patient: Um, you think it may have spread elsewhere?

Doctor: I don't know if it's spread elsewhere. So then we have to find that out and um, to do that, the first thing I'd like to do is just go over how you've been feeling in general the last little while. For example, how's your appetite been?

Patient: Well, this past week has been terrible. Uh, my husband's away and my only child, I have a daughter who's pregnant. I haven't told any of them about this. So, I'm not sleeping. I'm not eating and I feel terrified...

(The doctor asks about cough, shortness of breath, nausea, vomiting, bowel movements, and pain in the abdomen.)

Patient: Um, my stomach hurts all the time.

Doctor: Any particular place?...

Patient: I, I really don't know. What does this got to do with any of this?

Doctor: Well, it's important to know the state of your health. So that's what I'm trying to establish so that we can go ahead and determine the best way to treat you. Um, Alright. You know when we're finished discussing these issues, I'm going to examine you. But um, in the mean time I think it's important we get some further tests and try and...once we do that we can discuss the treatment.

Patient: Treatment...What do you mean treatment?

Doctor: Well treatment for your cancer. A lot will depend on whether it's localized or whether it's spread out.

Patient: Okay. Um, are you sure there's nothing else I can be doing right now? This is all so hard. I, I wasn't prepared for this. Is there something I could have done differently to have prevented this?

Doctor: There's nothing you can do to prevent this. Nothing you can do to prevent anyway. The important thing is to find out exact state of the cancer so that we can determine optimal treatment. And that's

Patient: Are you talking about chemotherapy again?

Doctor: Ah, well chemotherapy is possible. It depends on where the tumour is. And we really prematurely discussed that and I just want to establish we don't know. There's so many treatment options depending on the nature of the cancer. And we don't know that.

Patient: I don't want to die right now. I have a granddaughter coming and I want to do things with my husband. I, I just don't want to die right now.

Doctor: Mrs. Collins, of course you don't. I think what you really need is to get some help. And I have here a couple of organizations that can be very helpful for you. The Canadian Breast Cancer Foundation, got their phone number. The Canadian Cancer Society has a self help group. Why don't you take these brochures and give them a call and um forget the tests. I'll get my secretary to book them. And I'll see you as soon as we get them.

Patient: Okay.

Doctor: So, all clear now?

Patient: I suppose so.

The Patient-Centered Approach

Doctor: Good morning Mrs. Collins.

Patient: Good morning Doctor.

Doctor: This must have been a terrible week for you.

Patient: It's been dreadful, absolutely.

Doctor: Can you tell me a bit about it?

Patient: Well, of course, Dr. Armstrong gave me the news last week.

Doctor: Yes, I know.

Patient: And, ah, I wasn't expecting this, but, ah three years ago I went through it and I guess this is my worst nightmare. I, I'm a wreck. I haven't slept, I haven't eaten. Sam's in Europe on business. I haven't talked to Helen, I don't want to upset her, she's four months pregnant. And I just feel like my world is falling apart.

Doctor: Have you talked to Sam?

Patient: No I haven't, ah, other than on the phone. I haven't told him. I haven't told him...I don't want to worry him I guess. There's no point. He's got things to do.

Doctor: But if he had cancer, wouldn't you want to know?...

Patient: Perhaps, perhaps you're right. Listen um, during this week though, because I'm at home alone, I've been doing some reading and doing some internet searches and there's a lot of talk in alternative medical circles about shark's cartilage, perhaps too much fat in the diet. Is there something I could have done, is there something I can do now, um, is there anything at all I can do to feel like I am in some control here?

Doctor: Okay. So you've been doing a lot of reading and been preparing stuff over the internet

Patient: Yeah.

Doctor: Look, ah with respect...I don't think you've done anything to bring this on. The issue of alternative medicine and what to do about it is not something that I'm very familiar with but I think that at times it's very helpful to people. But I would suggest we might just put this on hold for a short period of time until we really clarify what's going on.

Patient: Okay.

Doctor: I think we could, because I think the issue now is as you know, the biopsy showed that the cancer had reoccurred on the chest wall.

Patient: Yeah.

Doctor: And one of the issues that we have to address is, has it spread anywhere else? Now it may well not have...but I think it's important that we make sure because how we treat you is going to depend on the results of that sort of...

Patient: Treatment, what do you mean?

Doctor: Well, there are a variety of ways of treating breast cancer which has recurred...(Pause and seeing her shoulders slump). That is certainly not the kind of thing I hope you have to have.

Patient: (Crying) I just don't know why?

Doctor: I know.

Patient: This is just so wrong. It's just the wrong time. I don't want to die. I, I want to live to see my grand daughter. I want to retire with my husband. I want to do everything that I've worked all my life to do.

Doctor: Mrs. Collins, I wish I could tell you 100% that you are not going to die of this cancer. And even if we find out that the tumor has spread, there are excellent treatments that can give you many years of useable life. But I can't tell you that for sure or not because I don't know the extent of which the tumour has spread. If not

Patient: How do I find out the extent to which it's spread? What do we do?

Doctor: Well, we do three things...(Doctor enumerates the three things). But what I'd like you to do is tell me how you've been in general, not in the last week, because obviously the last week everything's been chaos. But before that, were you feeling reasonably well before you

Patient: Yeah, reasonably well.

Doctor: Okay. Had you lost any weight?

Patient: No, not that I, no I don't think so.

Doctor: Was your appetite okay?

Patient: Good, normal.

Doctor: No nausea or vomiting?

(Doctor covers the history and several tests.)

Doctor: Now, when is Sam coming back?

Patient: He should be by the end of the week.

Doctor: Why don't you call him? (pause) Or would you like me to call him?

Patient: Um, That might work better, I don't want to right now. (sigh) Oh, God, I'll do it. I'll do it.

Doctor: My guess is he will want you to share this with him and I'm sure he'll want to be here to help you out.

Patient: I guess I just kept hoping it would go away. Denial again I guess.

Doctor: Okay. Um, is there anything else right now that I can do to help you out?

Patient: Well, I guess just...no...I mentioned the alternative things and you said that we can proceed on some of that according to the results, is that...

Doctor: Well, yeah, I thought that when we...By all means, you know, look up what you want and if there's anything in particular that you wish to pursue, I'd appreciate if you'd bring it to me...

Patient: Okay...

Doctor: And, I'd really like to see you later this week. I won't have the test results but this is a pretty stressful time.

Patient: Yeah.

Doctor: I think it will help to talk a little bit more about how your feeling and what we can do about it.

Patient: Okay, thank you.

In the example of not being patient-centered, the physician initially cuts off the patient's ideas about alternative treatments. He states his agenda and preempts the patient's description of her terrible week, her isolation from her family, and her feelings of terror. When the patient questions the relevance to her concerns of the physician's history-taking, the physician ignores the cue and defends his approach, continuing to the end in an unfeeling manner.

In the patient-centered example, the physician immediately acknowledges the patient's suffering. The physician allows the consultation to be guided by the patient's issues, her husband's absence and her search for control through considering alternative treatments. He responds to her emotions, after which she expresses a readiness to discuss the history, tests, and treatment. He ends with an offer of a return visit to talk about her feelings.

The patient-centered approach is also illustrated in the following clinical example.

Case 8.1

An elderly woman complained of a suffocating feeling in the chest, occurring in the early hours of the morning, which was relieved to some extent by sitting by an open window. She first came in the middle of a busy office session when time was short. Given the above cues, the doctor formed a first hypothesis of nocturnal cardiac asthma, and after a physical examination revealed no signs to support the diagnosis, sent the patient for a chest X-ray. When this too was normal, he asked the patient to come in for a longer interview.

On this occasion he obtained the following history. Her main complaint was of very active peristalsis and abdominal discomfort occurring at night and keeping her awake. After lying awake for hours she would get more and more tense, get a suffocating feeling, and have to get up and go to the window. The abdominal symptoms had been present for 20 years, but the insomnia was of more recent origin. Many years previously she had had a cholecystectomy, which failed to relieve her symptoms, and a mastectomy for carcinoma. She had a fear of surgery and on direct questioning admitted to an anxiety that her abdominal symptoms might be due to cancer. She had been widowed several years and lived in an apartment by herself. Recently her landlord had raised her rent without giving her any notice. Her two children were both married and living away. Recently, her daughter had moved near to her after living away for some years. During the interview, she expressed hostility toward her landlord, who, she felt, had been very unfair to her.

The process in this case is shown as a flow diagram in Figure 8.2. In addressing the patient's agenda, the physician is formulating and testing hypotheses based on the cues he or she receives and on the previous knowledge of the patient or of the symptoms. To an experienced physician, some symptoms are associated with particular fears, such as the fear of cancer. This knowledge may enable the physician to identify the patient's fears very rapidly. But we must always guard against the fallacy of treating a hypothesis as an assumption. In the above example, the doctor-centered physician assumed without attempting validation that the main item on the patient's agenda was to follow-up on his surgery. This is a common pitfall with doctor-initiated visits of all kinds (Stewart, McWhinney, and Buck, 1979).

Five questions are commonly asked about the patient-centered clinical method. First, is it always necessary to use the method? Suppose the problem is very straightforward: an injury, for example, or an uncomplicated infectious disease. The answer is that we do not know unless we ask. Patients have fears and fantasies even about common and minor problems. In emergencies, of course, the medical priority must take precedence, as in the above clinical example. But when these needs have been met, no patient is in greater need of being listened to than the one with sudden and severe acute illness or trauma.

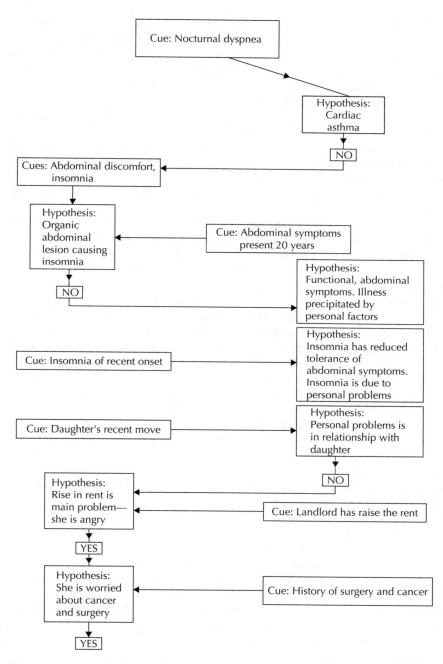

Figure 8.2   Flow diagram to illustrate hypothesis testing in Case 8.1.

Second, what if there is a conflict between the patient's expectations and the medical assessment? Suppose, for example, that a patient wishes to manage his diabetic ketoacidosis without admission to the hospital. The physician must then try to reconcile the two conflicting views. The more the physician can understand about the reasons for the patient's position, the more chance there will be of a satisfactory conclusion. The reluctance to go into the hospital, for example, may be caused by a feeling of responsibility for a child or elderly parent. In some cases, there will be an irreconcilable conflict, as in a demand for a narcotic drug, and the physician will have to refuse to meet the patient's expectations. In the more usual situation, doctor and patient have different interpretations of the illness or conflicting notions about its management. The patient, believing the pain indicates an organic disease, cannot accept the doctor's view that this is not the case. The doctor is reluctant to prescribe oxycodone tablets for a patient who finds they relieve his periodic headaches. Our contribution to reconciling conflicting views is threefold. First, we can acknowledge the validity of the patient's experience and take his or her interpretation seriously, even if we cannot accept it. Second, we can be aware of the danger that our own prejudice, rigidity, dogmatism, or faulty logic may be the cause of the difference. A mild narcotic used occasionally by a sensible person may be an appropriate remedy for headaches (see p. 282). The patient may actually be correct in saying that his symptoms are organic in origin. Third, we can make sure that the patient has all the information we can provide. Conversely, some humility may be called for, as when a very well-informed patient knows more than we do about his or her condition.

The third common question is, is there not a risk of invading the patient's privacy? Suppose the patient does not want to, or is not ready to, reveal her secrets? If privacy is invaded, then the method has been misunderstood. The essence of it is that the doctor responds to cues given by the patient, allows and encourages expression but does not force it. If cues are not given, feelings are explored with general questions that invite openness. If the patient does not wish to respond, the matter is not pursued. At least the doctor has indicated that such matters are admissible.

Fourth, what about the time problem? How can we afford the time to listen to the patient? It is difficult to answer this, because little research has been done on the relation between consultation time, clinical method, and effectiveness. From work done so far, we can say tentatively that patient-centered consultations take a little longer, but not much longer, than doctor-centered ones. Beckman and Frankel (1984) found that when patients are uninterrupted, their opening statements lasted only 2.5 minutes on the average. Stewart et al. (2003) reported that 9 minutes or more was the critical duration for patient-centered consultations. What we do not know is how much time is saved in the long run by an early and accurate identification of the patient's problems. Our hunch is that the patient-centered clinical method will prove to be a time-saver in the long run.

Fifth, what if the doctor opens up a host of psychological, emotional, and social problems that he or she is not able to deal with? This is closely related to the time issue, but it is also the case that sometimes physicians eschew emotionally laden encounters in the midst of a busy day. Physicians, by their nature feel compelled to offer an intervention, but for some human suffering, such as great and tragic loss, no effective intervention is available. In these situations, simply bearing witness to the suffering is what is needed.

It is important to distinguish between active and passive listening. Attentive listening, as described on page 128, is not a commitment to listen indefinitely to a rambling monologue. That would be passive listening. A flow of words usually expresses something, even if its significance is the feeling rather than the content. A response to the feeling may enable the patient to express herself in a different way. Making a home visit to a 90-year-old man with lung cancer, I (IRMcW) was detained by his wife, who went on at great length about what she tried to get her husband to eat. Eventually I broke off the conversation and left. As I was driving away, the penny dropped. Surely she was trying to express her feeling of impotence at being unable to care for her husband in the way she believed to be best.

Validation

The ultimate validation of a diagnosis in the conventional clinical method is the pathologist's report. In the clinico-pathological conferences modeled by *The New England Journal of Medicine*, a clinician is presented with a case report and develops a differential diagnosis, which is then confirmed or otherwise by a pathologist. The clinicopathological conference can be regarded as the quintessence of the conventional method. Other forms of validation are available, notably the response to therapy and the outcome of illness.

The ultimate validation of the patient-centered method is also the patient's report that his or her feelings and concerns have been acknowledged and responded to. This may be ascertained by qualitative studies and by periodic surveys of patients, using validated questionnaires such as the one produced by Stewart et al. (2000 and 2003). In the normal course of practice, validation comes from the natural history of the illness and the patient–doctor relationship. If common ground has been attained, therapy is likely to go more smoothly, reassurance to be more effective, and the relationship to be free from tension.

Physicians wishing to have some external validation of their clinical method may choose to have their consultations evaluated by an observer using one of the rating scales developed for this purpose (Stewart et al., 2003). If these are used as a basis for coaching by an experienced teacher, they can be a source of valuable insights. It is difficult for any of us to be fully aware of recurring faults in our clinical practice. Until the coming of audio and video recording technologies, the consultation—the central event of family practice—remained hidden from view. After-the-fact reporting of the process could not possibly convey its nuances. An observer in the same room was liable to change the process, and discussion afterwards was limited by the inability to verify the observer's recollection of the process by recourse to a recording. Thanks to the evolving technology, all of us can now develop as clinical artists in the way that artists have always learned—by submitting our work to the judgment of a respected teacher.

Learning the Patient-Centered Method

It is important to distinguish between the process by which physicians learn a clinical method and the process by which they practice it. To assist learning, the process is broken down into a number of rules, tasks, and stages. Learning these components is not the same as acquiring the process itself. No list of components can include all the tacit knowledge that can only be acquired by experiencing and "dwelling in" the process. One problem faced by the student is that it is impossible to be aware of the components and the whole process at the same time. Polanyi (1962) has clarified this issue by distinguishing between focal and subsidiary awareness. Focal awareness is awareness of the process as a whole. Subsidiary awareness is awareness of the components. Riding a bicycle can be described in terms of rules for correcting imbalance and of the adjustments made by the body in response to changes in equilibrium. Learning the rules, however, is not the same as riding a bicycle, because the rules cannot embody all the tacit knowledge involved in performing the task. To perform the task, one must be focally aware of the whole process while remaining only subsidiarily aware of the components. Focusing on the components may actually cause one to fall off the bicycle. Similarly, when practicing a clinical method, one cannot do so while trying to keep in mind the subsidiary rules and components. These can be learned beforehand and referred to afterwards, but in the performance of the task they must remain at the level of subsidiary awareness. The tension between these two levels of awareness, and the need to alternate between them, can be difficult for students at first. When the skill is acquired, the tension resolves. The doctor "dwells in" the process, and focal awareness is maintained throughout. Subsidiary awareness is brought into being only when teaching the skill to somebody else or when reviewing one's own process after the fact.

Case presentations are an important learning and teaching tool and were recognized as such in the late nineteenth century by Walter Cannon (1890). The traditional format of the case presentation has evolved over the century since that time, taking into account new and emerging ideas such as the problem-oriented medical record (Weed, 1969) and the biopsychosocial model of Engel (Engel, 1977). Presentation of case histories are an important part of the medical training of students and residents and it has been pointed out that the decision of what material to present and its organization are powerful reinforcements of a particular worldview (Anspach, 1988). Typically, the conventional case history leaves out the more personal aspects of the patient including the lived experience of the individual. There is an overwhelming focus on the disease to the exclusion of everything else. Attempts to correct this imbalance include the use of patient stories to increase physician empathy (Charon, 1986; Donnelly, 1989). Narrative-based medicine has developed an extensive literature (Greenhalgh and Hurwitz, 1998;

Charon, 2001). The Clinical Crossroads section of the *Journal of the American Medical Association* has been a welcome change to the usual case history and includes the patient's first-hand account (Winker, 2006). The patient-centered case presentation has been used to reinforce the patient-centered approach in the education of residents in family medicine (Freeman, 2003). It explicitly requires the presenter to address a couple of areas not found in the conventional case history. These include the patient's illness experience with an appropriate quotation, if possible, and comment on the patient–doctor relationship and whether common ground was achieved. By placing the patient at the core of the report, the patient-centered case presentation reinforces the primacy of the person rather than the disease. Without sacrificing the information found in the conventional case history, it supports the values inherent in the patient-centered method.

Case books are another way of describing and re-inforcing the principles of the patient-centered method (Borkan, Reis, Steinmetz, and Medalie, 1999; Brown, Stewart, and Weston, 2002).

Evaluation of the Patient-Centered Method

Some studies have been critical of the patient-centered clinical method, but have misunderstood the method. For example, in one study, patients were asked to choose their preference from several consulting styles, one of which was the patient-centered method. Patients were then numbered according to their preferred style. The authors inferred that: "some patients do not want the patient-centred clinical method." This is not correct. The physician conducts the consultation in accordance with the cues he or she receives from the patient. There are no "styles" of clinical method any more than there are styles of biomedical approach. Patients are not given a choice between what tests they have.

In contrast, Little et al.'s (2001a,b) series of studies in the United Kingdom revealed that over 75% of patients wanted a patient-centered approach. In addition, patients valued highly all three of the components studied.

Recent reviews of outcome studies of patient-centered care, measured in a variety of ways, have revealed benefits to the doctor, the patient, and the system. Benefits to doctors include higher doctor satisfaction, better use of time and fewer complaints from patients. Benefits to patients include higher patient satisfaction and better patient adherence (Stewart et al., 2003, Chapter 17). Benefits to the system include fewer diagnostic tests, fewer referrals (Stewart et al., 2000), and fewer return visits (Campbell et al., 2005).

However, the most stringent validation is the patient self-report and patient health status. Studies have found patient-centered care to correlate with patient self-report and patient health status in a cohort study (Stewart et al., 2000) and to influence patients feeling better in a randomized controlled trial (Stewart et al., 2007).

The systematic review by Griffin et al. (2004) found that most of the 35 interventions—to improve patient-centered care—increased scores on patient–doctor communication and slightly more than half improved patient's health such as: resolution of symptoms; headache; sore throat; anxiety distress; and physiologic status.

Furthermore, studies confirm the positive influence of patient-centered care internationally, in Spain (Moral, Almo, Jurado, and de Torres, 2001), South Africa (Henbest and Fehrsen, 1992) and China (Ge and Stewart, submitted and under review).

The Patient-Centered Method in Family Practice

Like the conventional method, the patient-centered method is applied somewhat differently in each field of medicine. Because family doctors are available for all types of problems, they can make no prior assumptions about why the patient has come (the reason for the encounter). Nor can they assume that the first problem presented is the main problem. In the early part of the consultation, therefore, they will be forming hypotheses about the patient's reason for coming and expectations and formulating the problem to be addressed. The hypotheses will be based on cues from the patient's expressions and body language, as well as any intuitions from previous knowledge of the patient. As the patient talks, the doctor will be assessing the significance of the presenting symptoms. On this assessment will depend hypotheses about whether the symptoms signify a minor clinical problem, a major clinical problem (perhaps urgent), a problem of living presenting as symptoms, or a need for reassurance.

Putting all these together into a global assessment, the physician should have an idea of what course the consultation is likely to take. The original hypotheses, of course, may be wrong and it may take an unexpected turn. In *Cases 8.1* and *10.1*, the initial hypothesis of an urgent clinical problem proved to be incorrect, and the focus shifted to the patient's emotions and relationships. In *Case 12.1*, the patient's story and expressive language correctly indicated emotional turmoil and traumatic life events. In *Cases 7.1* and *7.3*, the mode of presentation, together with the doctor's previous knowledge of the patient, pointed to emotional distress. In *Case 10.3*, the symptoms and the doctor's knowledge of the family correctly indicated stressful family relationships. In *Cases 10.2* and *13.1*, early hypotheses of a major psychiatric disorder proved incorrect on testing—one proving to be a marital problem, the other a carcinoma.

There is no predetermined order in the consultation. It does not flow in a uniform fashion from history of present condition through to systems inquiry and examination. The order is mutually guided by the patient's presentation and the doctor's response. It is an important principle of the patient-centered method that the doctor should in most cases allow the patient to determine the flow. "I think I can feel a lump in my breast" will lead very quickly to a history, and examination, followed by an exploration of the patient's feelings and fears. For a skin rash, history, examination, and exploration of feelings will probably occur together. In the case on page 273 the doctor simply let the patient tell the story of her headaches. The physical examination reveals more than physical signs. From the beginning of the consultation, the doctor is noting the patient's body language: posture, gait, movements, and facial expressions. Sometimes, the deepest feelings are not expressed until a painful area is palpated. Rudebeck (1992) writes,

When moving from dialogue to examination it is assumed that the symptom has been quite well defined by the doctor. However, the patient continues to present her symptoms by vegetative and muscular reactions, by the look of her face, by gestures and bodily posture.

It is not uncommon that spirit and meaning enter into communication precisely at the moment of examination. The doctor must not abandon the patient at this point and turn his attention to the possible disease.

Nor is therapy left only to the end. The whole consultation is part of the therapeutic process.

Symptoms

Symptoms are the patient's way of expressing his or her experience of the illness. A bodily sensation, with its affective coloring, is translated into language. Because patients describing their own symptoms are saying something about themselves, their language always has an expressive as well as a literal meaning. The important meaning may be the literal one, or the expressive one, or both. Symptoms that fit closely with a well-defined disease category have a literal meaning in terms of physical pathology. Experience that is difficult to articulate may only be understood by attending to the expressive language. A terminally ill patient's pain may be expressed only by a furrowed brow or a groan when the patient is turned. In a patient with headache, key information may be expressed by the quivering lip, which soon gives place to tears if the response is appropriate.

Rudebeck (1992) distinguishes between the symptom and the symptom presentation: "*Doctors do in fact judge 'symptom presentations' rather than symptoms.* Symptoms are abstractions. As such they are detached from the acts through which the patient presents them." Rudebeck postulates that the ability to grasp the meaning of the symptom presentation is a fundamental skill of general practice. A key element in general clinical competence, it is "a basic ability to grasp the character of patient's problems and needs, useful in a vast number of patient–doctor interactions." Symptoms described in medical textbooks are abstractions. The doctor does not face abstractions, he or she "faces a human being who in her *symptom presentation* tries to communicate an experience which is often quite personal, since body and self are inseparable. A symptom gives rise to reflections and fantasies, which in important ways decide how the symptom will be presented.... The first and very basic question of general practice is therefore: Who is this person presenting this symptom?... A symptom is no longer an evident expression of disease, but a bodily experience which might be an expression of disease."

Clinical Diagnosis in Family Practice: The Grammar of Clinical Problem Solving

This section deals with the physician's conventional task of clinical problem solving and decision making, with particular reference to family practice. Although discussed in this separate section, the process is integral to the patient-centered method described earlier.

Although the general principles of problem solving and decision making are the same in all branches of medicine, each discipline has its own way of applying them. The differences between disciplines are the result of differences in the problems they encounter and in their roles within the health-care system. The problem-solving strategies of family physicians have evolved in response to a number of special features of family practice. Some of these features are shared with other primary care disciplines, especially those providing continuity of patient care.

For many years, medical thinking about the diagnostic process was dominated by a fallacy. The fallacy was that physicians make diagnoses by collecting data in routine fashion, by history-taking and examination, then by making deductions from the data. Studies of clinicians' thinking have now shown that this is not how physicians solve clinical problems. They do it in the way everybody else solves problems, in science and in everyday life. Early on in the process, they form hypotheses based on the available evidence. They then proceed to test their hypotheses by the selective collection of data from the patient's history, clinical examination, and laboratory investigation. This is known as the hypothetico-deductive approach to problem solving. It may not be the only approach. In some situations, clinicians may use reasoning that is purely deductive, such as, "since this male patient is sixteen years of age, we need not consider prostatic hypertrophy as a reason for his urinary symptoms." We suspect, however, that this type of thinking plays a relatively small part in most fields of medicine.

Although clinical problem solving is better taught nowadays, some important aspects are still not made explicit. The setting in which instruction takes place is often the medical department of a tertiary-care hospital. It is natural for the student to assume that the methods appropriate to this setting can be transferred unmodified to any other medical context. As we will see, this is not the case. The sensitivity, specificity, and predictive value of clinical data and tests vary greatly with the prevalence and distribution of illness in the population, and therefore with the setting in which the physician is working. Moreover, how we perceive and interpret the world is shaped by our mental constructs. We see what we know. A student who learns clinical problem solving in a tertiary-care hospital will tend to have a frame of reference appropriate for patients with serious and well-defined diseases in their later stages. If the student uses this frame of reference for solving problems in family practice, he or she will get into difficulties, the kind of difficulties described so well by James Mackenzie many years ago:

I had not long been in the practice when I discovered how defective was my knowledge. I left college under the impression that every patient's condition could be diagnosed. For a long time I strove to make a diagnosis and assiduously studied my lectures and textbooks, without avail.... For some years I thought that this inability to diagnose my patients' complaints was due to personal defects, but gradually, through consultations and other ways, I came to recognise that the kind of information I wanted did not exist. (Mair, 1973)

A frame of reference will have to be learned, one which will take into account problems rarely encountered in the tertiary-care hospital. Learning a new frame of reference is one of the objectives of vocational or postgraduate training. Family physicians of previous generations did this by trial and error—slow and painful process. Thanks to progress in describing the principles and methods of family practice, it is now possible to acquire this knowledge in a much shorter time and with less risk to ourselves and our patients. Even so, the transition from one context to another can be difficult, as many residents find when they experience family practice for the first time. The trauma is lessened if a student's early experience of clinical problem solving has taken place in a variety of contexts ranging from primary to tertiary care.

This section takes an analytical approach to clinical method, including quantification in some places. One might question whether this is necessary or even wise. Medicine has had many brilliant diagnosticians who worked intuitively, without being able to make their thinking explicit. Is it necessary to understand the theory of diagnosis and decision making in order to be a good clinician? For most physicians, we believe it is. We learn and grow as clinicians mainly by examining our errors. Error, like uncertainty, is inherent in medicine. If we are going to learn from our errors, we need to be able to analyze our decision making so that we can pinpoint where the error occurred and why. It is rather like learning to write. We do not usually think in terms of grammar when we write something: as long as it reads well and expresses what we want to say, we do not need to. But if what we have written looks wrong or conveys the wrong meaning, then we have to get down to the business of analyzing our sentences and thinking about our tenses and subordinate clauses. The theory of clinical decision making is a grammar we can use to gain insight into our own thought processes, and to understand our errors so that we can avoid them in the future. It may be true to say that one can be a good intuitive clinician without having any insight into the clinical process. It is also true that the greatest clinicians in medical history—the Sydenhams, the Laennecs, the Oslers of medicine—have taken a deep interest in the theory of medicine.

There are other reasons for family physicians to take an analytical approach to clinical method. We sometimes receive well meaning but ill-conceived advice from physicians in other branches of medicine about adopting certain procedures into our practices. The advice is ill conceived if it falls into the error of extrapolating from one clinical context to the other without supporting data from family practice. When given this kind of advice, we usually feel intuitively that it is wrong. It is not easy, however, to put our feeling into words, particularly when the person offering the advice has all the authority of being an expert in the field. How much better, both for ourselves and for the expert, if we can say exactly why the advice is erroneous.

New tests, procedures, and therapies are constantly being introduced. We rely on specialists to recommend them to us, but we need also to be critical of them. We need to know what kind of questions to ask our colleagues. How will the test change the relative likelihood of the diagnosis in this patient? What is its predictive value? What is its risk?

The reader will notice that we tend to use terms such as problem solving and decision making rather than diagnosis. Diagnosis is a time-honored word, but it is—somewhat ambiguous. To some physicians, it has meant diagnosis of a disease; to others, diagnosis of a patient. In its modern sense, diagnosis is the assignment of the patient's illness to a category that links the symptoms with a pathological process and, in some cases, with a specific cause. It is in this sense that we will use the term here. Problem solving and decision making both have wider scope than diagnosis. The solution to a patient's problem may have very little to do with the diagnosis, as in the following example.

Case 8.2

Sarah is an 88-year-old woman who has been a widow for the past 20 years. She came to her family physician with complaints of frequent urination. A quick urinalysis noted that there was glucosuria and subsequent culture found no evidence of infection. A fasting blood sugar was undertaken and found to be 10 mmol/L. The results were explained to her and a treatment plan outlined to which she readily agreed. There were no other illnesses identified. Her family physician started her on metformin and made arrangements for her to attend a diabetic education clinic. A month later her blood sugars were normal, but on the follow-up visit, she discussed the need to dispose of her personal belongings and her desire not to have extreme measures taken in the event of a heart attack or stroke. Her physician noted the dramatic change in her normally optimistic demeanor and inquired about it. She related to him that she considered the diagnosis of diabetes to be fatal and that she recognized the need to "get things in order." Her physician emphasized that diabetes was a controllable chronic disorder that would require some changes in her life, but need not be considered fatal. Further discussion revealed that she had attended her older sister in the last year of her life as she died due to complications of diabetes. She and her physician discussed the differences between her sister's experience and the expectations of the course of events for her. In this case, the physician's perspective was that the disease was a manageable phenomenon. From the patient's perspective, it had grave symbolic significance. This was only understandable after learning of her previous experience with it.

Decisions have to be made at all stages of the clinical process. The process of making a diagnosis is itself a series of decisions. As well, decisions have to be taken before diagnosis and often without a diagnosis. For family physicians, one of the most common and most difficult decisions is the one demanded by a night call: should I see the patient now or give advice on the phone and see the patient in the morning? In family practice, as we will see, it may be necessary to go straight from assessment to decision making without diagnosis.

The Family Practice Context

The pattern of illness in family practice is similar to the pattern of illness in the community—not identical, but similar. This means that there is a high incidence of acute, short-term illness, much of it transient and self-limiting; a high prevalence of chronic illness; and a high prevalence of illness unrelated to identifiable organic pathology. Contrary to the conventional view, patients do not usually present with either physical or psychological problems; they come with problems that are often a complex mixture of physical, psychological, and social elements.

Diseases that are common in a referral practice or tertiary-care hospital may be rare in a general practice, and vice versa. It is often astonishing for new students in family practice to realize that they could go years without seeing a patient with leukemia or systemic lupus erythematosus. Put in technical terms, the population at risk for a family practitioner differs greatly from the population at risk for a referral specialist. The probability that the family physician will encounter certain diseases differs greatly from the probability that the specialist will encounter them. In technical terms, again, the prior probabilities of diseases are very different in family practice. This does not mean that family physicians never think of uncommon diseases. Under certain conditions—given certain presenting symptoms—a rare disease may be the first hypothesis. It does mean, however, that other things being equal, they will usually consider the most likely disease first. This may sound obvious, but it is important. Failure to think in this way can result in unnecessary and inappropriate investigation.

Because of their role as primary physicians, family practitioners tend to encounter illness in its earliest stages. Early diagnosis is a special responsibility, especially in those diseases where early treatment makes a difference to prognosis. The family physician, therefore, has to be especially alert to the clinical data that distinguish serious and life-threatening illness in its early stages from less serious illness. This presents a problem. The symptoms, signs, and tests that identify diseases in their early stages are often different from those that identify them in their later stages. The sensitivity and specificity of signs and tests varies with the stage of the disease. As we will see later, this creates pitfalls for those beginning in family practice after experience limited to in-hospital medicine. Textbooks of medicine are of little help, for they do not usually tell one how to diagnose disease in its earliest stages.

The differences in prevalence of disease between family practice and specialized practice have another consequence. The predictive value of a test varies with the prevalence of the disease in question. Why this is so will be explained later (p. 175). It means that the same test may be useful for diagnosis in tertiary care, but useless—and perhaps harmful—in family practice, and vice versa.

Another feature of the family practice context is that the illness encountered is usually undifferentiated and unorganized. By an undifferentiated illness, we mean one that has not previously been assessed, categorized, and named by a physician. In the process of diagnosis, the physician interprets the raw data presented by the patient, adds the data acquired by his or her own search, and tries to fit the illness into a disease category within his or her own frame of reference. In this way, many patients presenting to family physicians have their raw illnesses differentiated into well-known disease categories.

On the other hand, many patients have illnesses that defy this kind of differentiation. There are at least five reasons why this should be so. First, an illness may be transient and self-limiting, creating a functional disturbance that clears completely, leaving no evidence on which a diagnosis can be based. These illnesses are usually brief, but not invariably so. Sometimes a patient may suffer for months from an illness that eventually clears without ever having been diagnosed. Second, an illness may be treated so early that it is aborted before it reaches the stage of a definitive diagnosis. Many cases of pneumonia are probably aborted in this way by giving antibiotics to patients with fever, cough, and minimal chest signs.

Third, there are, at the edge of every disease category, borderline and intermediate conditions that are difficult or impossible to classify. Because family physicians see all variants of disease, they are especially liable to encounter milder variants and borderline conditions that may never reach the specialist.

Fourth, an illness may remain undifferentiated for many years before its true nature unfolds in time. It may be years before a transient blurring of vision is followed by other evidence of multiple sclerosis.

Fifth, an illness may be so closely interwoven with the personality and personal life of the patient that it defies classification. Patients with chronic pain are often examples of this type of illness.

Estimates of how much illness in family practice remains undifferentiated—even after assessment—vary from 25% to 50%. The exact figure will obviously vary with the duration of observation and the criteria adopted for differentiation.

The fact of persistently undifferentiated illness has many implications for the clinical method in family practice. The key to its understanding may be the diagnosis of the patient as a person or the patient–doctor relationship, rather than of the disease. Hence the importance of the patient-centered clinical method. The importance of time in revealing a diagnosis makes clinical observation an important tool in the family physician's armamentarium, and one that he or she has excellent opportunities to use. The elusiveness of diagnosis, moreover, faces the family physician frequently with the question "When do I stop the investigation?"

The concept of the organization of illness is an important one for family medicine. As we have seen in Chapter 7, when patients first present their problems to a physician, they often do so in a fragmented and oblique manner. Several problems are often presented at one visit; the most important one for the patient may not be presented first; for many reasons, problems may be expressed in indirect rather than in direct literal language. Although the patient may have his or her own explanation for the illness, it is probably not organized in terms of a medical frame of reference. Once the patient has been through the physician's assessment process, all this changes. Unless the patient's own frame of reference is very resistant to change, he or she will tend to see his illness in a different light. Instead of having troublesome pain, the patient will now have a gallbladder problem or a duodenal ulcer. By the very direction of the inquiry, the doctor will have taught the patient which symptoms are medically significant and which are not. This is an illustration of the fact that one cannot observe nature without changing it. It is an awesome responsibility for the family physician. As the first doctor to see the patient, he or she has great power to change the way the patient perceives and organizes the illness.

Giving the illness a name has great symbolic significance. It may be a great relief for a patient to know that the illness is a familiar thing, not some vague menace. It may have an important legitimizing function. Patients with chronic fatigue syndrome describe receiving a diagnosis as a turning point in their illness. At last, their suffering is taken seriously by family and friends (see Chapter 13). On the other hand, the name given to the illness may be so terrifying that the word should not be spoken unless support is at hand.

Organizing and naming the illness (diagnosing the disease), when based on good clinical evidence, confers great benefits. It has great explanatory and predictive power, adding meaning to the patient's experience. On the other hand, diagnosis based on spurious clinical evidence has potential for harm in fostering somatic fixation.

We must also consider the importance of time in the family practice context. The patient–doctor relationship is usually a long-term one. This makes for pitfalls that are less of a problem in other fields of medicine (see Chapter 7). It also has many advantages. Observation of the patient over time can be a powerful test of clinical hypotheses, provided, of course, that there is no risk attached to waiting or that the risk of waiting is less than the risk of active investigation. Because the relationship is continuing, the family physician need not be in a hurry to solve all the patient's problems, unless, again, there is a risk attached to delay. The difference in the time scale between tertiary-care medicine and family medicine is one of the most difficult things for beginners in family medicine to grasp. The use of time to validate hypotheses can save many unnecessary investigations in self-limiting illnesses.

Classification

One of the objectives of the clinician is to place the patient's illness into its correct disease category. In modern times, in fact, this has been viewed as the chief objective. Classification has five very important results:

1. By using their knowledge of the natural history of the disease category, clinicians can predict the outcome of the illness, if untreated.
2. They can make inferences about the cause or causes of the illness.
3. Armed with this knowledge, they can prescribe the specific therapy for the disease.
4. They can make inferences that go beyond the evidence of their senses—for example, about the state of the internal organs.
5. By using the common nomenclature of medicine, they can communicate their findings to other clinicians and provide the patient with a name for his or her disease.

If, for example, a patient with fatigue, pallor, and loss of weight is classified as having pernicious anemia, the clinician can predict that he or she will die if untreated and will respond rapidly to injections of vitamin B_{12} and can infer that he or she is deficient in intrinsic factor.

Classification is a very powerful tool. The successful application of technology to medicine depends on it, for unless we can predict the outcome of untreated illness, we cannot know whether our interventions are effective. Unless we can classify illness correctly, we cannot be specific in our application of therapeutic technologies.

Disease categories vary greatly in their predictive power. In giving pernicious anemia as an example, I chose a particularly powerful one. Others have very little power. "Low back syndrome," for example, tells us very little about the prognosis of the condition or its pathological basis. Such categories are sometimes no more than a restatement of the patient's symptoms. As we have seen, our system for classifying diseases is based on the linkage of symptoms and signs with pathological data. Our categories are mental constructs that we create for their explanatory and predictive power. As our investigative and therapeutic technologies become more precise and effective, some of our old categories change and some new ones are called into being. It is only since the advent of coronary angiography and bypass surgery that we have had a precise anatomical classification of ischemic heart disease. The category "polymyalgia rheumatica" was unknown until the 1950s, when steroids had recently become available. One sometimes reads editorials in medical journals that ask whether or not such-and-such a category is an "entity." This question betrays confusion about what a disease category is; the questioner is guilty of the fallacy of treating a mental construct as if it had a concrete existence. The question should be "Does such-and-such a category have good predictive and explanatory power?"

Besides using the common disease categories, family physicians use other types of category to help them in dealing with early and undifferentiated illness. In a patient with acute abdominal pain, for example, the doctor's first task may be to place the patient into one of two categories: "probably acute abdomen" or "not acute abdomen." If the latter, then the physician can discontinue the search and observe the patient, expecting the illness to be minor and self-limiting. In these cases, the physician can achieve the objective by defining what the patient does *not* have—the so-called eliminative diagnosis (Crombie, 1963).

Other clinical dichotomies are exemplified in Figure 8.3. Although patients may be usefully categorized in this way, one must always bear in mind that the patient's problems may fall in both categories; for example, upper and lower respiratory tract infection. It need hardly be said that such categorization is only a starting point, leading to further steps toward a more precise clinical diagnosis or a better understanding of the patient. One thing to remember about these binary categories is that the tests that are useful for distinguishing between them are different from the tests that are useful for making more precise diagnoses. This is often forgotten in the teaching of clinical method. The erythrocyte sedimentation rate, for example, is a very useful test in family practice for assessing patients with aches and pains and older patients with headache (see p. 277). It is of little or no value in distinguishing between different categories of inflammatory disease of connective tissue.

Another use of categorization by family physicians is the movement from assessment to decisions, without an intervening stage of diagnosis in the

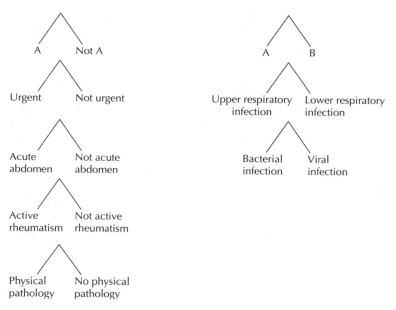

Figure 8.3   Examples of broad categories used in family practice.

conventional sense. Howie (1973) has described how family physicians base their management decisions in acute respiratory illness on the presence or absence of certain clinical features rather than on the diagnostic label applied. His study encompassed 62 practices and 1,000 patients with respiratory illness. Cough and chest signs were present in 163; of these, 152 (93%) received an antibiotic. The presence of cough and chest signs had, therefore, a predictive value for antibiotic treatment of 93%. Twelve different diagnostic labels were applied to the 163 patients. Five of the labels had a predictive value of only 45%. It appears that the physicians were placing the patients into one of two treatment categories (antibiotic/no antibiotic) based on clinical data. The actual name given to the condition was comparatively unimportant and probably given as an afterthought.

In dealing with this type of illness, the strategy used by the physicians makes a lot of sense. The distinction between different types of respiratory illness in their early stages (tracheitis, laryngitis, bronchitis, coryza) is arbitrary and of little value. Waiting for definitive pneumonia or bronchitis to develop may lead to a more precise diagnosis but is not good medical practice.

While maintaining a proper respect for the power of diagnostic categories, we should also not become their prisoners. Some categories in common use have very little predictive value. An example given in Chapter 12 is the distinction between common migraine and tension headache. Rather than spending time trying to make this distinction, we might be better employed in listening to the patient. We must also keep in mind the limitations of classification. Categorization is a

generalizing process that works by ignoring individual differences. Precise categorization is not a substitute for understanding the individual features of the
patient and his or her illness.

The Problem-Solving Process

Figure 8.4 shows a model of the process of clinical problem solving based on the
work of Elstein, Shulman, and Sprafha (1978), with modifications. When presented with a problem, the clinician responds to cues by forming one or more
hypotheses about what is wrong with the patient (Figure 8.5). The clinician then
embarks on a search (the history, examination, and investigation) to test the
hypotheses. In the course of the search, he or she looks for positive (confirming) and negative (refuting) evidence. If the evidence refutes the hypothesis, it is
revised and the search begins again. The process is a cyclical one, the clinician
constantly revising, testing, and further revising the hypothesis, until it is refined
to the point at which treatment decisions seem justified. Even after this point,
the clinician must still be prepared to revise the hypothesis if the progress of the
patient is not as predicted.

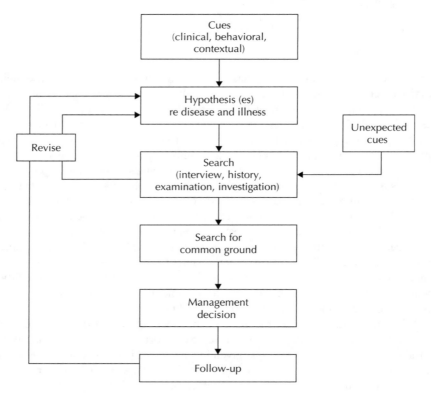

Figure 8.4   A model of the diagnostic process.

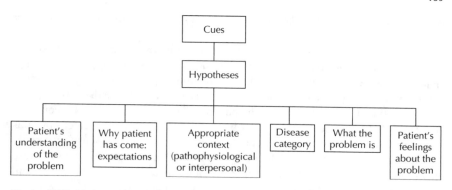

Figure 8.5 Variety of hypotheses formed by the family physician.

Cues

When a patient presents his or her problem, the physician is faced with a plethora of data: from what the patient says, from the physician's own observations, from his or her previous knowledge of the patient, from the relatives, from other physicians who have seen the patient, or from other members of the health-care team. There is so much information that the physician cannot deal with all of it. Moreover, the different items of information are not of equal value. The physician therefore responds to certain items of information that have a special meaning for him or her. We call these cues. The information in the cue may be useful for a number of reasons. It may help the physician to identify and solve the patient's problem; it may help him or her to understand the context of the problem; or it may help him or her to understand the patient.

A cue may be a symptom, sign, statement, or an aspect of the patient's behavior. It may be something that is known about the patient, such as age, previous history, or ethnic origin. It may be a contextual cue, such as when a teenaged girl is accompanied by her mother or a patient tolerates a symptom for 20 years before presenting it. It may be a subjective cue, arising from the doctor's personal feelings, such as "This patient makes me feel depressed."

As well as identifying cues, the physician also assesses their significance; he or she attempts to grasp the meaning of the symptom presentation. The physician responds not only to individual cues, but to patterns. The patient's symptoms form patterns or clusters that the physician can relate to similar patterns presented by patients in his or her past experience. For the experienced clinician, pattern recognition is an important factor in the formation of hypotheses.

Cues may be certain or probabilistic. A certain cue enables the physician to say with certainty what is wrong with the patient. This is what we usually mean by a spot diagnosis. The rash of herpes zoster is an example. Certain cues are rare in family practice, as they are in most fields of medicine. Most cues are probabilistic; that is, they may indicate a number of different conditions with varying probabilities. The physician can therefore only formulate hypotheses about what is wrong with the patient. The hypotheses then have to be tested by a search for further information.

Of all the cues presented to family physicians, symptoms are the most frequent. In the early stages of illness, and in the varieties of illness seen by the family physician, signs are less frequently available. The family physician is especially concerned with two aspects of a symptom: first, its capacity to bring the patient to see the doctor (i.e., its significance for the patient). This has been called by Feinstein (1967) the "iatrotrophic stimulus." For example, hemoptysis has greater power as an iatrotrophic stimulus than does cough. Also important are the sensitivity, specificity, and predictive value of the symptom in the early stages of illness. These terms will be defined later in this chapter when we discuss the search. All of them are measures of how effective a symptom or test is in identifying a disease and in discriminating between it and other diseases or a state of health.

Hypotheses

Investigators of the clinical process have found that clinicians form their first hypothesis very soon after the patient has presented the first problem (Elstein, Shulman, and Sprafha, 1978). Hypothesis formation is a mark of the clinician's creativity. We do not know how clinical hypotheses are generated, any more than we know how they are generated in scientific discovery. They are certainly not the result of linear logic; they seem to spring into consciousness as we respond to the cues. Experience is certainly a factor; the incoming information is matched with other information stored in our mind's filing system. Generally speaking, the greater the clinician's experience in his or her field, the more powerful will the hypotheses be. It does depend, however, on what use the physician has made of his or her experience. There is a well-known comparison between a physician with 20 years of experience and one who has 1 year of experience twenty times.

The clinician usually has between two and five hypotheses at any one time; to handle more than six is difficult for the human mind. As old hypotheses are discarded and new ones called up, the clinician can consider many more in the course of the investigation.

The hypotheses are placed in ranking order, based on two main criteria: probability and payoff. Payoff is an indication of the consequences of diagnosing or not diagnosing a disease. The more serious a disease and the more amenable to treatment, the greater the positive payoff of making the diagnosis and the greater the negative payoff of missing it. If a disease has a high payoff, it may be ranked high on the clinician's list, even though it has a low probability. In a child with abdominal pain, for example, acute appendicitis may be ranked high—even though of low probability—because of the high positive value of an early diagnosis.

If considerations of payoff do not arise, the hypotheses are ranked in order of probability. Note that this is not the prior probability (the prevalence of the disease in the practice population) but the conditional probability (the probability of the disease, given the patient's symptoms). A synonym for conditional probability is predictive value: the predictive value of symptom x for disease A. As we have seen on page 150, predictive value varies with prevalence. Because of differences in disease prevalence, there may be a big difference between the predictive values of the same symptom in family and specialty practice. For example, in a patient with fatigue but with no other presenting data, the first-ranking hypothesis would usually be depression. For a hematologist, the first-ranking hypothesis might be a blood disorder. Each would be correct in its own context, given the differences in predictive value of the symptom fatigue. Similarly, our first-ranking hypothesis in a patient with headache might be different from that of a neurologist.

How much does the ranking order matter? It matters because the order of hypotheses determines the search strategy. If depression is the first-ranking hypothesis, we would begin by seeking evidence of depression. If our hypothesis is supported, one would test it further by ruling out other causes of fatigue— usually by a few simple and economical tests and by continuing observation over time. If the first hypothesis is a blood disorder, one would begin by seeking evidence for this and consider depression as part of the routine inquiry. Again, each search strategy would be appropriate in its context. However, a search strategy based on erroneous ranking (assuming payoff factors are not operative) can lead to waste of resources and—here tests carry a risk—harm to the patient.

Before we leave hypotheses, two fallacies must be mentioned. The first is that the family physician always thinks of common diseases first. This is not necessarily so; it depends entirely on the cues. If the cues are highly probabilistic, such as fatigue, this will hold true. If, on the other hand, the cue indicates a rare disease with relative certainty, this will be the physician's first hypothesis. If a hypertensive patient complains of attacks of sweating and flushing, for example, the first hypothesis may be pheochromocytoma, even though the physician may see only one case in his or her whole lifetime.

The second fallacy is that diagnosis in family practice is different from diagnosis in other fields of medicine because it is probabilistic. All clinical diagnosis is probabilistic. Where family practice differs is in the relatively low levels of probability at which many decisions have to be made. This is because of the early stage at which disease is seen, not—as sometimes suggested—because of lack of time to pursue a more specific diagnosis.

The Search

The purpose of the search is twofold: to test and validate the physician's hypotheses, and to bring to light new and unexpected cues. These purposes are fulfilled respectively by the directed and the routine search.

The Directed Search

Because the purpose of the directed search is to test the physician's initial hypothesis, it follows that the search strategy will vary with the hypothesis. In selecting a search strategy, the family physician has to make two kinds of choices: which tests to use and what the extent of the search should be.

The word *tests* embraces history questions, items of physical examination, and laboratory and imaging investigations. Tests are selected according to two kinds of criteria. First, the capacity of the test to change the prior or pretest probability that the patient has or has not the disease in question; second, the risks and benefits of doing the test. The measures used to determine the usefulness of a test are its sensitivity, specificity, and predictive value.

One way of understanding these indices is by means of a 2 × 2 table, illustrated in Table 8.2.

Patients with the disease (infectious mononucleosis) are in the two left-hand boxes, those without the disease in the two right-hand boxes. Patients testing positive (with the monospot test) are in thev upper two boxes, those testing negative in the lower two boxes. The boxes are identified from the upper left as *a*, *b*, *c*, and *d*. Box *a* contains those patients who have the disease and who test positive (true positives). Box *b* contains those without the disease who test positive (false positives). Box *d* contains those without the disease who test negative (true negatives). Box *c* contains those with the disease who test negative (false negatives).

With the help of the table, we can now look at the meaning of the three indices.

Sensitivity

Sensitivity is the proportion of patients with the disease who have a positive test result, which has been called "positivity in disease" (Galen and Gambino, 1975). In the table, boxes *a* + *c* give us those patients with the disease and box *a* gives

Table 8.2 Sensitivity, specificity, and predictive value of the monospot test for infectious mononucleosis (IM) in patients with sore throat (prevalence of IM in patients with sore throat = 20/1000)

		Infectious Mononucleosis	
		Present	Absent
Monospot Test	Positive	17 *a*	69 *b*
	Negative	*c*	*d*
		3	911
		20	980

$$\text{Sensitivity} = \frac{a}{a+c} \times 100 = \frac{17}{20} \times 100 = 85\%$$

$$\text{Specificity} = \frac{d}{b+d} \times 100 = \frac{911}{69+911} \times 100 = 93\%$$

$$\text{Predictive Value Positive} = \frac{a}{a+b} \times 100 = \frac{17}{17+69} \times 100 = 19\%$$

us those with the disease who test positive. Sensitivity expressed as a percentage is therefore

$$\frac{a}{a+c}\times100$$

Another way of putting this would be

$$\text{Sensitivity} = \frac{\text{True positives (TP)}}{\text{True positives (TP)} + \text{False negatives (FN)}}\times100$$

In Table 8.2, the boxes have been completed for the monospot test in infectious mononucleosis. The sensitivity of the test is

$$\frac{17}{17+3}\times100 = 85\%$$

Some things about sensitivity are especially important for family physicians. A highly sensitive test is very good for ruling out hypotheses. If we have a test that is 100% sensitive and the patient tests negative, we can say with confidence that the patient does not have the disease. Because the test is 100% sensitive, we know that there are no false negatives. A positive test, however, is not so helpful, because we do not know whether it is a true or false positive. If a test is 100% sensitive it will certainly not be 100% specific, and there will be some false positives. Let us consider some examples.

In a study of headache in family practice, we found that tenderness on pressure over the sinuses was 100% sensitive for sinusitis. Absence of tenderness ruled out sinusitis. Presence of tenderness, however, was of little value because so many patients without sinusitis tested positive. In headache patients over the age of 50, an erythrocyte sedimentation rate of greater than 50 mm in 1 hour was 100% sensitive for cranial arteritis. This is very tentative because the disease is rare and there was only one case among the 272 patients in the study. There was also only one false positive, a patient who turned out to have pernicious anemia. Our study supported a clinical impression that the test is very useful for ruling out cranial arteritis.

As we have seen, sensitivity varies with the stage of the disease. Failure to understand this can lead to difficulties for the newcomer to family medicine.

Case 8.3

A second-year resident saw a 12-year-old boy in the office during his morning session. The boy had complained of continuous central abdominal pain for several hours. On examination, there was no abdominal tenderness and the temperature was normal. Because there was some frequency of micturition, the resident diagnosed a urinary infection. That same evening, the mother called the doctor on duty because the pain was worse and the boy was vomiting. Examination of the abdomen showed tenderness and muscular rigidity in all areas. A perforated appendix was diagnosed and the boy made a full recovery after emergency surgery.

The pitfall here was that abdominal tenderness and pyrexia, although sensitive signs in the later stages of appendicitis, are not 100% sensitive in the early stages.

The family physician cannot, therefore, rely on these for ruling out appendicitis. In this case, the history of continuous abdominal pain should have been sufficient to require reexamination of the patient within 4 hours. An additional error was to make urinary infection a top-ranking hypothesis, because it is uncommon in males of this age and not usually associated with continuous abdominal pain.

There are many examples of this variation of sensitivity with evolution of a disease: the chest X-ray in pneumonia, lung cancer, and pulmonary embolus; the ECG in myocardial infarction; and splenic enlargement in infectious mononucleosis, to mention some of them. Few are well documented; textbooks are not written about the early stages of illness.

Specificity
Specificity is the proportion of patients without the disease who have a negative test result. This is sometimes referred to as "negativity in health" (Galen and Gambino, 1975), but note that absence of the disease in question is not synonymous with health. The patient may have some other disease. In Table 8.2, boxes *b* and *d* give us those patients without the disease, and box *d* gives us those without the disease who test negative. Specificity, therefore, expressed as a percentage is therefore:

$$\frac{b}{b+d} \times 100$$

Another way of putting this would be

$$\frac{\text{True negatives (TN)}}{\text{True negatives (TN)} + \text{False positives (FP)}}$$

In Table 8.2, the specificity of the monospot test is:

$$\frac{911}{69+911} \times 100 = 93\%$$

A highly specific test is very good for ruling in hypotheses. If a test is 100% specific and the patient tests positive, we can say with certainty that the patient has the disease. Because the test is 100% specific, we know that there are no false positives. The test is diagnostic. A negative test, however, is less helpful, because we do not know whether it is a true or false negative. If a test is 100% specific, it will almost certainly not be 100% sensitive.

Predictive Value
As we have seen, sensitivity tells us nothing about the false positives and specificity tells us nothing about the false negatives. Yet it is important for us to know about them. The trouble with false positives and false negatives is that both carry penalties for the patient. A false positive can be hazardous in two ways: by imposing a disease label on a healthy person and by exposing him or her to risky investigations and therapies. A false negative carries a penalty because it misses the

diagnosis in a sick patient. Thus, we need a measure that tells us about the false positives and negatives. The predictive value does this.

The positive predictive value is the proportion of positive test results that are true positives:

$$PV^+ = \frac{TP}{TP + FP} \times 100$$

The negative predictive value is the proportion of negative test results that are true negatives:

$$PV^- = \frac{TN}{TN + FN} \times 100$$

The denominator in each case is the number of positive or negative test results, rather than the number of patients with or without the disease. In Table 8.2, the positive predictive value is:

$$\frac{a}{a + b}$$

the negative predictive value is

$$\frac{d}{c + d}$$

Synonyms for positive predictive value are the conditional probability of a positive test result, and the post-test probability of disease following a positive result. Synonyms for negative predictive value are the conditional probability of a negative test result, and the post-test probability of no disease following a negative result.

In Table 8.2, the predictive value positive of the monospot test is

$$\frac{17}{17 + 69} \times 100 = 19.7\%$$

The negative predictive value of the monospot test is

$$\frac{911}{3 + 911} \times 100 = 99\%$$

The predictive value is a key index, for it tells us the power of a test to change the probability that the patient has the disease in question. There is, however, something very important to bear in mind. We have already mentioned it: *the predictive value varies with the prevalence of the disease*. Let us see how this works in the case of the monospot test. In Table 8.2, the prevalence of mononucleosis in patients with sore throat is 2%. In Table 8.3, the prevalence is 10%. This could be the difference between a family practice and a student health service practice. The effect of this is to increase the predictive value positive to 58%, while the sensitivity and specificity remain virtually the same. The reason is that as the

Table 8.3 Sensitivity, specificity, and predictive value on the monospot test for infectious mononucleosis (IM) in patients with sore throat (prevalence of IM in patients with sore throat = 100/1000)

		Infectious Mononucleosis	
		Present	Absent
Monospot Test	Positive	86 *a*	63 *b*
	Negative	*c* 14	*d* 837

$$\text{Sensitivity} = \frac{a}{a+c} \times 100 = \frac{86}{86+14} \times 100 = 86\%$$

$$\text{Specificity} = \frac{d}{b+d} \times 100 = \frac{837}{63+837} \times 100 = 93\%$$

$$\text{Predictive Value Positive} = \frac{a}{a+b} \times 100 = \frac{86}{86+63} \times 100 = 58\%$$

prevalence increases, the proportion of people with the disease increases and the number of false positives decreases.

As we have seen, the variation of predictive value with prevalence can mean that a routine test that may be indicated in a specialty clinic may be contraindicated in family practice. An example of this is given in Chapter 14, where we see that the prevalence of correctable secondary hypertension in family practice is so low that the benefits of screening for renovascular causes with ultrasound, MRI angiography or spiral CT, to the small number of patients with true positives is outweighed by the risks and costs of the test and subsequent investigations to those with false positive results.

Having said that predictive value varies with prevalence, we must go on to say that there is one exception. If the sensitivity of a test is 100%, the predictive value of a negative test does not vary with prevalence. There are no false negatives, and the predictive value negative is also 100%. Conversely, if the specificity of a test is 100%, the predictive value of a positive test does not vary with prevalence. There are no false positives, and the predictive value of a positive test is also 100%. Unfortunately, there are not many tests that reach 100% for either sensitivity or specificity. Those that we have we treasure for their capacity to rule out or to rule in a diagnosis.

For the more common tests with sensitivity and specificity of between 80% and 95%, the variation with prevalence is important. Table 8.4 shows how predictive value changes with prevalence for a test that has 95% sensitivity and specificity. As prevalence falls, positive predictive value falls, and negative predictive value rises. Note that a test has greater power to change the pretest or prior probability in the middle ranges of prevalence (40%–60%).

Table 8.4 The effect of prevalence on the predictive value of an excellent sign, symptom, or laboratory test

Prevalence (Pretest likelihood or prior probability of disease)	99%	95%	90%	80%	70%	60%	50%	40%	30%	20%	10%	5%	1%	0.5%	0.1%
Predictive value of a positive test (Posterior probability of disease following a positive test result)	99.9%	99.7%	99.4%	99%	98%	97%	95%	93%	89%	83%	68%	50%	16%	9%	2%
Predictive value of a negative test (Posterior probability of *no* disease following a negative test result)	16%	50%	68%	83%	89%	93%	95%	97%	98%	99%	99.4%	99.7%	99.9%	99.97%	99.99%
(Posterior probability of disease following a negative test result)	84%	50%	32%	17%	11%	7%	5%	3%	2%	1%	0.6%	0.3%	0.1%	0.03%	0.01%

Both sensitivity and specificity equal 95% in every case.

From Sackett et al., Little Brown and Co., Copyright 1985. Reprinted by permission.

When we get to prevalence rates of 95% and 5%, the test does not help us much. Whether or not this makes the test justifiable depends on the payoff of the diagnosis and the risk of the test. A disease may be so devastating if undiagnosed, and so amenable to treatment, that we do the test even though the disease has a very low prevalence. The test for phenylketonuria is an example of this.

A reminder is in order here. Remember that our definition of test includes elements of the history, examination, and investigation. The experienced clinician selects questions and items of physical examination for their capacity to change the prior probability. Even before the clinician starts, the patient's presenting symptoms have changed the prior probability in some way.

Despite the panoply of investigations available to us, the history and physical examination—in family practice, especially the history—are still the most effective ways of increasing the probability. Let us see how this works in the case of a patient with chest pain.

Suppose we have a middle-aged man who presents with a typical history of angina of effort: tight substernal pain coming on after a fixed amount of exertion and relieved within 5 minutes by rest. The probability of coronary disease, given these symptoms (conditional probability), is about 90% (Diamond et al., 1979). By taking the history alone, we have raised the probability from the prevalence of coronary disease in males of his age group in our practice (about 5%) to 90%. Now, will an exercise ECG help us? The predictive value positive at this prevalence rate is 98%, a small increase on the previous figure; the predictive value negative is 20%; that is, even if the test is negative there is still an 80% probability of coronary disease. The sensitivity of the test is 60%, the specificity 91%.[4] Let us apply the acid test for an investigation: Will it change our approach to the patient whatever the result? In this case the answer is no. If the test is positive, we will still be certain of our diagnosis; but we were already certain. If the test is negative, it will not make any difference, because we will still go by our clinical assessment; with a 60% sensitivity, the rule-out value of the test is low.

Now suppose we have a 40-year-old man with vague left-sided chest pain, unrelated to exercise, but worse on some movements of the chest wall. The history is suggestive of intercostal muscle pain and has no features to indicate coronary disease, although the patient is worried about his heart. The probability of coronary disease in this patient is about the same as any other male of his age in the practice population—about 5%. The predictive value positive of an exercise ECG at this prevalence rate is only 26 percent. The predictive value negative 98 percent, so only 2% of the negatives will be false negatives. Will an exercise ECG help us? A negative result will reinforce our opinion that the patient does not have coronary disease. A positive test will not help us, because 74% of positives will be false positives. In fact, it will probably do harm because it will make it more difficult to reassure the patient that he does not have coronary disease—a big price to pay for a marginal benefit. The physician will do better to have confidence in his or her own clinical judgment.

Now suppose we have a middle-aged man with attacks of substernal pain for several months, occurring at rest and lasting from a few minutes to half an hour,

sometimes related to exertion but not relieved by rest, with no tendency to worsening since the onset. The pretest probability of coronary disease in a patient with
this history is about 50%. At this prevalence rate, the predictive value positive of
the test is 87%—a big increase in probability of coronary disease. The predictive
value negative is 69%, so 31% of negatives will be false negatives, a reduction of
19% in the pretest probability. If positive, the test does help to clarify the management options. The physician will feel justified in treating as ischemic heart disease with appropriate drugs and reduction of risk factors, and referral for further
investigation if there is a poor response or if the pain progresses. If negative, the
test is less helpful.

In all these patients, the history alone has been enormously effective in assessing the probability of coronary disease. It has provided the family physician with
virtually all that is needed for making good management decisions, and the exercise ECG has very little to add.

Before leaving the question of how to select tests, mention must be made of
two other tools for helping us to make choices: likelihood ratios and decision
analysis. As a tool for helping us with decisions about individual patients, decision analysis has little application in family practice. It comes in useful mainly in
developing optimal strategies for complex clinical conditions.[5] Sackett, Haynes,
and Tugwell (1985) define decision analysis as "a method of describing complex
clinical problems in an explicit fashion, identifying the available courses of action
(both diagnosis and management), assessing the probability and value (or utility)
of all possible outcomes, and then making a simple calculation to select the optimal course of action." For a description of how it works, see Sackett, Haynes, and
Tugwell (1985).

Likelihood Ratios
Likelihood ratios are another way of expressing how good a test is for increasing the probability of a diagnosis. The calculation of the ratios uses indices with
which we are already familiar: sensitivity and specificity. The likelihood ratio
for a positive result is the odds that a test will be positive in a patient with the
disease, in contrast to a patient without the disease. The likelihood ratio for a
negative result is the odds that a test will be negative in a patient with the disease,
contrasted with a patient without the disease.

The first figure in the likelihood ratio positive (positivity in disease) is the sensitivity of the test. The second figure (positivity in nondisease) is 100 minus the
specificity (expressed as a percentage). For example, the likelihood ratio of a positive monospot in infectious mononucleosis (from Table 8.2) is

$$\frac{a}{a+c} \times 100 / 100 - \left(\frac{d}{b+d} \times 100\right)$$

That is,

$$85/7 = 12:1$$

The odds of a patient with a positive test result having the disease are 12 to 1. By multiplying the ratio with the pretest odds, we can arrive at the post-test odds for the diagnosis. The pretest odds are calculated as pretest probability/1−pretest probability. Pretest probability is calculated as a+c/a+b+c+d. For our example in Table 8.2, pretest probability = 20/1000 or 0.02. Hence, the pretest odds are 0.02/1 − 0.02 or 0.02. The pretest odds on a patient having infectious mononucleosis were 1:50 or 0.02:1. The post-test odds with a positive test are therefore 0.02:12, or 0.24:1. If we prefer to think in probabilities, odds can be converted to probabilities, and vice versa. To convert odds to probability, we divide it by itself plus one. The post-test odds on infectious mononucleosis becomes a post-test probability of

$$\frac{0.24}{0.24+1} = 0.19 \text{ or } 19\%$$

To convert probabilities to odds, we divide the probability by its complement (one minus itself). The post-test probability of 19% becomes a post-test odds of

$$\frac{0.19}{1-0.19} = \frac{0.19}{0.81} = 0.23$$

In this example, we have treated the test as if the result will be either positive or negative, rather than a continuous variable. It is also possible to express likelihood ratios for different levels of a test result that varies over a range. For the serum uric acid, for example, we can express the likelihood ratio for gout at 7.0, 8.0, and 9.0 mg/100 mL.

Because likelihood ratios are calculated from sensitivity and specificity data, they do not vary with the prevalence of the disease. Like sensitivity and specificity, however, they do vary with the stage of the disease.

As time goes on, information about the likelihood ratios and predictive values of tests will probably become increasingly available. As family physicians, we should not only get to know these indices for the symptoms, signs, and tests we use ourselves, but also become accustomed to asking our consultants for the likelihood ratios or predictive values of tests they recommend to us. As our patients become more informed, we may also find that they begin to ask these questions themselves.

In testing a hypothesis, the clinician seeks both positive and negative evidence. He or she seeks not only to support it but also to refute it, to rule it in, and to rule it out. Suppose that the first two hypotheses in a patient with weight loss are thyrotoxicosis and diabetes. Suppose that the search has yielded evidence in support of thyrotoxicosis. The clinician will then proceed with tests such as urine and blood glucose, which should be negative if the first hypothesis is correct (unless both conditions are present). Studies of problem solving have shown that clinicians, like problem solvers in other fields, show a marked preference for positive over negative evidence. They would much rather try to support their hypothesis than to refute it. As Elstein, Shulman, and Sprafha (1978) have observed, this is an experimental confirmation of an observation made centuries ago by Francis Bacon: "It is the peculiar and perpetual error of the human intellect to be more moved and excited by affirmatives than by negatives." The testing of hypotheses raises the difficult question of when the directed search should be ended. When have we collected enough evidence? What is the appropriate level of probability?

The Last Part of the Search

This brings us face to face with the problem of uncertainty and with the potential conflict between precision on the one hand and the patient's well-being on the other. Uncertainty is inherent in medicine. The data we collect are of uncertain value; the observations we make and the tests we perform are subject to error; our diagnoses are probabilistic; both the outcome of the patient's illness and the results of treatment are to varying degrees unknown. The main purpose of our search is to reduce uncertainty. The problem comes when we have to balance the pursuit of greater precision against the risk of further testing. In modern times, precision in medicine has been the overriding value. It is of course a great good and a worthy objective. But greater precision does not necessarily reduce uncertainty. The quest for precision can become mindless, as in the inexorable search for a diagnosis in a patient who is already recovering from an illness. The quest for precision can become a false trail when the true need is to gain a better understanding of the patient.

Until recently, an excessive pursuit of precision did not carry many risks. Now the technology of investigation has advanced so rapidly as to create many hazards, not to speak of enormous expense. Not the least of the hazards is that of finding a spurious abnormality, with all the attendant risks of inappropriate treatment.

Sometimes a test does not carry a hazard by itself but rather because it may unleash a succession of investigations, the so-called cascade effect (Mold and Stein, 1986). The physician may feel that he or she can maintain control, but this is sometimes easier said than done. The process can become inexorable.

Case 8.4

A 79-year-old man was known to have had liver metastases from a carcinoma of the colon for 12 months. He was also known to have gallstones. He eventually developed obstructive jaundice, which was thought to be caused by the tumor. Because he continued to be quite active, it was suggested to him that he should have an ultrasound to try to rule out a stone in the common duct. The result was equivocal, and the radiologist reported that the issue could only be resolved by a transcutaneous cholangiogram, or an endoscopic cholangiogram.

This was put to the patient with the recommendation that no further tests be done. However, he requested a surgeon's opinion and this led to an endoscopic cholangiogram. He found the procedure extremely unpleasant. The X-ray showed multiple intrahepatic obstructions. One of these was bypassed by a tube that drained some bile through the nasogastric tube. He requested that the tube be removed the following day. The same day, he developed septic shock and died within 72 hours.

The End Point in Family Practice

Traditionally, the end point of the search has been a diagnosis. In family practice, however, this is not always realistic. For reasons already discussed, many of the illnesses seen in family practice do not have a diagnosis in the strict sense of the term.

The illness may be at too early a stage for definitive diagnosis; it may clear spontaneously before diagnosis is possible; or it may be so interwoven with the personal life of the patient as to defy categorization.

In all patients, however, decisions have to be made, even if no diagnosis is possible. It is more helpful, therefore, to describe the end point in terms of a treatment decision. The end point of the search on any particular occasion is the point at which enough information is available for an informed decision to be made without avoidable risk to the patient.

It is important to understand that end points are often different in family practice than in referral specialties. A consultant seeing a referred patient will probably feel the need to make a definitive diagnosis before referring the patient back to his or her own physician. A family physician is not under the same constraint. The continuing relationship with patients means that all problems do not have to be solved right away. Because the relationship itself has no formal end point, the search can be discontinued and resumed according to need. In this sense, there is no final end point; the family physician should always be ready to revise the hypothesis if new evidence becomes available.

Family physicians, because of their role, make two types of decisions that do not arise as often in other branches of medicine:

1. The decision to wait. In making this decision, the physician is using the evolution of the illness over time as a test of the hypothesis. It is obviously inherent in this decision that no extra risk should be incurred by waiting. The use of time to validate hypotheses in this way can make many investigations redundant. One example of this decision is the eliminative diagnosis referred to earlier, in which the physician decides that the illness is transient and minor, then waits for the hypothesis to be verified.

2. The decision to refer. The end point of a search may be the decision to consult with or refer to another physician. This decision may have to be made before a definitive diagnosis is arrived at, for example, with a severely ill baby or a patient with an acute abdomen. It is clear that the objective of the family physician in these cases is different from that of the specialist. The family physician has fulfilled his or her obligation if the referral was made in time for the patient to receive effective treatment. The physician has failed to fulfill his or her obligation if the outcome of the illness was worsened by delaying referral in an effort to provide a more definitive diagnosis.[6]

The Routine Search

This comprises the routine systems inquiry and physical examination. The chief aims of the routine part of the search are to prompt alternative hypotheses by bringing to light cues that have not emerged in the directed part of the search, to collect baseline and background data on the patient, and to screen for symptomless conditions such as hypertension.

The routine search is sometimes referred to as a complete history and physical. This is a misnomer, for even the routine search is a selection from a much larger number of possible tests. As in the directed search, the tests are selected for their usefulness in achieving the objective. Internists would probably include ophthalmoscopy in their routine but not laryngoscopy—for the very good reason that ophthalmoscopy is more useful in generating new cues in patients seen by internists. For similar reasons, otolaryngologists would probably make the opposite choice. For four reasons, the family physician tends to make different use of routines than some other clinicians. First, because the patient is usually well known to the family physician, he or she may already have all the baseline data needed. Second, in minor and transient disorders, little in the way of a routine search is required. Third, because the family physician deals with such a wide range of clinical problems, from minor to life-threatening, no single routine is appropriate for every patient. He or she therefore develops different routines for different problems: one for sore throat, one for fatigue, one for dyspepsia, and so on. Finally, the affective component is so important that some question about feelings is routine unless covered earlier in the process.

The Search for Common Ground

Common ground between doctor and patient about the definition of the problem, the goals of treatment, and the care plan is a key element in the patient-centered clinical method. The search for common ground is a process of clarifying the issues, encouraging the patient's questions, and seeking his or her agreement with the plan. The whole consultation is an exchange of meanings between patient and doctor, culminating in an interpretation of the illness that is a joint creation of doctor and patient. The contribution of the patient will vary with the nature of the problem and the patient's expectations. In family practice, the process often will not have led to a high degree of certainty. Nevertheless, collaborative decisions have to be made, even if the decision is to wait.

The Care Plan and Therapy

We make a distinction here between a care plan and therapy. A care plan may or may not include therapy. Even if, at the end of a consultation, there is no specific therapeutic plan, it is still necessary to have a care plan, including arrangements for follow-up, further investigation, and reporting back. It is misleading to think of therapy only in terms of decision making. Therapy includes decision making but much more. Therapy that heals requires a deep involvement of the physician and a close attention to all the patient's needs and as much common ground as can be attained. The whole consultation is potentially therapeutic.

Case 8.5

A married woman in her mid-forties, a professional pianist and accompanist, was struck with a severe constricting chest pain while playing the piano. She was taken directly to the hospital and discharged a few days later with a diagnosis of angina. She said later that she left the hospital with the feeling that a sword of Damocles was hanging over her. She returned to work with some trepidation and had a recurrence of severe pain. This time she had angiograms, followed by coronary bypass surgery. From that day onwards, she referred to this as her "open heart operation."

She made a good recovery and was discharged home 2 weeks later. During this time each member of the family—patient, husband, and son—kept his or her own counsel, each thinking that one or both of the others knew something he or she did not know. No one addressed this problem and each withdrew into his or her own way of dealing with the crisis. The patient changed from being a talkative, rather exuberant woman to being quiet and depressed. She looked fragile and lost weight. Her husband and son saw this as a portent of a tragic outcome, and neither of them knew what to do. When the family were together, the subject was avoided. In the 3 months after the patient's discharge, she had frequent chest pain. Any attempt to play the piano resulted in pain. She paid frequent visits to her physician, who at each visit did an ECG, reassured her that it was all right, and reminded her to be careful. She was given quinidine, which made her think of herself as in danger of heart irregularities. The drug also gave her diarrhea and abdominal distress. Antidepressives and benzodiazepines were prescribed but did not help. She was advised also to give up her attempts to play the piano.

At this point, she came under the care of another physician, introduced by a mutual friend who was concerned for her life and health. She was depressed, in poor physical condition, and having frequent pain. She said that she wanted to feel better but was not interested in a long life if its quality could not be improved. Her inability to play the piano was a great loss to her and she did not know whether she wanted to live without her music.

In the course of several visits over the next few weeks, the following needs were identified and addressed: (1) The need for a definitive cardiac assessment. A cardiologist was consulted and gave her an excellent prognosis, with assurance that her chest pain was not cardiac. It was agreed that he would see her once a year for reassessment, but that apart from this, no further ECGs would be done. (2) The need to reduce and discontinue all medications, because they were not helping. This was done over the course of 2 months. (3) The need for physical rehabilitation. A physiotherapist experienced with cardiac patients was found. The patient embarked on a program of relaxation, pain control, and muscle strengthening. (4) Her need to play the piano. She was encouraged to sit at her piano and run her fingers over the keys. At first she could tolerate only a few minutes of this, but as her muscular strength increased, she was able to play for increasing periods. She was angry and frustrated with her playing at first, but was determined to play as well as ever. (5) Her need to understand how all this came to happen to her. This took weekly visits over many months. (6) Her family also had the need to understand what had happened, especially to appreciate the effects on the patient of their withdrawal and silence.

Within a year, the patient had recovered. She was free from pain, off all medication, and playing the piano for 2 to 3 hours a day. She had become her normal talkative self again.

No single individual would have been able to meet all this patient's needs. Each had to play his or her part: the family physician, the cardiologist, the physiotherapist, and the family. More than this, each needed to understand how their part fitted with the others. They had to work as an orchestra, rather than a number of soloists. The family physician was the conductor of the orchestra but also provided a *sine qua non* of the therapy: a belief in the patient's eventual recovery. The family physician helped the patient to understand her illness and to believe in recovery. She also selected a cardiologist and a physiotherapist who were appropriate for the patient's needs. If either had been ill-chosen, the therapy might have failed.

Much of diagnosis is a categorizing, generalizing process. A collaborative care plan is a synthesizing, individualizing process. The approach to care is probably more individualized in family practice than in any other field of medicine. It has much in common with the approach described by occupational therapists (Mattingly and Fleming, 1994). Obviously, the more precisely defined the problem, the less scope for variation in treatment. If a patient has pernicious anemia, the treatment in all cases is vitamin B_{12}. Even in this case, however, there may be aspects of management that if neglected can lead to failure of treatment. How likely is the patient to comply, for example? What is to be done to ensure that the patient is followed up? Few problems in family practice are as easy to define as pernicious anemia.

The complexity of problems, the frequent difficulty in achieving diagnostic precision, and the close personal knowledge of patients all combine to make therapy the most challenging and the most rewarding part of family practice. Gayle Stephens (1975) has called it "the quintessential skill of clinical practice and the ground of what family physicians know that is unique."

In a study of decision making in general practice, Essex (1985) identified 10 categories of factors affecting decisions.

Health problem (urgency, seriousness, natural history, etc.)

Patient (expectations, culture, compliance, etc.)

Family (impact on, requests from, etc.)

Other people (person accompanying patient, effect of problem on others, etc.)

Doctor (communication difficulties, experience with problem, knowledge/ignorance, mental state, workload, uncertainty, etc.)

Investigations (indications, reliability, results)

Resources (availability, constraints)

Time factors

Ethical and medicolegal factors

Management (indications and contraindications, drug side effects and interactions, risks and benefits of therapy, etc.)

In a qualitative study using semistructured interviews with general practitioners, Jones and Morrell (1995) found that the doctors frequently used personal background knowledge of patients in decision making. Four areas of knowledge were described: patient's coping abilities; social supports and stressors, especially in the family; social circumstances; and the doctors' feelings about the patients. Jones interviewed doctors about patients they had seen the same day, with the patients' records to assist their recall. The knowledge used was mainly of the tacit kind (Polanyi, 1962) and clearly had an affective component.

The result of all these interacting factors is that two patients with the same condition may be treated quite differently. Consider the example of two mothers phoning in the early hours of the morning about a sick child. One is well known to you, has good coping skills but tends to be overanxious, and is able to give a good clinical description of the child from which it appears that there are no indications of serious illness. The other is an immigrant who is not well known to you, has difficulty with the language, gives equivocal answers to your questions, and leaves you uncertain about the child's level of consciousness. The decision will probably be to see the second child at once and to reassure the mother of the first, with arrangements to see the child later. Patients with the same kind of acute sore throat may be treated differently if one is a student with an exam the next day, one a married office worker with no children, and another a single mother on welfare with no transport who has three young children.

As we have already seen, family physicians in some cases proceed directly from assessment to treatment, without going through a stage of specific diagnosis. The need for this is dictated by the conditions of family practice, with its early stages of disease, undifferentiated illness, and high level of uncertainty.

It is in arriving at a collaborative care plan with the patient that the family physician has the greatest scope for creativity. How a patient's problem is addressed depends on how it is perceived. Failure to understand the context of a problem will limit the range of decision alternatives. It is in this area that family medicine demands that a physician be skilled at synthesis rather than analysis. The following case vignette illustrates the relationship between perception of the problem and choice of management.

Case 8.6

A 19-year-old woman injured her knee while playing baseball and was admitted to the hospital for surgery. When seen for follow-up by Dr. A, she showed weakness and muscle wasting in the leg and complained of a number of general symptoms (fatigue, sweating, and pain in the neck). When Dr. A suggested that she was not doing her exercises, she became hostile and angry. Eventually she saw another doctor (Dr. B), who found her with severe muscle wasting in the leg and still complaining of the same general symptoms. After excluding some physical causes of her symptoms, Dr. B invited her to talk about the impact of her injury on her life. It turned out that the injury, by forcing her to cease her athletic pursuits, had, at a critical stage in her life, removed the main basis of her self-esteem. Given some insight into the problem, and the opportunity to discuss it with the doctor, she made a gradual recovery from her illness and returned to full activity.

Dr. A saw a hostile and uncooperative patient with an injured knee; Dr. B saw a patient with an injured knee and a life crisis.

The approach preferred by the physician may not be in accordance with the patient's expectations; it may even be in conflict with the patient's wishes. This is a challenge to the physician's skill in finding common ground. Therapy that the patient does not agree with is very unlikely to be beneficial. If the clinical method has been patient-centered, a search for common ground should have preceded treatment decisions.

Extraneous Factors in Clinical Decision Making

It is important to recognize, however, that factors outside the clinical situation may have a powerful influence on the process. Some of these factors are as follows.

Clinical Practice Guidelines (CPGs). One product of the evidence-based medicine movement has been a proliferation of CPGs that frequently target family practitioners. Increasingly, measures of practice quality use adherence to guidelines as one metric. Evidence-based guidelines are based on studies involving large numbers of patients who may or may not be similar to one's practice population casting doubt on their applicability. Nevertheless, they have a strong influence on decision making in family practice, more so when tied to remuneration mechanisms.

Institutional. In deciding on a search strategy, a physician may be heavily influenced by the rules of the institution. With the growth of managed care, there is an increasing tendency to standardize care. The clinical guidelines published by expert committees may become institutional rules rather than general statements requiring interpretation for individual patients.

Patients' expectations. As a result of reading medical articles in the press, or of hearsay, or of a need to take action in their care or need to exercise some control over their care, patients may ask questions about or request tests that the physician my find difficult to resist, even though there is no logical justification for them.

Fear of litigation. The prevalence of malpractice suits has had a powerful influence on the search strategies of physicians, the effect being to encourage defensive medicine.

Physician factors. Another influence on the diagnostic process is the physician's own personality, feelings, and experience. Physicians who feel insecure or who cannot tolerate uncertainty tend to carry out more tests than those who feel secure and tolerate uncertainty well. A physician's strategy may be influenced by feelings of anxiety about a particular patient or type of problem. If the physician feels he or she has made past errors with a patient, or with a particular problem, for example, he or she may tend to be overmeticulous in investigations or especially liable to refer the patient to a specialist.

The time factor. All physicians have to work within time constraints. Because workload is so unpredictable, this is particularly the case in primary medical practice.

Identification of Errors

As mentioned earlier, one of the reasons for knowing the theory of clinical decision making is that it enables the clinician to identify errors and thus to enhance his or her skills. Errors can be classified according to the level at which they occur: cues, hypotheses, search, or management. Some examples are given below.

Cue Blindness (Cutoffs)

This describes the situation where the clinician fails to respond to cues presented by the patient. We will give three examples, two from observation of trainees, one from (IRMcW's) own practice.

A resident saw a number of patients in one morning session, all with malaise, fever, and aches and pains. They all appeared to be suffering from a mild epidemic virus infection. One of them, however, when describing his symptoms, said "...and my water is like tea." The resident did not respond to this cue but, after prompting, obtained a urine specimen that was strongly positive for bile.

A resident was about to see a 19-year-old unmarried woman with a sore on her lip. When asked about what question was in his mind, he said, "Why has she come with this minor problem?" When the resident opened the interview by saying "How are you?" the patient replied "Okay, I guess." In the local idiom, this actually means not okay. The resident did not respond to this cue and went on to examine the lesion—a herpes simplex infection. He then asked her about her expectations, to which she replied: "I want to get rid of it—fast." The resident assured her that it would soon go away and did not require any treatment. However, the patient did not look pleased as she left the room, and the resident admitted to feeling dissatisfied with the interview. By cutting off two cues to her feelings, he had missed the opportunity of learning about her fears. Because his reassurance was not based on knowledge, it was ineffective.

The patient from my own practice (IRMcW) was a 65-year-old man with a fever of unknown origin and a very high erythrocyte sedimentation rate. Although his temperature was swinging between normal and 103°F, he was not ill enough to suggest an infection. All investigations for infection, autoimmune disease, and malignancy were negative, and an internist I consulted could not suggest a diagnosis. Some time after the onset of the illness, the patient mentioned that he was getting headaches, to which I did not pay much attention, regarding them as a result of his fever. Eventually, I consulted a second internist who immediately focused on the headaches as a significant cue. He diagnosed cranial arteritis, and the patient responded dramatically to prednisone. This is an example of a common pitfall—the cutting off of a cue that does not appear until later in the course of the illness. It is also relevant that the second consultant had seen many cases of cranial arteritis and had published one of the largest series in the literature.

Another reason for cutting off cues is the mental set of the clinician. The following story was told by a resident about a clinician he was working with. The patient suffered from anterior chest pain, and the clinician was taking a history with a diagnosis of ischemic heart disease in mind. Suddenly the patient interjected, "and I feel like crying all the time." The clinician failed to respond to this cue and continued to ask questions about his pain. The eventual diagnosis was depression. In this case, the clinician had a "set" on a certain line of inquiry, which blinded him to the most valuable cue of all.

Premature Convergence on a Hypothesis

In the early stages of hypothesis formation, it is important for the clinician's thinking to be lateral and divergent, considering many possible explanations for the patient's symptoms. One common error at this level is premature convergence on a hypothesis of viral infection in a patient with a mild febrile illness. This leads to failure to test such alternative hypotheses as urinary infection.

Errors in the Search

Two opposite errors are common in the search strategy. The first is redundancy. In this case, investigations are continued far beyond the point necessary for making an informed decision. Overinvestigation is perhaps the most common error in medicine today. Sometimes it is due to the inexorable search for a diagnosis in a patient who is already recovering from the illness. Another example of this error, often found early in the family medicine residency, is the use of investigations when clinical observation would provide a better search strategy. For many illnesses encountered in family practice, such as the preeruptive pain of herpes zoster, clinical observation is the only way of making the diagnosis.

A second common error is inadequate testing. Sometimes very simple procedures will increase the validity of a diagnosis without additional risk or expense: an erythrocyte sedimentation rate in a patient with fatigue and depression, a rectal examination in a patient with abdominal pain, a urine analysis in a patient with fever. Yet these opportunities for validation are often not taken if the clinician feels that he or she has good positive evidence for a hypothesis. This is an example of the well-known preference of all problem solvers for positive rather than negative evidence.

A third type of error, already described on page 173 is the premature ruling out of an important diagnosis because of reliance on a test with low sensitivity in the early stages of illness.

Management Errors

A common fault in management is failure to consider some of the important variables that should enter into the decision, such as the risks of treatment or the ethical issues. Another is the failure to consider the effect of management on the ecology of the family, as in the following example:

Case 8.7

An 87-year-old woman was seen at home by her family physician for acute low back pain. Apart from loss of central vision due to macular degeneration, she was in good health for her age. She and her 89-year-old husband were living independently and just managing to cope with the daily household tasks. The doctor ordered 2 weeks of complete bed rest and, because he arranged for no home help, the whole burden of care fell on the shoulders of the husband.

Because the patient's husband was unfamiliar with the household tasks he was assuming, he had to ask his wife repeated questions about them and was unable to understand her answers from the bed because of his deafness. This produced great anxiety and feeling of helplessness in his wife, which was exacerbated by her blindness.

While resting in bed, the patient developed frequent loose stools and began to lose weight rapidly. Carcinoma of the colon was suspected, and she was admitted to the hospital for investigation, which proved to be negative. At this point, her daughter arrived from a distance and stayed for 6 weeks. Under her daughter's care, the patient gradually recovered. The old couple lived on into their nineties in good health.

The doctor's chief error here was in not foreseeing that his management strategy would put an intolerable strain on a precariously balanced system. The strain produced acute anxiety, with psychogenic diarrhea and wasting. Moreover, complete bed rest was probably not good treatment for back pain in an 87-year-old. Even if it had been correct, it could only have been carried out by mobilizing a home support system. If the patient-centered method had been followed, the management plan would not have been implemented without seeking the response of the patient and her husband. Even if they had agreed, an exploration of the patient's feelings at a follow-up visit would have disclosed her anxiety and made clear the harmful consequences of the therapy.

References

Anspach RR. 1988. Notes on the sociology of medical discourse: The language of case presentation. *Journal of Health and Social Behavior* 29:357–375.

Balint M. 1964. *The Doctor, his Patient and the Illness*. London: Pitman Medical Publishing.

Beckman HB, Frankel RM. 1984. The effect of physician behavior on the collection of data. *Annals of Internal Medicine* 101:692.

Borkan J, Reis S, Steinmetz D, Medalie J. 1999. *Patients and Doctors: Life-Changing Stories from Primary Care*. Madison, WI: The University of Wisconsin Press.

Brown J, Stewart M, McCracken EC, et al. 1986. The patient-centered clinical method. II. Definition and application. *Family Practice* 3:75.

Brown J, Stewart M, Weston W. 2002. *Challenges and Solutions in Patient-Centered Care: A Case book*. Oxford: Radcliffe Medical Press.

Campbell K, Wulf Silver R, Hoch JS, Osbyte T, Stewart M, Barnsley J, et al. 2005. Re-utilization outcomes and costs of minor acute illness treated at family physican offices, walk-in clinics, and emergency departments. *Canadian Family Physician* 51:82–83.

Cannon WB. 1890. The case method of teaching systematic medicine. *Boston Medical Surgery Journal* 142:31–36.

Charon R. 1986. To render the lives of patients. *Literature and Medicine* 5:58–74.

Charon R. 2001. The patient–physician relationship. Narrative medicine: A model for empathy, reflection, profession, and trust. *Journal of the American Medical Association* 286(15):1897–1902.

Crombie DL. 1963. Diagnostic methods. *Practitioner* 91:539.

Crookshank FG. 1926. The theory of diagnosis. *Lancet* 2:939.

Diamond GA, Forrester JS, Hirsch M, et al. 1979. Application of conditional probability analysis to the clinical diagnosis of coronary heart disease. *New England Journal of Medicine* 300:1350.

Donnelly WJ. 1989. Righting the medical record: Transforming chronicle into story. *Soundings* 72(1):127–136.

Elstein AS, Shulman LS, Sprafha SA. 1978. *Medical Problem-solving: An Analysis of Clinical Reasoning*. Cambridge, MA: Harvard University Press.

Engel GL. 1977. The need for a new medical model: a challenge for biomedicine. *Science* 196:129.

Engel GL. 1980. The clinical application of the biopsychosocial model. *American Journal of Psychiatry* 137:535.

Essex BJ. 1985. Decision analysis in general practice. In: Sheldon M, Brooke J, Rector A, eds., *Decision-making in General Practice*. London: Macmillan.

Fabrega H. 1974. *Disease and Social Behavior*. Cambridge: MIT Press.

Feinstein AR. 1967. *Clinical Judgment*. Baltimore, MD: Williams and Wilkins, pp. 74–77.

Freeman TR. 2003. The case report as a teaching tool for patient-centered care. In: Stewart M, Brown JB, Weston WW, McWhinney IR, McWiliam CL, Freeman TR, eds., *Patient-centered Medicine: Transforming the Clinical Method*, 2nd edn. Oxford UK: Radcliffe Medical Press, chapter 14.

Galen RS, Gambino SR. 1975. *Beyond Normality: The Predictive Value and Efficiency of Medical Diagnoses*. New York: John Wiley.

Ge B, Stewart M. Comparison of clinical communication patterns of internists in outpatient departments of teaching hospitals and general practitioners in community-based clinics in Beijing. Submitted and under review.

Gombrich EH. 1960. *Art and Illusion: A Study in the Psychology of Pictorial Representation*. Princeton, NJ: Princeton University Press.

Greenhalgh T, Hurwitz B. 1998. *Narrative Based Medicine: Dialogue and Discourse in Clinical Practice*. London: BMJ Books.

Griffin SJ, Kinmonth AL, Veltman MWM, Gillard S, Grant J, Stewart M. 2004. Effect on health-related outcomes of interventions to alter the interaction between patients and practitioners: A systematic review of trials. *Annals of Family Medicine* November/December; 5(2):595–608.

Henbest RJ, Fehrsen GS. 1992 Patient-centredness: Is it applicable outside the West? Its measurement and effect on outcomes. *Family Practice* 9(3):311–317.

Howie JGR. 1973. A new look at respiratory illness in general practice: A reclassification of respiratory illness based on antibiotic prescribing. *Journal of the Royal College of General Practitioners* 23:895.

Jones J, Morrell D. 1995. General practitioners' background knowledge of their patients. *Family Practice* 12(1):49.

Kleinman A, Eisenberg J, Good B. 1978. Culture, illness and care: Clinical lessons from anthropologic and cross-cultural research. *Annals of Internal Medicine* 88:251.

Levenstein JH, McCracken EC, McWhinney IR, et al. 1986. The patient-centered clinical method. I. A model for the doctor–patient interaction in family medicine. *Family Practice* 3:24.

Little P, Everitt H, Williamson I, Warner G, Moore M, Gould C, et al. 2001a Observational study of effect of patient centredness and positive approach on outcomes of general practice consultations. *British Medical Journal* 323:908–911.

Mair A. 1973. *Sir James Mackenzie, M.D., General Practitioner*. 1853–1925. Edinburgh: Churchill Livingstone.

Marinker M. 1983. Communication in general practice. In: Pendleton D, Hasler J, eds., *Doctor–Patient Communication*. London: Academic Press.

Mattingly C, Fleming MH. 1994. *Clinical Reasoning: Forms of Inquiry in a Therapeutic Practice*. Philadelphia, PA: F.A.Davis Company.

Miller WL. 1992. Routine, ceremony or drama: An exploratory field study of the primary care clinical encounter. *Journal of Family Practice* 34(3):289.

Mold JW, Stein HF. 1986. The cascade effect in the clinical care of patients. *New England Journal of Medicine* 314:512.

Moral RR, Almo MM, Jurado MA, de Torres LP. 2001. Effectiveness of a learner-centred training programme for primary care physicians in using a patient-centred consultation style. *Family Practice* 18:1:60–63.

Polanyi M. 1962. *Personal Knowledge*. Chicago, IL: University of Chicago Press.

Rudebeck CE. 1992. General practice and the dialogue of clinical practice. *Scandinavian Journal of Primary Health Care*, Supplement 1.

Sackett DL, Haynes RB, Tugwell P. 1985. Clinical epidemiology: A basic science for clinical medicine. Boston, MA: Little, Brown.

Stephens GG. 1975. The intellectual basis of family practice. *Journal of Family Practice* 2:423.

Stewart MA, McWhinney IR, Buck CW. 1979. The doctor–patient relationship and its effect upon outcome. *Journal of the Royal College of General Practitioners* 29:77.

Stewart M, Brown JB, Donner A, McWhinney IR, Oates J, Weston WW, et al. 2000. The impact of patient-centered care on outcomes. *Journal of Family Practice* 49(9):796–804.

Stewart M, Brown JB, Weston WW, McWhinney IR, McWilliam CL, Freeman TR. 2003. *Patient-Centered Medicine: Transforming the Clinical Method*. Oxford, UK: Radcliffe Medical Press Ltd.

Stewart M, Brown JB, Hammerton J, Donner A, Gavin A, Holliday RL, et al. 2007. Improving communication between doctors and breast cancer patients. *Annals of Family Medicine* September/October; 5(5):387–394.

Tait I. 1979. The history and function of clinical records. M.D. thesis, University of Cambridge.

Weed LL. 1969. *Medical Records, Medical Education, and Patient Care*. Chicago, IL: Year Book Medical Publishers

Winker MA. 2006. Clinical crossroads: Expanding the horizons. *Journal of the American Medical Associaton* 295(24):2888–2889.

Notes

1. See Chapter 5, p. 77.

2. See Chapter 5, p. 61.

3. Used with permission of M. Stewart, Principal Investigator of the project Communicating with Breast Cancer Patients, Centre for Studies in Family Medicine. See related paper Stewart M et al., 2007.

4. We have based this example on cases described in Sackett DL, Haynes RB, Tugwell P. 1985. *Clinical Epidemiology: A Basic Science for Clinical Medicine*. Boston, MA:Little, Brown.

5. See Chapter 11 for its application to acute sore throat.

6. See Chapter 18 for a more extensive discussion of referral.

9

The Enhancement of Health and the Prevention of Disease

Family physicians are in an unrivaled position for helping their patients to maintain and improve their health. They see each of their patients, on the average, three or four times a year. Many of these visits are for self-limiting problems in healthy people. They provide, therefore, an excellent opportunity for health counseling and the early detection of disease. Because of their personal knowledge of patients and their families, family physicians may be aware of resources, both inner and outer, that are important for the maintenance or recovery of health. In secondary prevention, they can take responsibility for the whole process, from case finding through investigation to the approach to the problem.

General Principles

By convention, preventive practice has been divided into three categories:

1. Primary prevention increases a person's ability to remain free of disease.
2. Secondary prevention is the early detection of disease—or precursors of disease—so that treatment can be started before irreversible damage has occurred.
3. Tertiary prevention is the management of established disease so as to minimize disability.

All these refer to preventive services for individuals. Measures to maintain health are also applied to communities and populations. They may involve clean water, food inspection, sanitation, waste disposal, pollution control, accident prevention, or social services that relieve poverty, protect children, and improve access to health care. Even though in many societies a dependable infrastructure can be relied on for the basic protection of public health, family doctors rooted in their communities may encounter hazards to public health at any time through the experience of their patients. An outbreak of food poisoning in an institution may point to poor food hygiene. A local cluster of cases may raise suspicions of environmental pollution, as in the case of the Love Canal (see p. 14). In some communities, the health problems may require an approach at both individual and population levels. For family doctors in many Native North American communities, the epidemic of diabetes calls for work at the community level as well as the care of individual patients. The same applies in the central areas of large cities, where individual prevention may be vitiated by social breakdown. In poor countries, the lack of infrastructure may render individual prevention ineffective. For example, a reliable supply of electricity is necessary for the refrigeration of vaccines.

Promotion of Health versus Prevention of Disease

The categorization of preventive activities into primary, secondary, and tertiary was intended to apply to specific diseases. Health promotion is the development of a person's general resistance resources (GRR) (Antonovsky, 1979). Health is attained through a healthy environment, balanced diet, and physical fitness as well as the fostering of coping skills, self-confidence, and self-control. Antonovsky has described this approach as salutogenesis. To provide a more inclusive nomenclature of preventive services, the Canadian Medical Association uses the following categories (CMAJ, 2001 www.cma.ca/index.cfm/ci_id/3391/la_id/1.htm):

1. Health enhancement: counseling and information
2. Risk avoidance: ensuring that people at low risk remain at low risk—for example, immunization, accident prevention
3. Risk reduction: identification of individuals at high risk for disease in order to help them reduce the risk
4. Early identification of disease at the presymptomatic stage (equivalent to secondary prevention)
5. Complication reduction in patients with established disease (equivalent to tertiary prevention)

What Is Health?

The meaning of health has always proved to be elusive. According to the Constitution of the World Health Organization, health is "a state of complete physical, mental and social well-being and is not merely the absence of disease or infirmity." For the great majority of people this represents an impossible ideal. In the words of René Dubos (1980) "positive health is not even a concept of the ideal to be striven for hopefully. Rather it is only a mirage, because man in the real world must face the physical, biological and social forces of his environment, which are forever changing, usually in an unpredictable manner and frequently with dangerous consequences." In the words of Gordon (1958),

The "positiveness" of health does not lie in the state, but in the struggle—the effort to reach a goal which in its perfection is unattainable.... the words health and disease are meaningful only when defined in terms of a given person functioning in a given physical and social environment. The nearest approach to health is a physical and mental state fairly free of discomfort and pain, which permits the person concerned to function effectively and as long as possible in the environment where chance or choice has placed him.

Health and "normality" always have to be defined in terms of a particular person or group in a particular environment. The person's values must also be taken into account. Health is a value, and to some it may not be the highest value. It is sometimes sacrificed in the service of others. It is sometimes squandered in the pursuit of pleasure, fame, or fortune.

Value judgments also enter into physicians' concepts of health, especially when they concern human behavior. In accepting unthinkingly the norms of his or her own class and culture, the physician may not even realize that a value judgment is being made. It is important, therefore, to be clear about what normal means.

The Meaning of Normal

To identify individuals at high risk requires an understanding of the meaning of normal. In the history of medicine, few errors have led to so much harm as the failure to be precise about the meaning of the term. Although present when the physician is assessing and treating illness, the risk of harm is especially great in preventive medicine, for here the physician is identifying abnormalities in patients who have not come for treatment of symptoms or who have come with symptoms that bear no relation to the identified abnormality. Identification of the abnormality may then lead to treatment that has risks and costs. At the very least the patient will have an anxiety he or she did not have before.

To think clearly about normality, the physician must have an appreciation of human variability. Two types of variability are found in humans, the first of which is individual variation. In a given person, physiological values vary widely from minute to minute, hour to hour, day to day, week to week, and so on. These variations are manifestations of the adaptability of the organism to environmental change. Variations occur within a certain range compatible with life. Variations outside this range, if sustained, lead to pathological change and perhaps death of the organism.

The other kind is variation between individuals. Physiological values vary between one individual and another. If a value is plotted in a population, the result is a distribution curve with most members of the population having values about the middle of the range and smaller numbers at the two extremes. This type of variation is partly genetic but also partly the result of adaptation of individuals to different environments.

Variations resulting from adaptation are particularly noticeable when two populations from different environments are compared. The distribution of blood pressure and blood cholesterol in certain African tribes is quite different from their distribution in North Americans. The intestinal mucosa of an average Thai peasant has the same appearance as the mucosa of a North American with sprue. What we have said about physiological variables is equally true of cultural and behavioral variables. There are vast differences in what is considered normal behavior between different cultures and between subcultures and social classes of the same society. A degree of aggressiveness that is normal in the white North American may be considered pathological in a Pueblo Indian. A European who complained of being under a spell would be considered delusional; a rural African might be providing an explanation of symptoms consistent with his or her view of the world.

The history of medicine is full of examples of unnecessary suffering imposed on patients because they have been erroneously classified as abnormal. Some dubious practices—the wholesale removal of large tonsils for example was in vogue until after the mid-twentieth century. One that is of particular interest to family physicians is the practice, common in the late nineteenth century, of keeping young people with sinus arrhythmia in bed for months on end. This particular error was rectified by James Mackenzie, the British GP who showed the harmlessness of sinus arrhythmia by following a group of patients for 15 years.

John Ryle (1948) wrote

Each new instrument has left a trail of faulty diagnoses in its wake. The stethoscope, through misinterpretation of natural sounds or innocent murmurs, at one time created its thousands of cardiac invalids. The sphygmomanometer—through unfamiliarity with normal ranges and fluctuations of blood pressure—has created blood pressure invalids in a similar fashion. The gastroscopist who did not sufficiently recognize that the gastric mucosa, like the face, was responsive to normal stimuli, at first, exaggerated the importance of gastritis. Many laboratory methods have also been liable to misinterpretation through failure to study the limits of variability which are observable in health.

Mitral valve prolapse (MVP) provides a more recent example. Prolapse of the posterior leaflet of the mitral valve was first recognized during angiography and a relationship with late systolic click and murmur was noted. The development of echocardiography aided recognition of the condition and it became a common finding in patients without abnormal clinical features. As availability of this technology increased, recognition of MVP became more common. Soon the finding of MVP by echocardiography was being taken as an explanation for a whole range of signs and symptoms, including atypical chest pain, arrhythmias, syncope, dyspnea, panic and anxiety, numbness or tingling, effort syndrome, and skeletal abnormalities. MVP syndrome became a popular and overused diagnosis.

In 1983, the results of a study of the Framingham population became known. Echocardiography was done on 4,967 people, 5% of whom hadMVP. In women, the prevalence declined from 17% in their twenties to 1% in their eighties. In men the prevalence remained between 2% and 4% in all age groups. A systolic click or murmur was found in only five people out of the 208 with echocardiographic MVP. Symptoms of chest pain, dyspnea, and syncope were no more common in the 208 with echocardiographic prolapse than in those without. Only half the people with systolic clicks have echocardiographic prolapse. Subsequent studies have demonstrated a much lower prevalence of MVP with values typically in the range of less than 1% up to 2.4%. In a study of 24,265 (12,926 females and 11,339 males) echocardiograms carried out for clinical reasons the prevalence of MVP was found to be only 0.4% in women and 0.7% in men (Hepner, Ahmadi-Kashani, and Movahed, 2007). In a study of the offspring cohort of the Framingham Heart

Study, the prevalence of MVP was 2.4%, with 1.3% showing classic prolapse and 1.1% nonclassic prolapse. Complications such as heart failure, atrial fibrillation, cerebrovasular disease, and syncope were no more common in those with prolapse than in those without. Also, the frequencies of chest pain, dyspnea, and electrocardiographic abnormalities were the same in those with and without prolapse (Freed et al., 2002). It thus appears thatMVP, found only on echocardiography, is, like sinus arrhythmia, a variant of normal. Confirmation of this will await the follow-up of this cohort of people. This normal variant can now be distinguished from the MVP with mitral regurgitation found in those over 50 years of age.

How have these examples happened? Several recurring errors can be identified.

1. The distinction between normality and abnormality is regarded as an either/ or question. A person is either hypertensive or not hypertensive, diabetic or not diabetic, mentally retarded or not mentally retarded. This kind of thinking flies in the face of the truth. Variables such as blood pressure and blood cholesterol are continuously distributed in the population. They are also continuously related to mortality and other undesirable outcomes. It is difficult to identify a point at which blood pressure suddenly becomes associated with an increased risk of dying. A person with a diastolic blood pressure of 100 mm Hg has a greater risk of dying than one with a diastolic blood pressure of 90 mm, one with 90 mm has a greater risk than one with 80 mm, one with 80 mm a greater risk than one with 70 mm. Statements about the normality or abnormality of a continuously distributed variable are meaningless unless they are combined with a quantitative statement about the implications of the result. The implications will obviously depend on a number of other variables, including age, sex, existence of other diseases, and environment.

2. The term *normal* is confused with *average*. This is exemplified by the practice of plotting the results of a test in a representative population and arbitrarily defining as abnormal all results that lie outside two standard deviations from the mean. A moment's thought is enough to demonstrate the inadequacy of this concept in clinical medicine. Conditions such as abnormally low blood pressure and abnormally high intelligence are quite compatible with excellent health. Some conditions that are average are unhealthy— dental caries before fluoridation, for example. A condition may be accepted as healthy in one population because it is average, even though in another population the distribution of the variable may be quite different. We may question, therefore, whether the "normal blood pressure" in North America should be considered normal when compared with the level attained in other communities. Values within the normal range cannot be taken as an indication of health, nor can values outside this range be taken as an indication of disease. The fallacy in this approach is graphically illustrated by the probability of finding an abnormal result when multiple tests are done (Table 9.1). If enough tests are done, almost everybody is "abnormal." This

Table 9.1 Probability of obtaining an abnormal result when multiple tests are done

Number of Independent Tests	Percentage of Times an Abnormal Result Is Found
1	5
2	10
4	19
6	26
10	40
20	64
50	92
90	99

Source: Galen and Gambino, 1975.

Table 9.2 Referent values for serum uric acid (usual range 3–6 mg/dL)

Referent Value	Diagnosis	Predictive Value (%)
7.0	Gout	21
8.0	Gout	35
9.0	Gout	82

Source: Galen and Gambino, 1975.

had led Edmond Murphy (1976) to define (in jest) a normal person as "one who has been insufficiently investigated." There are several ways of guarding against this error. One is to report data in percentiles, as in the percentile growth charts we use to assess the development of infants and children. The percentile chart tells us how unusual the data for an individual child are in terms of the reference population that was used to compile the chart. The percentile chart is a very useful tool for clinicians, provided they do not equate deviation with disease and average growth with normality. The chart must obviously be used in conjunction with other criteria: the child's general health, other manifestations of disease, and whether or not the deviation is also a deviation in the child's own growth curve.

Another way of avoiding this error is to use referent values rather than the normal range as our criteria. The referent value relates the result of a test to its predictive value for a particular disease. Referent values for a particular test in a particular disease will vary with age, sex, and other population characteristics. The use of referent values is illustrated by Table 9.2. This tells us that 82% of subjects with a serum uric acid level of 9 mg/dL or higher subsequently develop gout.

3. The criteria of abnormality for a new test may be arrived at by testing an unrepresentative sample of the population, such as people admitted to hospital or attending a particular clinic. After a time a random sample of the

population is tested and the criteria are corrected. When data are collected to establish the normal range for any variable, great care has to be taken to ensure that the sample chosen is truly representative of the whole population.

4. Physicians reflect the cultural norms of their own society and social class and they may, therefore, classify as abnormal or unhealthy some behaviors that are only unfashionable or unpopular. Sexual behavior is especially likely to be treated in this way. It is not long since masturbation was classified as a disease and treated with severe measures. In the present moral climate, sexual activity is unlikely to be classified as abnormal, but the opposite error has taken its place. By unintentional and unconscious signals, physicians can convey to patients that they consider them abnormal for not being sexually active.

What are the implications of these observations for the family physician?

1. In judging the significance of a finding, it is important to ascertain that the result is not one extreme of an individual variation. A good example of this is the tendency of blood pressure to be higher at the first than at subsequent readings. Hence the need to establish the patient's normal range of variation before embarking on treatment for hypertension.
2. In using percentile charts as the criterion for normality (in developmental assessment for example), the physician should bear in mind the meaning of "normal" and "abnormal" results.
3. In judging the abnormality of a result, rather than using the statistical average or normal range as a standard, the physician should, where it is available, use the reference value.
4. Because of the long-term relationship with patients, the family physician is in a good position for obtaining baseline values from patients. This enables the physician to compare subsequent readings on the same patient with this baseline value—a potentially much more useful comparison than that with a "normal range." For example, if the physician knows that a woman's usual systolic blood pressure is 100 mm Hg, the fact that her blood pressure at 28 weeks of pregnancy is 120 mm Hg will warn of the possibility of preeclampsia, even though her reading is well within the normal range.
5. Because they care for more or less unselected populations, family physicians are in an excellent position to determine the range of normality for many kinds of variables. This is one of the most useful kinds of research a family physician can undertake.
6. Family physicians should be constantly aware, when dealing with family and personal problems, that it is very easy to convey value judgments without knowing that they are doing so.

Salutogenesis

The concept of salutogenesis switches our perspective from the causes of disease to the maintenance and improvement of health. It recognizes that stressors are universal and omnipresent, but not necessarily pathological. Their pathogenicity depends on the character of the stressor and the resources available to the individual. Research is focused on the sources of successful resistance. Antonovsky (1987) attributes successful resistance to a sense of coherence (SOC) that has three core components:

Comprehensibility. Stressors, either internal or external, should make cognitive sense to the person.

Manageability. To cope with the stressors, resources should be available either to the person or his or her supporters.

Meaningfulness. The person should feel that the experience is congruent with his or her beliefs and values.

The SOC is an expression of the fit between an individual and his or her social environment. The person must feel that he or she is valued and rewarded at home, at work, and in other social contexts. The inner and outer resources are mutually interactive. Inner self-confidence is increased by a sense of belonging, and the increased confidence leads to stronger social integration. A strong supportive network may balance weaker inner resources, and vice versa.

Siegrist (1993) emphasizes the importance of the emotions in an individual's response to experience. The response is not cognitive alone. The affective response to stressful experience often bypasses or overrides the cognitive. The devastating effect of unemployment, for example, can lower a person's feeling of self-worth, reduce the sense of belonging, and cut him or her off from a major source of social approval. Unemployment is associated with high rates of illness and increased death rates.

Self-Assessed Health and Mortality

The association between self-assessed health and mortality was first reported in an analysis of the Manitoba Longitudinal Study on Aging (Mossey and Shapiro, 1982). The self-assessments were given in response to the question "For your age, in general, would you say your health is excellent, good, fair, poor, or bad?" The answers proved to be better predictors of survival during the follow-up period than the extensive data on respondents' health from the Manitoba Health Insurance Plan. The data recorded diagnoses and utilization of medical services. Respondents with poorer subjective health status experienced greater mortality throughout the 7 years of the study. The finding has since been replicated in five other studies (Idler, 1992). How can we explain this surprising fact? Respondents may have been intuitively aware of their bodily state in a way that was not reflected in the objective evidence of health status. Alternatively, their assessment may have reflected a sense of coherence, or lack of it, which exerted an independent effect on their subsequent health. Self-assessment of health covaries with education, marital status, and income. For any given level of objective health status, those who have less education, lower income, and who are unmarried have poorer self-assessments of health.

The implication for family physicians is that what people say about their health should be taken seriously even if it contradicts other evidence. Hollnagel and Malterud (1995) have drawn attention to the lack of research on patients' healing potentials in general practice and on the lack of any system for recording patients' resources in primary care classification systems. Giving people confidence and supporting them in a sense of control is associated with better health and improved function. Sobel (1995) says, "There is a biology of self-confidence." Giving patients prescriptions for lifestyle and behavior changes that are difficult to achieve may only increase their sense of failure. A sense of being in control gives patients the confidence to set their own goals. Achieving the goals, even if they are limited, further increases the feeling of confidence. For example, Lorig, Mazonson, and Holman (1993) reported that the best predictor of improvement by participants in an arthritis self-management course was the patient's self-assessment of how likely they were to improve.

The Health Enhancement Continuum

The enhancement of health covers a spectrum from environmental and social policies at one end to good clinical practice at the other (Table 9.3). The environmental determinants of health create the conditions for enhancement of health at the personal level. Although family physicians in industrialized countries do not usually have primary responsibility for environmental health, they can often identify local health problems in the course of their work. In poorer countries where public health services cannot as readily be taken for granted, family physicians may have a more direct responsibility for this aspect of health.

Social class is one of the strongest predictors of health and disease. Even in countries with universal access to health services, and an effective social safety net, lower income and social status are associated with poorer health. The association has not been fully explained. It is likely that social status is a surrogate for several determinants of health, such as nutrition, housing, quality of environment, education, work satisfaction, control over one's life, and attitudes to prevention.

The next part of the spectrum concerns the identification of strengths and the enhancement of general resistance resources in individuals, followed by risk assessment and reduction. Prevention merges with clinical diagnosis and management in presymptomatic and early diagnosis, management, and rehabilitation. Measures for the enhancement of health are not limited to one part of the spectrum. General resistance resources (GRR), for example, are important both in the maintenance of health and in the recovery from disease. Assessment of GRR is an aspect of patient-centered medicine.

Identification of risk factors may be followed either by treatment (e.g., for hypertension) or by counseling in behavior change (e.g., for smoking). Because this involves either treatment of people without identified disease or interference in a person's way of life, it is only justified when supported by strong evidence (see following text).

Table 9.3 The health enhancement continuum

Environmental and Social Policies	Assessment of General Resistance Resources (G.R.R.)	Enhancement of G.R.R	Risk Assessment	Risk Reduction	Presymtomatic Diagnosis	Early Diagnosis	Rehabilitation to Enhance Recovery	Care and Support of Patients with Chronic Disease and their Families to Maintain Function and Reduce Complications
Housing	Self-assessed health status	Support	Smoking-related diseases	Smoking cessation	Screening and case finding	Prevention of complications by early diagnosis of serious treatable disease	E.g. industrial injuries	E.g. Diabetes
Electric power	Confidence	Health education and counselling (e.g., nutrition, exercise, sexuality, accident)	Substance abuse	Reduction of alcohol intake	Hypertension	e.g., meningitis cranial arteritis	Stroke	Hypertension
Clean air	Coping ability	Immunization	Coronary heart disease	Reduction of serum cholesterol	Cervical cancer	myocardial infarction	Accidents	Breast cancer
Clean water	Social support	Family planning	Family violence	Nutrition education	Breast cancer	major depression	Musculoskeletal disorders	Multiple sclerosis
Parks and recreation	Family function	Prenatal care	Accidents in aged	Accident prevention				COPD
Nutrition education	Work satisfaction	Child care	S.T.D.	Referral to social services				Chronic arthritis
Food inspection	Exercise		Teenage pregnancy	counselling				Schizophrenia
Occupational health and safety	Immunization status							Chronic depression
Insect control	Income security							Alzheimer's disease
Accident prevention	Knowledge of hygiene							
Child support and protection								
Access to health services								
Unemployment insurance								
Health education								
Social stability and law enforcement								

Health education is the provision of information, advice, and sometimes training in activities that can promote health. There are numerous examples: prenatal classes, preparation for parenthood, family planning, prevention of accidents in children, advice on seat belts and crash helmets, prevention of falls in the elderly, and information for travelers. Education for new experiences such as childbirth and parenthood is based on the principle that coping ability is enhanced by preparation. Health education is an activity for the whole health-care team, including nurses, occupational therapists, physiotherapists, and nutritionists. Brochures, books, and videotapes are a valuable resource. Health education can also play a part in tertiary prevention. Counseling before surgery can reduce postoperative pain and time in the hospital. Video presentations can help patients to make choices between alternative therapies—for example, when facing a decision about prostatectomy.

A screening procedure is one that is applied to an unselected population to identify those members who are either diseased or at risk for a disease. For example, the population of a factory or a town may be screened for hypertension. In case finding, a person is identified as diseased or at risk by the physician responsible for his or her health care. For example, a patient may be identified as hypertensive while attending for skin infection. It will be clear that case finding rather than screening is the method used in family practice. The family physician is responsible for the identification of the abnormality, its investigation and treatment, and follow-up.

Motivational Interviewing

Motivational interviewing techniques take into account that patients make significant changes in lifestyle in stages. These stages consist of pre-contemplation (no particular thoughts or intent to change), contemplation (thinking about making changes), preparation (getting ready to make changes), action (changes in behavior are made) and maintenance (changes achieved are consolidated and measure taken to prevent relapse) (Prochaska, 1979). Health promotion interventions are tailored to the particular stage of the patient. In the pre-contemplation phase it may consist of increasing a person's awareness of the problem and providing education about known consequences of it. If a patient is in the contemplation phase the physician encourages discussion about the patient's perception of the pros and cons of undertaking the needed change and validates the reasons for it. When a patient is in the preparation stage and has made a commitment to it, the intervention consists of supporting self efficacy, identifying and assisting problem solving, and encouraging small initial steps. Once a major change has been made, it is important to provide supportive follow-up and discuss coping strategies for relapse. This last step is important since, in its absence, an individual will tend to view any relapse as a failure and reason to give up rather than an expected event that can be made into a positive step.

By tailoring a health promotion or preventive intervention to the stages of change, the practitioner's and patient's time and the effectiveness of the intervention are made optimal. This approach has been shown to be useful in smoking cessation and other addiction counseling, and making lifestyle changes including diet and exercise (Burke, Arkowitz, and Menchola, 2003).

The Evaluation of Screening and Case Finding

To justify the application of a screening or case-finding procedure, the following conditions should be fulfilled:

1. The disease in question should be a serious health problem.
2. There should be a presymptomatic phase during which treatment can change the course of the disease more successfully than in the symptomatic phase.
3. The screening procedure and the ensuing treatment should be acceptable to the public.
4. The screening procedure should have acceptable sensitivity and specificity.
5. The screening procedure and ensuing treatment should be cost-effective.

Severe hypertension fills these criteria because if untreated, it is associated with a higher mortality rate from stroke and heart disease; because the detection procedure has high specificity and sensitivity; and because treatment before end organ damage has occurred has been shown by randomized trial to increase survival. On the other hand, prostate-specific antigen fails by these criteria as a screening test for prostate cancer, because of relatively low sensitivity (87%) and specificity (80%) and controversy over whether early prostatectomy increases survival (Fradet, 2007; Labrecque, Legare, and Cauchon, 2007). Moreover, there is no evidence from randomized controlled trials that prostatectomy for early carcinoma increases survival.

The efficacy of screening is sometimes accepted on evidence that fails to take account of certain pitfalls. First, patients who volunteer for screening programs are often those who are destined for favorable outcomes for other reasons. Second, the increased survival demonstrated as a result of screening may be only the longer time the disease is known to exist. And third, screening programs will tend to identify slowly progressive variants of disease since these are more likely to have a long presymptomatic phase. For example, a very malignant carcinoma is unlikely to be identified by screening because it is likely to cause symptoms early in the course of the disease. For all these reasons, the best evidence on which to base a screening procedure is that obtained by a randomized, controlled trial, with mortality, rather than duration of survival, as the end point. The increasing availability of screening tests has made it essential that decisions on screening should be made only after rigorous and critical examination of the evidence. As we will see in the next section, this is often not the case.

Problems in the Interpretation and Application of Evidence

Even when the evaluation has been conducted by experts in the field, there have been many examples of failure to apply rigorous standards to evidence.[1] Indeed, the involvement of experts carries its own risks, since deep involvement in an issue can generate so much enthusiasm for promoting it that contrary evidence is ignored.

The following are some examples:

Ignoring Contrary Evidence

On the basis of a trial showing that lowering blood cholesterol with cholestyramine reduced the rate of heart attacks in middle- aged men with high cholesterol levels, the National Cholesterol Education Program (NCEP) in 1988 published its recommendations for screening. All adults were recommended to have blood cholesterol levels checked every 5 years. Levels were defined for high (240 mg/dl or above) and borderline high cholesterol (200–239 mg/dL). Those with high levels, and those with borderline levels and either heart disease or two other risk factors were recommended to have their level of low density lipoprotein (LDL) determined. Recommendations were then made for the reduction of LDL cholesterol by diet, with the addition of cholesterol-lowering drugs if the LDL level was high enough, and was not lowered by diet alone.

Since one quarter of the adult population of the United States has cholesterol levels of 240 mg/dL or above, the implications were huge. It has been established that, after implementing the recommendations, 36% of the adult population would require dietary or drugs (Russel, 1994). Even when these recommendations were made, it was known that while lowering cholesterol reduced the rate of heart disease, it did not increase survival. This was because the reduction in death from heart disease was balanced by an increase in deaths from other causes. Subsequent trials have confirmed this result. Only in persons who already have coronary heart disease have trials shown that lowering cholesterol level increases survival. Thus, recommendations with implications for the whole population were based on a selective assessment of the evidence. Results that should have suggested caution were downplayed—an instance of the human tendency to prefer positive to negative evidence (Russel, 1994).

Assuming That the Relation between Test Results and
Mortality Is Continuously Graded

Through the relationship between borderline and high cholesterol level and death from heart disease is continuously graded (the higher the level, the more deaths), it cannot be assumed that the same continuous grading is present at lower levels. Indeed, this is not the case. The death rate does decline until the level reaches about 180 mg/dL, but then begins to rise again. For men with levels below 160, the extra deaths are due to cancers other than colon cancer, respiratory disease, digestive disease, and trauma.

In spite of this, the NCEP in 1991 recommended that all Americans over the age of two restrict fat intake to 30% of calories or less. The fact that this may reduce those who already have a natural low level of cholesterol to even lower levels does not necessarily mean that they will experience the same increased risk of death as those with naturally lower levels. Nevertheless, the possibility is there. A seemingly harmless intervention may prove to be harmful to some people.

Failing to Take into Account the Impact of False Positive Tests

Tests like Papinicolou smears, mammograms, and prostate-specific antigen are initial screens which, if positive, require additional tests to confirm the result. When the number of false positive screening tests is high, large numbers of normal people are subjected to these further tests, with their attendant risks, and to the anxiety caused by the process.

One cervical screening program reported a striking increase in minor smear abnormalities to 10% (Raffle, Alden, and Mackenzie, 1995). At this rate, the number of false positives far outnumbers the number of true positives. When the test involves human judgment, as does the Pap smear, the stresses on laboratory workers can affect the false positive rate. Since the penalties for a false negative ("missing" a case) are much greater than for a false positive, there is a natural tendency to err on the side of identifying abnormalities. The investigation of false positives also adds greatly to the cost of the program and has to be factored into the economic analysis of health benefits.

The Ritual of Annual Testing

Once a screening test is introduced there is a tendency to advocate annual testing, even though the advantage over less frequent testing is only marginal. Doing Pap tests every 3 years reduces the incidence of invasive cervical cancer by 90.8%. Increasing the frequency to annual smears only reduces the incidence of invasive cancer by another 2.7% (Russel, 1994, p. 14). Those who argue that even marginal improvements are worth the cost should logically not stop at annual tests, since increasing the frequency to 6 monthly or 3 monthly might produce additional marginal improvements. As the frequency of testing increases, so does the likelihood of a false positive result during a woman's lifetime.

Many women in the United States are having annual Pap smears. At the same time, a quarter report no test in the previous 3 years (Russel, 1994, p. 16). The greatest impact on the incidence of the disease would come from testing women who are at present not being tested. For the individual practitioner, greater benefits will come from screening the women in the practice who do not attend than from increasing the frequency of screening in those who do.

The Chimera of Universal Consensus

When all the evidence has been considered, decisions about screening still depend on judgment. There is no single correct answer to questions like the cutoff point between "normal" and "abnormal," the level at which treatment is indicated, or the frequency of testing. The answers vary from one country to another, depending on cultural and economic factors. After reviewing cholesterol guidelines in six countries, Rosser et al. (1993) concluded that policy and guidelines tended to be more influenced by political and economic factors than by evidence of health benefit. The assessments produced by the international Cochrane project will probably be interpreted differently in each national jurisdiction.

Extrapolation to Beyond the Group Investigated in the Trial
When a trial has established that a screening test is justified in one age and sex group, there is a tendency to assume that the evidence also justifies the procedure in other groups such as females and the elderly of both sexes. This cannot be taken for granted since biological differences between males and females, and between children, mature adults and the elderly, make it very likely that different criteria will apply. Most of the research on cholesterol and heart disease has been conducted on middle-aged men. More than 10,000 men with preexisting coronary disease have enrolled in trials of cholesterol reduction but only just over 400 women—too few for definitive results (Rich-Edwards, Manson, Hennekens, and Buring, 1995). Only 5,800 of more than 30,000 people enrolled in primary prevention trials of cholesterol reduction have been women—not enough to obtain the necessary statistical power. Clinical trials may include balanced numbers of both sexes, but may not report the results separately. Trials also tend to recruit people with fewer coexisting diseases than the general population.

The Concept of Risk

The identification of risk factors has become a major objective of epidemiological research and an increasing number of reports are appearing in major medical journals (Skolbekken, 1995). Much of this research has been criticized for its conceptual confusion (Hayes, 1992) and lack of rigor (Feinstein, 1988). Many studies do not begin with a hypothesis based on clinical observation. The factors to be tested for association with the target disorder are therefore not determined in advance. Instead, large numbers of variables are subjected to statistical manipulations that are easily done with modern computers. When a statistically significant relationship comes out, it may be wrongly interpreted as a causal relationship. Rarely a week passes without one of these findings being reported in the media, raising public anxieties and undermining peoples' confidence in their ability to lead a healthy life. Reports with major methodological errors have been accepted by leading medical journals. More than 80,000 articles on risk were published between 1987 and 1991 (Skolbekken, 1995).

The identification of a causal factor, such as smoking for lung cancer, usually begins with a clinical observation or a hypothesis based on some logical connection between factor and target disorder. A cohort of patients with the target disorder is assembled with special care to avoid selection bias. A matching group without the target disorder is obtained, again with care to match the groups for all variables which could influence the factor in question. The groups are then compared for the presence of the factor. For any factor which depends on self-reporting, such as diet or smoking, great care must be taken to validate questionnaires and avoid recall bias. Many studies do not follow this procedure. Since there is no hypothesis to guide the formation of a cohort, a convenience cohort, selected for some other purpose is used. The investigators thus have no control over the way data was collected, either at entry to the study or afterwards. To avoid selection bias, it is crucial that the target disorder should be sought with equal thoroughness in groups with and without the disorder, so that "silent" cases in the latter group will not be missed. For example, the apparent association of alcohol and breast cancer could be explained if heavy drinkers were more likely to be diagnosed because of increased medical attention, or if moderate drinkers were of a different social class from abstainers, and more likely to attend for screening.

Even when well-designed studies have shown a causal relationship between factor and target disorder, and randomized trials have shown that modification of the factor can change the outcome, unjustified extrapolations may be made to groups of people not represented in the cohort. Studies of men may be extrapolated to women, or studies of younger people extrapolated to the elderly (McCormick, 1994).

Flawed methodology leads to the accumulation of "risk factors" that are no more than statistical associations between observations. More than 300 risk factors for coronary disease have been identified (Skrabanek and McCormick, 1990). The term "risk factor" covers a number of quite different concepts of risk. It does not distinguish between factors which are causal, such as smoking for lung cancer, and those which are contingent, such as age and sex for coronary heart disease. Nor does it distinguish between factors which are unalterable and those which can be changed. Whether a risk factor is called a disease or a cause of disease is a matter of convention. Blood cholesterol above a critical level is called a risk factor for coronary heart disease. Blood sugar above a critical level is called a disease— diabetes mellitus—even if there are no symptoms. Symptomless carcinoma of the prostate, discovered at transurethral prostatectomy is called a disease, not a risk factor, even though it may not progress to the stage of symptoms.

Foss and Rothenberg (1987) maintain that risk factors tend to be called causes if they fit with the prevailing mechanistic paradigm; behavioral factors are still called "risk factors" even when they have a causal relationship with disease. Skrabanek and McCormick (p. 94) believe that risk factors should be called "risk markers" to emphasize that they are associated with altered probability of developing disease rather than necessarily being causally related.

Epidemiology came of age when the doctrine of specific causation held sway. Infectious diseases provided the model for diseases to be defined in terms of single causal agents, even though multiple factors in host and environment contributed to the web of causation. The factor isolated as the cause was the one "necessary" for a case to be classified as an example of the disease. With the infectious diseases of the nineteenth century the doctrine worked well. Now, infectious disease is often nosocomial and the "cause" has to be sought in some change in the host. The doctrine of specific causation does not work well for chronic diseases, which cannot usually be classified in terms of a single necessary cause. Epidemiology is thus becoming a probabilistic science. Identification of factors strongly associated with disease is a valid procedure, provided that they are treated as hypotheses to be tested. If a prospective study shows a causal relationship, then the factor should be classified as a cause. The magnitude of its contribution to the causal web should also be expressed in terms of probability.

The necessity of having a hypothesis should not blind us to the importance of unexpected findings. Many important discoveries have been the unexpected result of research done for some other purpose. The usual course of events is that the finding is confirmed by a study in which the unexpected finding becomes a new hypothesis.

Perception of Risk from Relatives' Knowledge of Their Family Histories

Risk perceptions have been shown to be held by people with a family history of breast cancer, colon cancer, diabetes, and heart disease (Walter and Emery, 2006). Understanding of familial risk may be influential in motivating preventive measures and healthy behavior. Structured models have been developed to integrate different health beliefs and to understand their role in predicting health related behavior.

Levanthals' Common Sense Model of Self-Regulation of Health and Illness (CSM) (Leventhal et al., 2003) arose from the observation that biomedical symptoms (or identity) represented only one type of perceptual information needed to appraise a health risk situation. Other attributes of threats used in the CSM. were as follows (Walter and Emery, 2005):

1. Identity: internal or external sources of information of a relative's illness (e.g., a symptom of information that a relative has a disease)
2. Time scale of the threat (timeline)
3. Potential to affect life expectancy or quality of life
4. Perceived cause of the illness
5. Controllability: the possibility of coping with the illness

In their study, Walter and Emery used the framework of the CSM to compare and contrast perceptions about family history among primary care patients with a family history of cancer, heart disease, or diabetes.

Participants were recruited from two general practices and the sampling strategy aimed to gain as broad a range possible of age, gender, educational levels, and degree of family risk. Semi-structured qualitative interviews were conducted by one person (F.M. Walter), mainly in the interviewees' homes and lasted about an hour. Flexibility allowed for discussion of important issues.

At the time of writing, Walter and Emery's study is the first to examine inter-disease variations in perceptions of their family history among a primary care sample. It demonstrates some benefits of obtaining the relevant data in this way. From the scientific point of view the lengthy interchange between interviewee and investigator allows for accuracy of the data. For the family practitioner it obtains this important data at first hand and can enter into the patient's chart (Neither of the investigators were members of the two practices). Walter and Emery present their results in comparison with the CSM categories of *Consequences and timeline, cause, controllability and relative threats of cancer, heart disease and diabetes.* In each case, interviewee's comments are quoted verbatim and together with the investigator's findings.

Before the abovementioned publications, Fiona Walter and her colleagues had published two other papers on the same theme.

Walter and Emery write: "The family history is becoming an increasingly important feature of health promotion and early detection of common chronic diseases in primary care. Previous studies of patients from genetics clinics suggest a divergence between how persons with a family history perceive and understand their risk and the risk provided by health professionals . . . what exactly constitutes having a family history of an illness varied among participants. The development of a personal sense of vulnerability to the illness in the family depended not only on the biomedical approach . . . but also on an interplay of other factors." These included: the emotional impact of witnessing the illness in the family, members' personal relationships in the family, and different beliefs about the contribution to illness of nature and nurture.

Absolute Risk, Relative Risk, and the Number Needed to Treat

The family physician needs some way of applying epidemiological data to individuals and of explaining their implications to patients. The "number needed to treat" is a way of conveying both statistical and clinical significance. It is defined as the number of patients the physician will need to treat to prevent one adverse event. For patients, it is much easier to understand than percentages. We have to remember that many of our patients have difficulty with percentages, even to the extent of reckoning the amount of a waiter's tip.

Research findings are often expressed in terms of the relative risk reduction. This has no bearing, however, on the probability that an individual will acquire the disease. If the absolute risk is very small, the increase in risk, though relatively high, may in fact be very small. The 30% greater risk of lung cancer in passive smokers, compared to other non-smokers, moves them from a probability of 0.09 per 1,000 to 0.12 per 1,000 (Skrabanek and McCormick, 1990, pp. 40–41).

The number needed to treat is the reciprocal of the absolute risk reduction (Laupacis, Sackett, Roberts, 1988). Cook and Sackett (1995) use data from a recent review of antihypertensive therapy (Collins et al., 1990) as an illustration. Patients with mild hypertension receiving placebo had a 1.5% expectation of a stroke over 5 years, compared with 0.9% in those receiving antihypertensive drugs, giving a risk reduction of $0.015 - 0.009 = 0.006$. The reciprocal of this number is about 167, so that 167 patients would need to be treated for 5 years to prevent one stroke. This assumes that the individual patient's baseline risk is the same as the baseline risk of patients in the trial, which may not be the case. If the baseline risk of a patient is higher by a factor f times the risk of patients in the trial, the new number needed to treat is the original number divided by f. If the patient's baseline risk is estimated to be twice the risk of those in the trial, the number needed to treat would be 167/2 or 83.

This could be explained to a patient with the same baseline risk as the trial patients in the following way. If 100 men like you are followed for 5 years, about two will have a stroke, 98 will not. We do not know whether you are one of the two or one of the 98. If you reduce your blood pressure by taking antihypertensive medication, you can jump to another group. Then out of 100 men like you, one will have a stroke, 99 will not. We still do not know whether you are the one, or one of the 99. Which group do you wish to belong to: those who accept the status quo, or those who take medication?"

Clinical Guidelines

The sheer volume of evidence now available makes it impossible for any one physician to base his practice on his own critical review of the literature. To meet this need, institutions, academic bodies, professional groups, and others have started to develop recommendations or guidelines on matters such as diagnostic tests, management of disease, and preventive procedures. The process varies from one group to another. Sometimes the guidelines are developed by a group of experts on the subject in question. The problem with this is that experts develop enthusiasms for their subjects and may be inclined to brush aside critical evidence. Even when dissenting voices are raised, they may find it difficult to gain a hearing. An example is given on page 205. The process is "top down." Recommendations are handed down to practitioners without the opportunity of feedback while the guidelines are being developed. This may set the stage for disputes between practitioners and experts as occurred in the case of cholesterol screening in Ontario.

The process designed by the Dutch College of General Practitioners (NHG) is an example of the opposite "bottom up" approach, in which practitioners initiate and participate in the whole process. The aim is to achieve a balance between evidence-based guidelines and guidelines that are feasible in practice (Grol, Thomas and Roberts, 1995). An independent advisory board of experienced practitioners selects the topic. A working party of four to eight family physicians is appointed, representing a mix of scientific and practical experience. The group analyses the literature, explores clinical experience, and builds a consensus leading to draft guidelines. Since scientific evidence is often lacking or conflicting the discussions are often extensive. Only 5% to 10% of guidelines can be based on scientific evidence (Grol, Thomas, and Roberts, 1995).

The draft guidelines are sent for comment to 50 randomly selected general practitioners and to external reviewers who are usually experts in the subject. After this review, the working party has to defend its guidelines before a critical group of general practitioners with high academic and professional standing. The definitive guidelines are then published in the scientific journal for Dutch family physicians and educational programs are developed. Finally, the impact of the guidelines is assessed by surveys and updates are provided when new evidence becomes available. About half the members of working groups are general practitioners with academic appointments, some of whom have done research on the subject of the guidelines. The Dutch system would only be possible in a country where general practice research and academic general practice are well supported.

With the growth of managed care, there are fears that guidelines will eventually become mandatory, thus limiting the clinical freedom of physicians to apply them with discretion. There is a fear also that, in legal cases, failure to follow the guidelines may be used as evidence of malpractice.

Preventive Methods in Family Practice

The source of a family doctor's effectiveness is his knowledge of the strengths and vulnerabilities of individual patients and their families. Statistical probabilities and authoritative recommendations always have to be applied to an individual. A heavy smoker should be counseled to stop, but what if he is a chronic schizophrenic who derives from smoking one of his few comforts? Amniocentesis should be offered to pregnant women aged 35 or over, or if her risk of having a Down's syndrome child is similar to that of a 35-year-old woman. But what if she is a 33-year-old single mother with poor coping skills and doubts about her ability to raise a Down's syndrome child, or if she is a married woman whose husband is ambivalent about parenthood? Family doctors' knowledge of their patients can enhance their effectiveness in other ways: interventions can be made when patients are most receptive to them, and opportunities can be taken to increase patients' confidence in their health.

For many years one of the mainstays of preventive medicine in family practice has been the annual physical examination, at which a history and physical examination are combined with a battery of screening tests. The practice of applying a package of screening tests to a population is also called "multiphasic screening." Experimental evidence available has failed to show that the type of multiphasic screening applied during an annual physical examination has an impact on overall mortality rates (Holland et al., 1977, Dales, Friedman, and Collen, 1979). These studies failed to demonstrate any statistically significant differences in the overall death rates between the treatment and control groups. However, in one study (Dales et al., 1979) mortality from some of the diseases to which screening was directed showed significantly improved rates in the screening group. These findings indicate that screening programs must be evaluated by specific as well as overall mortality.

As a preventive strategy for family practice, the annual physical examination is also open to a number of other objections:

1. It bears little relation to the specific needs of different age groups.
2. Because of the global nature of the complete physical examination, it often includes tests that fail to fulfill the criteria for acceptance of a screening or case finding procedure—electrocardiography, for example.
3. Tests may be repeated at yearly intervals when a much lesser frequency would be equally effective.

4. In most practices complete physicals are given only to that section of the population who demand it or at least are compliant. If every member of a practice of 2,000 patients had a 20-minute annual health examination it would occupy the physician full time for 22 weeks of every year.

In other words, the annual physical is a poorly thought-out strategy for applying modern knowledge of preventive medicine in family practice.

The approach to prevention called "the periodic health examination" provides a more rational strategy for family practice. It is based on the following principles:

1. Tests and procedures are repeated at intervals determined by epidemiological evidence, not by arbitrary choice.
2. Where feasible, these are grouped into "packages," so that the number of visits the patient has to make are reduced.
3. Maximum use is made of the opportunity for case-finding provided by visits for all purposes. In 1 year, 70% of the practice population is seen at least once. The average number of visits for each patient is about four per year. In the course of 5 years, virtually the whole population of the practice will pass through the physician's office. A relatively straightforward procedure like detection of hypertension can be performed almost entirely as a case-finding maneuver.
4. Screening tests and procedures are not included unless there is good evidence for their effectiveness. For example, there is no justification for including a chest X-ray.

Since the periodic health examination makes a more efficient use of time and resources than the annual examination, the strategy can be applied to the whole practice population. The whole practice team, including family practice nurse and public health nurse, can participate in the process.

The Organizational Tools

To practice preventive medicine in an organized way, the practice needs a well-designed record system. Two types of records are required:

1. For the individual patient. If all visits to the physician are to be used for case-finding, the physician should be able to see at a glance from the patient's record which preventive procedures the patient has had and which procedures are needed in any particular year. This can be done by means of a flow chart. Different types of flow charts can be used for different age and sex groups.
2. For the whole practice population. Unless there is some system for monitoring preventive procedures in the whole population, there will be no way of knowing whether the practices' preventive targets have achieved or not. There will be no way of knowing which children remain unimmunized, which adults have not had a blood pressure reading, which women have not had a pap smear or mammography, or which diabetics have not attended for follow-up.

Record keeping in family practice has progressed rapidly with the increasing use of electronic record systems. It remains true, however, that some practitioners have not completed the transition to these systems and remain with paper-based records. Even with simple paper records many useful tools have been developed to enable tracking of preventive medicine procedures. One useful system is the practice age/sex register. A simpler method is to attach a colored tag or sticker to the chart when a particular procedure has been done. A red tag on the chart could mean that the blood pressure had been recorded in the years 2006 or 2007. By quickly looking through all the charts at the end of 2008, one could then identify those patients who had not had a blood pressure reading done in the previous 2 years. This method can also be used for identifying patients who are at special risk.

Computerized record systems used in family practice have made possible preventive medicine reminders tailored to the patient to appear on the screen at the time of the visit. So, for example, if a woman has not had a mammogram in the recommended time frame, when she is visiting for a prescription renewal, a prompt appears on her electronic record and the physician is able to use the visit to remind her of the importance of having the test done.

Electronic patient records also make it easy to derive aggregate data from a practice population, fulfilling the second requirement mentioned. Family physicians with such systems are able to quickly obtain a list of all diabetic patients in their practice and even display the average hemoglobin A1C for that cohort of patients. Insurance companies and government health insurance plans are using the achievement of preventive medicine benchmarks, such as this, to provide incentives to practitioners. In addition, a family physician can introduce a program to increase the uptake of, for example, influenza vaccinations and measure the degree of success by comparing practice-based immunization rates before and after.

Preventive Procedures for Specific Conditions

Excellent online resources detailing recommended preventive procedures are available from the Canadian Task Force on Preventive Health Care (www.ctfphc.org/) and the U.S. Preventive Services Task Force (www.ahrq.gov/clinic/uspstfix.htm). These databases are updated and are relevant to family physicians.

References

Antonovsky A. 1979. *Health, Stress and Coping.* San Francisco, CA: Jossey-Bass.
Antonovsky A. 1987. *Unravelling the Mystery of Health.* San Francisco, CA: Jossey-Bass.
Burke BL, Arkowitz H, Menchola M. 2003. The efficacy of motivational interviewing: a meta-analysis of clinical trials.*Journal of Consulting and Clinical Psychology* 71(5):843–871.
The Canadian Guide to Clinical Preventive Health Care. 1994. The Canadian Task Force on the Periodic Health Examination. Ottawa: Health Canada.

Canadian Medical Association Office for Public Health. (2001). *Health Promotion and Injury Prevention*. Retrieved August 8, 2008, http://www.cma.ca/index.cfm/ci_id/3391/la_id/1.htm

Collins R, Peto R, MacMahon S, Herbert P, Fiebach NH, Eberlein KA, et al. 1990. Blood pressure, stroke, and coronary heart disease. II. Short-term reductions in blood pressure: overview of randomized drug trials in their epidemiologic context. *Lancet* 335:827–838.

Cook RJ, Sackett DL. 1995. The number needed to treat: A clinically useful measure of treatment effect. *British Medical Journal* 310:452–454.

Dales LG, Friedman GD, Collen MF. 1979. Evaluating periodic multiphasic health check-ups: A controlled trial. *Journal of Chronic Disease* 32:385.

Dubos R. 1980. *Man Adapting*. New Haven, CT:Yale University Press.

Feinstein AR. 1988. Scientific standards in epidemiologic studies of the menace of daily life. *Science* 2(242):1257–1263.

Foss L, Rothenberg K. 1987. *The Second Medical Revolution: From Biomedicine to Infomedicine*. Boston, MA: Shambhala.

Fradet Y. 2007. Should Canadians be offered systematic prostate cancer screening?: YES. *Canadian Family Physician*, June 53(6):989–992.

Freed LA, Benjamin EJ, Levy D, Larson MG, Evans JC, Fuller DL, Lehman B, Levine RA. 2002. Mitral Valve Prolapse in the general population: The benign nature of echocardiographic features in the Framingham Heart Study. *Journal of the American College of Cardiology* 40(7):1298–1304.

Galen RS, Gambino SR. 1975. *Beyond Normality: The Predictive Value and Efficiency of Medical Diagnoses*. New York: John Wiley.

Gordon I. 1958. That damned word health. *Lancet* 2:638–639.

Grol R, Thomas S, Roberts R. 1995. Development and implementation of guidelines for family Practice: Lessons from the Netherlands. *Journal of Family Practice* 40(5):435–439.

Hayes MV. 1992. On the Epistemology of risk: Langauge, logic and social science. *Social Science Medicine* 35(4)401–407.

Hepner AD, Ahmadi-Kashani M, Movahed MR. 2007. The prevalence of mitral valve prolapse in patients undergoing echocardiography for clinical reason. *International Journal of Cardiology* 123(1):55–57.

Holland WW et al. 1977. A controlled trial of multiphasic screening in middle age: Results from the SE London screening study. *International Journal of Epidemiology* 6:357.

Hollnagel H, Malterud K. 1995. Shifting attention from objective risk factors to patients' self-assessed health resources: A clinical model for general practice. *Family Practice* 12(4):423–429.

Idler EL. 1992. Self-Assessed Health and Mortality: A review of studies. In: Maes S, Leventhal H, Johnston, M. eds., *International Review of Health Psychology*. John Wiley & Sons Ltd., pp. 33–54.

Labrecque M, Légaré F, Cauchon M. 2007. Should Canadians be offered systematic prostate cancer screening?: NO. *Canadian Family Physician*, June 53(6): 989–992.

Laupacis A, Sackett DL, Roberts RS. 1988. An assessment of clinically useful measures of the consequences of treatment. *New England Journal of Medicine* 318:1728–1733.

Leventhal H, Brissette I, Leventhal, EA. 2003. The common-sense model of self-regulation of health and illness. In: Katouzian, HD, Cameron LD, Leventhal H. eds., *The Self-regulation of Health and Illness Behaviour*. London: Routledge, chapter 13.

Lorig K, Mazonson PD, Holman HR. 1993. Evidence suggesting that health education for self-management in patients with chronic arthritis has sustained health benefits while reducing health care costs. *Arthritis and Rheumatism* 36:439–446.

McCormick J. 1994. Health promotion: The ethical dimension. *Lancet* 344:390–391.

Moore WS, Barnet HJM, Beebe HG, et al. 1995. Guidelines for carotid endarterectomy: A multidisciplinary consensus statement from the Ad Hoc Committee, American Heart Association. *Stroke* 26:188–201.

Mossey JM, Shapiro E. 1982. Self-rated Health: A predictor of mortality among the Elderly. *American Journal of Public Health* 72(8):800–808.

Murphy EA. 1976. *The Logic of Medicine*. Baltimore, MD: Johns Hopkins University Press.

O'Connor A, Tugwell P. 1995. Making Choices: Hormones after the menopause (cassette and booklet). University of Ottawa.

Prochaska JO 1979. Systems of Psychotherapy: A Transtheoretical Analysis. Homewood IL: Dorsey Press..

Raffle AE, Alden B, Mackenzie EFD. 1995. Detection rates for abnormal cervical smears: What are we screening for? *Lancet* 345:1469–1473.

Rich-Edwards JW, Manson JAE, Hennekens CH, Buring JE. 1995. The primary prevention of coronary heart disease in women. *New England Journal of Medicine* June:1758–1766.

Rosser WW, Palmer WH, Fowler G, Lamberts H, et al. 1993. An international perspective on the cholesterol debate. *Family Practice* 10(4):431–437.

Russel LB. 1994. *Educated Guesses*. Berkley, CA: University of California Press.

Ryle J. 1948 The meaning of normal and the measurement of health. Chapter 6 in: *Changing Disciplines*. New York: Oxford University Press,pp. 66–83.

Siegrist J. 1993. Sense of coherence and sociology of emotions. Comment on Antonovsky. *Social Science and Medicine* 37:974–979.

Skolbekken JA. 1995. The risk epidemic in medical journals. *Social Science and Medicine* 40(3):291–305.

Skrabanek P, McCormick J. 1990. *Follies and Fallacies in Medicine*. Glasgow: The Tarragon Press.

Sobel DS. 1995. Rethinking medicine: Improving health outcomes with cost-effective psychosocial interventions. *Psychosomatic Medicine* 57:234–244.

U.S. Preventive Services Task Force. 1996. *Guide to Clinical Preventive Services*, 2nd edn. Baltimore, MD: Williams and Wilkins.

Walter, Fiona and Emery J. 2005. Coming down the line-patient's understanding of their family history of chronic disease. *Annals of Family Medicine* September–October 3(50): 405–414.

Walter FM, Emery J. 2006. Perceptions of family history across common diseases: A qualitative study in primary care. *Family Practice* 23(4):472–480.

Notes

1. For additional reading see the excellent series of articles in the *Canadian Medical Association Journal* (Marshall KG. 1996: May 15, June 15, July 15, and August 15).

2. I am indebted to Professor Hanne Hollnagel for this way of explaining risk reduction.

10

The Family in Health and Disease

The importance of the family to family physicians is inherent in the paradigm of family medicine. Family medicine does not separate disease from person or person from environment. It recognizes the strong connection between health and disease, and personality, way of life, physical environment, and human relationships. It understands the strong influence that human relationships have on the outcome of illness and recognizes the family as the crucible of the development of the person.

Doherty and Baird (1987) describe four levels of physician involvement with families. The first is minimal involvement. The second is the provision of information and advice. To practice at this level, the physician has to be open to engaging families in a collaborative way, taking care to communicate medical findings and treatment options to family members, and listening attentively to their questions and concerns. This does not require special knowledge of family development or reactions to stressful experiences.

The physician at the third level includes the above, but also has an understanding of the affective aspects of family relationships. The physician is therefore able to provide emotional support and to help family members deal with the feelings aroused by having a family member with illnesses such as cancer, schizophrenia, diabetes, and physical disability. To practice at this level, the physician needs a knowledge of family development and of how families react to stressful experiences. He or she has to be a skilled listener, responsive to the subtle cues by which emotional needs are expressed. Also needed is enough self-knowledge to be aware of how the physician's own feelings affect his or her relationship with the patient and family.

At the fourth level, the physician can carry out a systematic assessment of family function and plan an intervention designed to help a family deal with its problems. This will often include reframing the family's definition of the problem and encouraging them to consider new ways of coping with their difficulties. To practice at this level, the physician needs an understanding of systems theory and the skills of convening and conducting a family conference. This may include engaging family members who are reluctant to participate and encouraging poorly communicating family members to express themselves.

Levels three and four must be distinguished from family therapy, which is based on the idea that the identified patient is a "symptom" of family dysfunction. Therapy is therefore directed toward the whole family system. At levels three and four, a member of the family is sick and the physician is helping the family to care for the patient. Of course, the levels may overlap with family therapy. A family with a sick member may also be dysfunctional; but family physicians will mostly be helping ordinary families mobilize resources to improve their coping skills.

Confusion has arisen from time to time between family medicine and family therapy. In family therapy, the physician can carry out a planned course of therapy for a dysfunctional family. The physician requires the insight and skill to intervene in such a way as to change the way the family functions. The few family physicians working at this level are trained family therapists who combine the roles of family physician and family therapist, some of them receiving referrals from other family physicians.

The therapist's aim is to change the way the family functions. He or she usually has no continuing commitment to maintain the health of individual members of the family. If change in the family is against the interests of an individual member, then the needs of the family may take precedence over the individual.

There are other differences between family therapist and family physician.[1] Therapists starting to work with a family are not usually encumbered by previous relationships with individual members. They begin as neutral and detached observers. Family physicians, on the other hand, will often be the object of different feelings in different members of a family. The physician may be seen, for example, as an ally by the wife, as an enemy by the husband, as an authoritarian parent by the children. Similarly, it is difficult for the family physician to avoid bias toward or against one or other member of the family. The family therapist has no other commitment to members of the family than to conduct family therapy. The family physician, even if trying to help a family to change, still has to treat the wife's urinary infection, the children's respiratory infections, or the husband's depression. At the end of therapy, the family therapist usually has no further responsibility to the family. The family physician's responsibility to its individual members is open-ended. The context in which the family physician works is worlds away from the working context of a family therapist. This does not mean that family physicians do not help families to change: it means that they do it in their own way, appropriate to their own context. Failure to understand this has led to disappointment in psychiatrists and behavioral scientists who have tried to teach family therapy to family physicians, and to family physicians who have confused their mission. It is yet another example of the truth that clinical methods cannot be transferred unmodified from one context to another.

Brennan (1974) has made the important distinction between "the person in the family" and "the family in the person." The person in the family represents the interpersonal relationships in the family group. The family in the person represents the individual's incorporated experience of his or her family of origin— an experience that profoundly affects self-concept and relationships with others. A person is raised and nurtured in a family for the early years of life, but the family remains "in" the person until his death.

Of course, family physicians are not the only clinicians who have this understanding of the family. Other physicians, especially those providing long-term care, may work with an awareness of the family context. Family physicians cannot claim to be the sole possessors of this knowledge. Whether a physician does so, however, is largely a matter of training. A physician who has not learned to "think family" in his training is not likely to "think family" in practice. The experience of one of the authors (IRMcW) provides an example. "My preparation for general practice was a year as resident in internal medicine, culminating in the Membership of the Royal College of Physicians (MRCP). When I entered practice I had no concept of the importance of the family in medicine. For example, I did not even make the connection between severe headaches in a young man and the fact that his child had muscular dystrophy. It was not for many years that, under the influence of academic family medicine, I developed some capacity for "thinking family." Other physicians can work with families, but the fact is that outside family medicine, few are trained to do so.

Although a clinician from another discipline may, by his ability to "think family," resemble a family physician, there remain some important differences arising from the fact that the latter often cares for several members of the family. First, this personal knowledge of individual members can give the physician the advantage of a knowledge of the family context that can be obtained in no other way.

Case 10.1

A young married woman with no children came to see me (IRMcW) with lower abdominal pains. Because she had previously had an ectopic pregnancy, this was suspected at first. Observation in the hospital was sufficient to exclude this diagnosis. The pains continued, however, and it became clear that the patient was going through a severe marital crisis. During the same week, her husband came to see me with intercostal muscle pain and her father attended with depression, neither of them connecting their problems with the family situation. The illnesses of husband and father took on a new meaning in the context of the crisis in the family. The crisis came to a head in the same week with the separation of husband and wife.

It could be argued that a physician caring for any one of these individuals could, by attentive listening, have obtained the same knowledge about the family. The knowledge, however, would have been of a different quality from that obtained through personal relationship with all three members and would probably not have been applied until extensive investigations had been done.

The picture of a family obtained through the eyes of one of its members is often very different from the picture obtained from the physician's personal knowledge of other family members. This derives from the reality that the family experience is different for each member of the family. Accepting without corroboration the

version given by one family member is one of the most common pitfalls for the
family physician.

Case 10.2

A man who was already a patient of the practice married a woman from another
town. Soon after their marriage the husband came to see me (IRMcW) because he
was worried about his wife's behavior. From his description I thought she might be
developing schizophrenia. I suggested that she herself should come to see me. She
did not come, but soon afterwards I was asked to see her at home because she was
vomiting. Her husband was there when I visited. It soon became clear that she had
hyperemesis gravidarum. I explained the problem and its management and arranged
for follow-up. Apart from some reticence, her behavior seemed normal. Shortly after
my visit, the husband told me that she had left him and returned to her home town.
I heard no more until she came to see me one day, late in her pregnancy. She came
to explain her sudden departure. Soon after her marriage she had developed a deep
antipathy toward her husband because of his behavior toward her. Shortly after my
visit things had come to a head and she had decided to leave him. She had returned
to her home town and made arrangements to have the baby there. There was no evidence of mental instability.

When the physician does have personal knowledge of all family members he or
she may be able to form hypotheses based on this personal knowledge.

Case 10.3

An elderly woman who shared a house with her sister had troublesome neuroderma-
titis and seemed anxious and tense. Her sister was also a patient and always produced
in me (IRMcW) a vague feeling of threat and uneasiness. I wondered if she was having the same effect on her sister. The response to the question "How do you get on
with your sister?" was an outburst of feeling.

The second advantage of caring for the whole family is the increase in management options available to the family physician. If, for example, the physician has
determined that the problem with a crying baby is the mother's exhaustion and
depression, attention can be turned to the mother.

Caring for more than one member of a family can lead the physician to some
ethical issues that do not arise in other fields of medicine. These issues arise when
the interests of different family members conflict. Dealing successfully with them
requires both moral awareness and a knowledge of pitfalls.

It could still be maintained that this knowledge and these skills are not unique
to family medicine. An internist could care for a family with adult members in
exactly the same way. Of course he could, and he would be functioning as a
family physician. The name and the academic pigeonhole are not really important. In practice, however, we still doubt whether many physicians outside family
medicine are trained to think and practice in this way.

Family Norms

In Western countries, we tend to assume that the norms we take for granted in
human development and family function are universal. Western assumptions

about the value of individual autonomy, and the need to raise children to be independent are foreign to the cultures of India, Japan, and many other countries. Child rearing in India and Japan, for example, fosters dependence and interdependence. India is a "high context" society (see p. 122). Roland (1988) observes that "contextualizing rather than universalising is central to Indian cognition.... Everything from the...time of day, which has its own moods and flow, to specific houses [and] landscapes...have their own substances, gross or subtle, which flow from their context to those around through permeable ego boundaries...everything in one's environment becomes personalised." These characteristics are compellingly captured in literature (Mistry, 2002).

Although the norms are so different between one culture and another, the importance of family relationships in health and disease is universal. Differences between cultures may have therapeutic implications. Family studies in the West and in India have shown that Indian families have a higher tolerance and acceptance of family members with schizophrenia, and are less likely to respond to them with negative emotions (Leff, 1989). While highly interdependent kinship groups may limit individual freedom, they can also provide strong support in illness and adversity. A high value placed on independence can lead to different needs in family members that are difficult to reconcile without conflict. In a culture of restrictive family relationships, individuals may be expected to sacrifice their own aspirations for the greater good of the family, and to stifle their feelings. Roland (1988) observes that Indian women who are obliged to bottle up their feelings often develop somatic symptoms. In contrast to people with similar illnesses in Western countries, however, Indians are more likely to understand the connection between their symptoms and the stresses of living in the extended family.

Among immigrant families, the first generation born in the new culture tends to adopt its values rather than those of their parents. The stage is then set for a stressful intergenerational conflict.

What Is a Family?

The changing nature of the family in industrial societies has led some to question whether the idea of a family physician is still appropriate. The error here is to identify "family" with a particular kinship group, such as the so-called nuclear family of father, mother, and children. If a family is defined as a group of intimates with both a history and a future (Ransom and Vandervoort, 1973), then the actual structure of the group may vary without changing its essential function. Any general practice is likely to contain family groups of different kinds. Most families will probably represent the common kinship group in the culture from which the practice population is drawn. This will vary in different parts of the world, according to whether the practice is in North America, Latin America, the West Indies, Africa, and so on. It may also vary within the same country, for example, if the practice has an immigrant, native, or inner city population.

Although most families in a practice will probably be conventional kinship groups, other kinds of family will almost certainly be represented. There is nothing new in this. When I (IRMcW) entered practice in the 1950s, these non-typical family groups were quite common: elderly women living together, often widowed or unmarried sisters; unmarried brothers and sisters; male or female couples living in stable relationships; elderly widowers with housekeepers who had become part of the family; and gay couples. We took it for granted that these groups functioned like families.

The decline of the extended family in many industrialized societies has been overemphasized. It is true that many families become widely scattered, but modern communications make it much easier for family members to remain in touch with each other, and to come together at times of crisis. It is not unusual nowadays for families to come together from the ends of the earth.

Recent Changes in the Structure and Function of the Family

Since the 1960s, big changes have occurred in the composition, activities, and economic status of families in most Western industrialized societies. Because many of the changes have been dislocating, their impact has been felt in the kind of health problems encountered by family physicians. Fragile families, buffeted by adverse social and economic forces, have become a source of the "new morbidity" (Haggerty, 1975): spousal and parental violence, sexual abuse, parental neglect, developmental and learning disabilities, substance abuse, emotional distress, eating disorders and premature parenthood. Domestic violence itself spawns or exacerbates many other health problems that present to family physicians (Heise, Pitanguy, and Germain, 1994; Day 1995).

In the United States, the poverty rate has declined from more than 20% in 1959 to 12.6% in 2005 (DeNavas-Walt, Proctor, and Lee, 2006). Nevertheless more than one in five children are now living in poverty, and the poverty rate exceeds one in four in female-headed households (Schor and Menaghan, 1995; U.S. Census Bureau, 2006). This is of great importance as poverty is a powerful determinant of health.

The United States has seen an increase in the average age at marriage and in families without children younger than 18 years. There is a greater proportion of births to women older than 30 years. The rate of births to unmarried women went from 5.3% in 1960 to 33.2% in 2000. Divorce rates have nearly doubled compared to the 1950s. Single parent families headed by women have experienced a growth of 131% since 1970, and these families report incomes that are only 47% those of married-couple families. As more women come into the workforce, there has occurred an increased demand for alternative childcare arrangements. There is a hidden cost to these arrangements as they lead to longer days for children and more exposure to infectious diseases. Care by baby boomers to their own parents has led to the designation "sandwich generation" as they try to balance the needs of elderly family with those of the younger generation. Children are increasingly raised in a media rich environment of television, computers, cell phones and so on, over which there seems to be little control. Not surprisingly, many parents express concerns about their own abilities to meet the competing demands and challenges represented by these changes (American Academy of Pediatrics, 2003). Pregnant teenagers are a particularly vulnerable group, tending to come from poorer families and to have poorer education and job prospects. In 1988, 61% of children lived with both biological parents, 19% with the mother only, 9% with mother and stepfather, and 11% in some other family arrangement. A much higher proportion of African-American families have a single parent, usually female.

There are links between economic trends and these changes in family composition and stability. High rates of unemployment and lower earning capacity among males are associated with lower marriage rates, more births to single women, and increased likelihood of marital disruption.

Poverty is the strongest predictor of poor health in children as indicated by mortality rates, activity limitations, and utilization of health care. The overwhelming majority of families who are failing to carry out their functions in child rearing are poor. In the United States, the Food Research and Action Center reported that about 5.5 million children had experienced hunger in the previous month (Community Childhood Hunger Identification Project, 1991). Residential fires are among the leading causes of death due to injury in children aged 1 to 5 (Baker, O'Neill, Ginsburg, and Li, 1992). Recent estimates of the number of homeless in the United States are that 744,000 people are in this situation. While the majority of these individuals are single adults, 41% were in families (National Alliance to End Homelessness, 2007).

The relationship between poverty and family function is a complex one. A strong family in a stable and supportive community can mitigate many of the adverse effects of poverty. On the other hand, poverty can weaken the ability of a family's ability to carry out its nurturing functions. Poverty is associated with pregnancy in poorly educated young single mothers, who have neither the earning capacity to provide for their children nor the parenting skills to care for them. Far from having supportive communities, they are condemned by their poverty to living in violent and socially disorganized neighborhoods.

Family physicians can do little to remedy these social ills in their relationships with families in their practice. Nevertheless, there is much they can do to mitigate their effects in collaboration with nurses and social workers. Family doctors are often aware of vulnerable families whom they can support and put in touch with social agencies. They can be sensitive to the cues to family violence and competent in bringing it to notice and dealing with it. They can be especially attentive to the needs of children and adolescents from poor, unstable, or abusive families.

What It Means to "Think Family"

A family is a social organization or system and has features in common with other social systems. A system, it will be recalled, is defined as a number of parts and processes standing in mutual interaction with each other. The family system changes over time as its members grow older. Part of "thinking family" is an awareness of the challenges faced by a family in adapting to these changes.

Any change in one part of the family system has repercussions for the whole family. A major change—birth, death, marriage, divorce, disability, loss of job—has profound effects. A family physician has to be attentive to the needs of family members affected by the misfortunes of their relatives: the children of divorced couples; the siblings of a disabled adolescent; the widows and widowers; the wife of an unemployed man.

Social systems depend for their proper functioning on information and communication. Problems in the family are often due to remediable difficulties in communication, especially the communication of feelings. "Thinking family" is being aware of a physician's responsibility for providing good information, and being vigilant for communication blocks within a family.

"Thinking family" is being sensitive to the unmentioned family stresses that often lie behind depression and somatic symptoms such as headaches, dyspepsia, or recurrent abdominal pain. It is also being aware of the effects on the family system of the physician's own actions—admitting somebody to the hospital, making a serious diagnosis. The case described on page 189 is an example of the failure to "think family."

"Thinking family" is being aware of some of the traps that await the unwary physician: being enlisted by one side of a family conflict, accepting the family's views of a troublesome adolescent, and disclosing to other family members information that should be confidential.

The Influence of the Family on Health and Disease

The family has six main effects on the health of its members.

Genetic Influences
Every individual is a product of the interaction between his genotype and the environment. Recent advances in describing and understanding the human genome makes it more important that family physicians be conversant with and able to communicate the significance of the results of genetic counseling to patients and their families.

The Family Is Crucial in Child Development
Although children have a remarkable capacity for overcoming early difficulties, there is a large body of evidence supporting the relationship between family dysfunction and childhood disorders—both physical and behavioral.

Parental deprivation for prolonged periods is associated with psychological problems, including suicide, depression, and personality disorder. The relationship is by no means constant, and the outcome depends on individual factors such as the previous parent–child relationship and the availability of parent substitutes. The evidence is sufficiently suggestive, however, for the family physician to advise parents to avoid separation from the child whenever possible in the crucial stage between 3 months and 4 years. When separation is unavoidable, as in the serious illness of mother or child, care should be taken to minimize the trauma by providing a good mother-substitute or by keeping the child's time in the hospital to a minimum.

The Newcastle-upon-Tyne "Thousand Families" study (Miller, Court, Walton, and Knox, 1960) is one of the few long-term studies of families designed to explore the relationship between child health and family function. A group of 1,142 infants was enrolled at the beginning of the study in 1947. These children and their families were observed and examined over a 15-year period by a team of health visitors (public health nurses) and pediatricians. By 1962, 763 children remained in the study. The results are generally applicable to any industrial community, although allowances must be made for the preponderance of working class families and the comparative poverty of the community in the early years of the study.

Respiratory disease was the most common health problem. In the first 5 years it accounted for half of all the illness and two-thirds of all infections. The frequency and severity declined during the school years, but the ratio of respiratory to total illness remained. At all ages the incidence and severity of lower respiratory infection was strongly related to adverse family factors. In 1961, 45 children had some disability due to respiratory disease: 6 had suppurative otitis media, 11 recurrent bronchitis, 10 asthma, 6 allergic rhinitis, and 4 bronchiectasis.

Intestinal infections were strongly related to inadequate housing, overcrowding, and poor maternal care. In 20 "streptococcal families" there were repeated streptococcal infections in different family members over months or years. In 25 "staphylococcal families" there was a similar pattern of repeated staphylococcal infections. Staphylococcal infection in preschool children was strongly associated with large families, overcrowding, and poor maternal care.

Nonfebrile convulsions were significantly associated with low social class, a family history of seizures, mental illness, parental deprivation, and defective child care.

Accidents in the first 5 years accounted for 8 percent of the total illness and nearly 50 percent of noninfectious illness. The peak incidence was in the second year. In this age group, more than half the accidents occurred at home. Accidents during the school years more commonly occurred away from home. At all ages there was a significant association with poor maternal care and low intelligence in the child.

Enuresis affected 18% of children at 5 years, 12% at 10, 6% at 13, and 2% at 15. Enuretic children were smaller than noneneuretic children, had a lower mean IQ, and more of them were maladjusted. Enuresis was associated with low social class, overcrowding, poor maternal care, and absence or ineffectiveness of the father. The authors conclude that "bedwetting is seen as a developmental disability, mainly determined by the interaction of adverse social, emotional and intellectual factors." Dysrhythmic speech was found in 43 children, and nine still stuttered at the age of 15. Stuttering was more common in children from families with adverse factors.

Children with behavioral disturbance (nearly 20%) were below the mean in height, weight, intelligence, school attainment, and ability to communicate. Their parents were younger, more recently married, often lived with relations, and tended to be dependent on their parents. A high proportion of mothers had a history of mental illness and had experienced severe stress during pregnancy. Miller and his colleagues conclude, "At the centre of maladjustment was a deeply unsatisfactory relationship between mother and child. Separation was a contributory factor, but mainly through intensifying preexisting family instability. The extent of maladjustment suggests urgent need for a critical study of existing methods of treatment and a more intensive search for rational ways of prevention."

Other work has continued to demonstrate the importance of parenting and the harmful effect of parenting failure on child development. Klaus and Kennell (1976) have demonstrated the importance of early postnatal bonding between mother and child, a relationship enhanced by breast-feeding but made more difficult by some of the procedures used in obstetric units.

Parental neglect, both physical and emotional, is considered to be the most common cause of failure to thrive. In emotionally deprived children, the secretion of growth hormone is reduced. Inadequate parenting has a range of effects on child development, from physical trauma at one end of the scale to mild behavior disorders at the other. What makes this doubly important is that children deprived of adequate parenting are likely to repeat the same pattern when they themselves become parents.

A number of longitudinal studies (Batty, 2004; Smith and Joshi, 2002), along with new knowledge from the neurosciences have provided important insights into the influence of early environment (biological, psychological, and social) and family life on later health. Life course research has begun to emphasize that many of the chronic diseases of adult life have their roots in early childhood. The concept of developmental "windows" for the optimal establishment of various human functions is important to understanding the impact of early family life on later health.

The Early Years Study (McCain and Mustard, 1999) summarizes the literature on environmental influences on the developing neuroarchitecture of children. The first few years of life represent a window of opportunity that, if missed because of poor nutrition, or physical and psychological stress, has an enduring impact. In this early time period, as neural connections are made and nurtured, the groundwork for functions such as binocular vision, emotional competence, habitual ways of responding, and language are laid down. After age 6 it becomes much more difficult to make changes in these areas. If the child receives inadequate or inappropriate stimulation during this period, he or she will be more prone to learning difficulties, behavioral and emotional problems later in life. For some this may include juvenile delinquency and crime. Further, poor nutrition in early life predisposes to later development of hypertension, diabetes, and obesity. The neural and endocrine responses to stress are determined during these early years and, in both animal and human studies, it has been shown that poor nurturing in this time period leads to prolonged hormonal responses, long after the original stimulation has subsided. This has negative long-term biological effects, for although stress hormones are a useful short-term adaptation, when prolonged they cause multiple deleterious effects. When there is a dysfunctional development of the limbic system and midbrain, it appears that children live in a constant state of low-grade arousal that may negatively impact on their learning capabilities. They become labeled as learning disabled and may resort to inappropriately aggressive behavior in order to cope with their stress.

Longitudinal studies have demonstrated that women who experience family disruption and conflict during their early years were more prone to depression and other mental health problems in adult life (Maughan and McCarthy, 1997). The advent of longitudinal studies has contributed to a new area of epidemiology called the *life history approach*. Emotional learning in early life happens implicitly, begins before birth and is shaped in the "limbic nexus" of family life. The concept of "limbic attractors" has been borrowed from systems theory to explain the tendency of repeating certain emotional behavioral responses, even when we desire a different outcome. This has been used to explain the observation that some individuals repeatedly enter into damaging relationships, for example.

Some Families Are More Vulnerable to Illness Than Others
In a long-term study of families in family practice, Huygen (1982) has described and analyzed his experience with families in a rural community in Holland over a period of more than 30 years. As one part of his study, he examined family influences on morbidity in samples of 100 young families and 100 older families. In the young families there was a significant correlation between morbidity rates in members of the same family. The correlation was greatest between mothers and children. The differences between families in frequency of illness tended to be stable over the years. Families with high morbidity rates tended to be high over the whole 20-year period, and those with low rates tended to be low over the whole period. The differences between families with high and low rates were not explained by factors such as hygiene, housing, and income. There were, however, significant relationships between emotional stability in the parents and family illness rates. Illness rates were higher in families where one or both parents were emotionally unstable and where there was marital discord.

In the older families, similar relationships were found. There was a familial incidence of disorders of the skin, respiratory tract, and gastrointestinal tract, and of nervous disorders, and accidents. In nervous disorders the correlations were significant only between father and mother, and there were no significant correlations between parents for accidents and gastrointestinal disorders. Further analysis showed that vulnerable families were susceptible to the whole range of these disorders, not one particular category. This is consistent with the finding of Hinkle (1974) that vulnerable individuals are susceptible to the whole spectrum of diseases "across the board," leading him to formulate the concept of "general susceptibility to illness."

Huygen found that members of the same family, although similar in their illness patterns, were not similar in their rates of patient–doctor consultations and admission to the hospital. This suggests that the similarities between family members were due to similar frequencies of illness rather than to similarities of illness behavior.

In 1970, Huygen and his colleagues carried out a cross-sectional study of 210 randomly selected families from his practice who had not been involved in the earlier studies. The children were between 12 and 22 years and the parents' ages ranged from 40 to 64. Medical students visited the families and collected data on sense of well-being, symptoms, medical knowledge, readiness to seek medical help, anxiety level, and experience with serious illness in their neighborhood. These data were related to the number of contacts with the family doctor and number of diagnoses between 1967 and 1970.

There were highly significant correlations between family members in their sense of well-being and in the number of symptoms experienced. Medical help was sought for less than 10% of all symptoms. There were significant correlations between family members in readiness to seek medical help and in contacts with the family doctor. Anxiety scores, however, showed little correlation between family members.

The psychological and social characteristics of parents showed a stronger relationship with the frequency of illness in their children than with their own. Children had more illnesses when

their parents tended to avoid conflicts;
their mother was little involved in social networks outside the family;
their parents were prone to somatic complaints;
their parents had less than average sense of well-being;
their mother was strongly inclined to accept the sick role;
there was a discrepancy in their parents' knowledge of the complaints of the spouse.

Huygen interpreted these results as supporting Balint's concept of "the child as a presenting symptom."

In a prospective study of the relationship of family structure and functioning, and life events, to the outcome of pregnancy, Ramsey, Abell, and Baker (1986) found that abnormal family functioning was a strong predictor of low birth weight. The abnormalities of function included disengagement, enmeshment, and both rigid and chaotic families.

Infectious Disease Spreads in Families
Streptococcal and staphylococcal family infections have already been mentioned. Meyer and Haggerty (1962) showed that streptococcal infection is related to acute and chronic family stress.

Virus infections have a strong tendency to spread from the index cases to other family members. In their study of family infections in Cleveland, Dingle, Badger, and Jordan (1964) found that infections were introduced into the home, in descending order of frequency, by schoolchildren under6, preschool children, schoolchildren over6, mothers, and fathers. Respiratory and intestinal infections decrease in frequency with increasing age. The number of infections is directly related to family size. Preschool children are the most susceptible to infections because they have not yet acquired immunity. Children starting school are more likely to bring infections home because they are exposed to other children at a time when their immunity is incomplete. The number of infections falls rapidly as immunity is acquired during the early school years.

The same infection may take different forms as it spreads through the family. A virus may produce sore throat in one member, diarrhea in another, cough and coryza in another. The mumps virus may produce parotitis in one member, orchitis in another.

Tuberculosis, venereal diseases, intestinal parasites, and skin infections must be included in any list of family infections.

Family Factors Affect Morbidity and Mortality in Adults

Mortality is significantly increased in widowers and widows in the first year after bereavement. This increase in mortality is not confined to one or two causes of death: it covers the whole range of diseases.

Mortality for most causes of death is much higher among widowed, divorced, and single people than among the married. Widowers are especially susceptible. Kraus and Lilienfeld (1959) have shown that young widowers (aged 25–35) have a mortality rate 12 times higher than the comparable married group for tuberculosis, eight times higher for vascular lesions of the nervous system, 10 times higher for hypertensive heart disease, eight times higher for influenza and pneumonia, and nearly five times higher for arteriosclerotic heart disease.

Bereavement is associated with an increase in consultation rate. This probably represents both a true increase in morbidity rate and an increased utilization of medical services.

In counties of North Carolina, stroke mortality in African-American males was significantly related to family disorganization as measured by rates of divorce, separation, and illegitimacy. In males between 35 and 44, mortality increased almost threefold as the level of disorganization increased from the lowest to the highest levels (Nesser, 1975).

Medalie and Goldbourt (1976) showed that males with severe family problems were three times more likely to develop angina than those with a low score for family problems. In males with high anxiety levels, the risk of developing angina was significantly lower in those who received much support and love from their wives than in those who did not.

For reasons that are little understood, husbands and wives are more often concordant for hypertension than would be expected by chance.

Family factors affect not only the occurrence of illness, but also the utilization of medical services. Utilization increases at times of family stress. Clustering of visits may be an important cue to family problems.

The Family Is Important in Recovery from Illness

Family support is an important factor in the outcome of all kinds of illness, but especially in chronic illness and disability. Pless and Satterwhite (1973) found that children with chronic disease fared better in well-functioning than in poorly functioning families.

When combined with the emerging understanding from the neurosciences, a picture is evolving that recognizes the impact of genetic endowment, prenatal and early childhood environment, on later physical and mental health and over the course of a person's lifetime. This begins to provide a unified vision of human health and disease for family practitioners. It fits well with the fundamental assumptions in the discipline of family medicine. When we confront an adult with a new diagnosis, we need to understand the entire history of the patient, not only current and recent life style choices. The physician who has attended a patient for a long period of their life time, perhaps including the prenatal period, delivery, and childhood, has an obvious advantage in coming to an insightful understanding and helping their patient cope realistically with the implications of a new diagnosis, illness, or life event. Indeed, such a physician has become an integral part of the patient's life history and vice versa. In addition, however, this new understanding of the importance of host factors in early life requires physicians to be advocates for measures that address negative environmental influences in early life.

The Family Life Cycle

An understanding of the family life cycle, together with an understanding of individual development, can help the physician form good hypotheses about the problems patients are experiencing. In the course of its development, the family goes through a number of predictable transitions: marriage, childbirth, school years and adolescence, school graduation and starting work or further education, children leaving home, involution, retirement, and widowhood. The physician, by using his insight into these transitions, can help families anticipate and prepare for them, and at the same time can enrich his or her own understanding of the context of illnesses.

Families also experience unexpected crises that demand adaptive responses: illnesses, accidents, divorce, loss of job, and death of a family member.

Duvall (1977) has developed an eight-stage schema of the family life cycle. Duvall's schema is reproduced in Figure 10.1, with the number of years an American family can be expected to spend in each stage. All families, of course, do not go through the complete cycle in sequence. One child may remain in the home after attaining adulthood and may stay there until the parents die. Divorced people with children, if they remarry, go through stages one and four at the same time.

Developmental Tasks

Developmental tasks are defined by Duvall as tasks that arise at a certain stage in the life of the individual or family, adaptation to which may lead to happiness and success with later tasks. Maladaptation to these tasks, on the other hand, may lead to unhappiness, disapproval by society, and difficulty with later tasks. In assuming a developmental task, an individual must (1) perceive new possibilities for his or her behavior, (2) form new conceptions of self, (3) cope effectively with

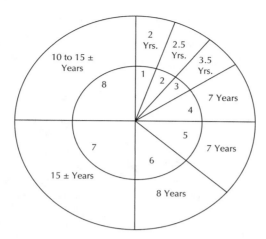

1. Married couples (without children).
2. Childbearing families (oldest child—30 months).
3. Families with preschool children (oldest child 30 months –6 years).
4. Families with school children (oldest child 6–13 years).
5. Families with teenagers (oldest child 13–20 years).
6. Families launching young adults (first child gone to last child leaving home).
7. Middle-aged parents (empty nest to retirement).
8. Aging family members (retirement to death of both spouses).

Figure 10.1 The family life cycle by length of time in each of eight stages. (From Duvall, 1977.)

conflicting demands, and (4) have the motivation to achieve the next stage in his development. Sometimes the developmental tasks of different family members are in harmony, as when a husband and wife are jointly learning to live in an "empty nest." Often, however, developmental tasks of family members are in conflict, and many of the tensions of family life are caused by these conflicts. The adolescent's need to achieve independence almost inevitably brings him into conflict with his parents' task of guiding his development to a responsible maturity. When husband and wife both have careers, their needs for education and career development can easily lead to conflict at some stage in the family life cycle.

Duvall's concept of the developmental tasks facing the family at each stage in its life cycle is shown in Table 10.1. The family's developmental tasks are centered on the family's most important function: the nurturing of children from birth to maturity. They obviously relate closely to the developmental tasks of individual family members.

In recommending the family life cycle and the concept of developmental tasks as a perspective for family physicians, a word of caution is necessary. Families

Table 10.1 Stage-critical family developmental tasks through the family life cycle

Stage of the Family Life Cycle	Positions in the Family	Stage-Critical Family Developmental Tasks
1. Married couple	Wife Husband	Establish a mutually satisfying marriage Adjusting to pregnancy and the promise of parenthood Fitting into a new kin network
2. Childbearing	Wife–mother Husband–father Infant daughter or son or both	Having, adjusting to, and encouraging the development of infants Establishing a satisfying home for both parents and infants
3. Preschool-age	Wife–mother Husband–father Daughter–sister Son–brother	Adapting to the critical needs and interests of preschool children in stimulating, growth-promoting ways Coping with energy depletion and lack of privacy as parents
4. School-age	Wife–mother Husband–father Daughter–sister Son–brother	Fitting into the community of school-age families in constructive ways Encouraging children's educational achievement
5. Teenage	Wife–mother Husband–father Daughter–sister Son–brother	Balancing freedom with responsibility as teenagers mature and emancipate themselves Establish postparental interests and careers as growing parents
6. Launching center	Wife–mother–grandmother Husband–father–grandfather Daughter–sister–aunt Son–brother–uncle	Releasing young adults into work, military service, marriage, etc., with appropriate rituals and assistance
7. Middle-aged parents	Wife–mother–grandmother Husband–father–grandfather	Rebuilding the marriage relationship Maintaining kin ties with old and younger generations
8. Aging family members	Widow–widower Wife–mother–grandmother Husband–father–grandfather	Coping with bereavement and living alone Closing the family home or adapting it to aging Adjusting to retirement

Source: Duvall, 1977.

have taken on many new dimensions including unmarried couples, single parent adoptions, permanent single parent households, and same sex unions with or without children. The expectations of individuals and families vary greatly between one culture and another. Other cultural groups, elsewhere in the world and even in North America, can be expected to have different norms. Family physicians should be aware of the cultural rituals that mark the major transitions of family life in their patients. Hence the importance for family physicians of learning the cultural norms of their patients. Whatever the cultural differences, however, it is probably a universal reality that family life is marked by crises and conflicts, adaptation and maladaptation.

The Traumas of Family Life

Besides the normal transitions, many families also face adverse conditions and go through traumatic episodes that may have profound effects on health (McEwen and Seeman, 1999). The cumulative effect of genetic endowment and environmental stress, or wear and tear, is known as the allostatic load and has been linked to the long observed, negative relationship between socioeconomic status and health.

The Effects of Inadequate Parenting

In all families, the arrival of children is a major change. In some it produces stresses that the system is too fragile to bear. The effects on the children can range from failure to thrive to physical abuse.

Family physicians are in a very good position to identify families that are at risk for these problems, especially if they are caring for the mother during pregnancy. No single cue is a certain indication that a problem exists. It only indicates a need for extra vigilance. Some situations are known to be associated with problems of parenting:

Parents: unsatisfactory childhood experience with their parents; early marriage; single parents; psychiatric illness; immaturity; prison record in father; alcoholic background in family of origin.

Children: prematurity; handicapped children; unwanted children; babies who cry a lot.

Problems of parenting need to be understood not as the result of single causes but as the result of mismatches between parent and child and to the stresses of a difficult environment. A mother who is able to cope with a normal child may become an abusing parent if her child is handicapped. The physician has to observe the interaction between parent and child rather than individual behavior. The prenatal and postnatal periods provide opportunities for making systematic observations of maternal and child behavior. Tables 10.2, 10.3, and 10.4 give warning signs that may be detected during pregnancy, delivery, and the postpartum period. Once a family has been recognized as vulnerable, they can be given additional support in the form of more frequent visits by doctor or nurse and extra time for dealing with problems.

Table 10.2 High-risk signals in the prenatal clinic setting

These are the indication of possible problems. A high-risk situation is created by varying combinations of these signs, the family's degree of emphasis on them, and the family's willingness to change. The interviewer must take into consideration the mother's age, culture, and education, as well as observations of her affect and the significance of her feelings. Many of these signs can be observed throughout the perinatal period; they are listed in this order because they are found most commonly at these times.

Overconcern with the unborn baby's sex.
　　Reasons why a certain sex is so important, e.g., to fill the mother's needs.
　　The mother's need to please the father with the baby's sex.
　　The quality and rigidity of these needs.

Expressed high expectations for the baby.
　　Overconcern with the baby's physical and developmental progress, behavior, and discipline.
　　The parents' need to have control over the baby's actions and reactions.
　　Is this child wanted in order to fulfill unmet needs in parents' lives?

Is this child going to be one too many?
　　Is there adequate spacing between this child and the next younger child?
　　During the pregnancy, has there been evidence of a disintegrating relationship with the older child(ren), e.g., physical or emotional abuse for the first time?

Evidence of the mother's desire to deny the pregnancy.
　　Unwillingness to gain weight.
　　Refusal to talk about the pregnancy in a manner commensurate with the reality of the situation.
　　Not wearing maternity clothes when it would be appropriate.
　　No plans made for the baby's nursery, layette, etc., in the home.

Great depression over the pregnancy.
　　Date of onset of depression to this pregnancy.
　　Report of sleep disturbance that cannot be related to the physical aspects of pregnancy.
　　Attempted suicide.
　　Dropping out socially.
　　Bland affect.

Did either parent formerly ever seriously consider an abortion?
　　Why didn't they go through with it?
　　Did they passively delay a decision until medically therapeutic abortion was not feasible?

Did the parents ever seriously consider relinquishment?
　　Why did they change their minds?
　　The reality and quality expressed in the change of decision.

Whom does the mother turn to for support?
　　How reliable and helpful are they to her?

(continued)

Table 10.2 Continued

Who accompanies the mother to the clinic?
Are any community agencies involved in a supportive way?
Is the mother very alone and/or frightened?
  Is this just because of the lack of education or understanding of pregnancy and
    delivery?
  Is she overly concerned about the physical changes during pregnancy,
    labor, and delivery?
  Do careful explanation, prenatal classes, etc., dissipate these fears?
  Does she tend to keep the focus of the interview on her fears and needs
    rather than any anticipation, excitement, or joy projected onto the new baby?
The mother has many unscheduled visits to the prenatal clinic or the emergency
  room.
  With exaggerated physical complaints that cannot be substantiated on
    physical examination or by laboratory tests.
  Multiple psychosomatic complaints.
  An overdependence on the doctor or nurse.
What are the patient's living arrangements?
  Are the physical accommodations adequate?
  Does she have a telephone?
  Is transportation available?
  Are there friends or relatives nearby?
The parents cannot talk freely on the above topics and avoid eye contact.
What can you find out about the parent's backgrounds?
  Did they grow up in a foster home?
  Were they shuffled from one relative to another?
  What type of discipline was used? (They may not see this as abusive.)
  Do they plan to raise their children the way their parents raised them?

Source: Gray, Cutler, Dean, Kempe, 1976. Reprinted with permission *from Child Abuse and Neglect: The Family and the Community,* copyright 1976, Ballinger Publishing Company.

Conflict

Some conflict occurs in all families. The ways in which conflict is handled and resolved is a measure of how well the family functions. Continuing, unresolved conflict between husband and wife, or between parents and children, may present to the family physician as depression in an adult or child, as physical injury in the wife, as somatic symptoms in adults or children, as school behavior problems, or as acting-out behavior in adolescents. Sometimes, the presentation is a cluster of illnesses in different family members.

Case 10.4

A 10-year-old boy was brought by his mother with aches and pains. No physical abnormality was found. A few weeks later his teenaged sister was admitted to the hospital with attempted suicide. On further inquiry, the mother revealed that

Table 10.3 High-risk signals in the delivery room

Written form with baby's chart concerning parents' reactions at birth.
    How does the mother look?
    What does the mother say?
    What does the mother do?

The following phrases may help in the organization of information regarding observations for the above-mentioned form.
    Does the parent appear sad, happy, apathetic, disappointed, angry, exhausted, frightened, ambivalent?

    Does the parent talk to the baby, talk to spouse, use baby's name, establish eye contact, touch, cuddle, examine?

    Does the spouse, friend, relative offer support, criticism, rejection, ambivalence?

If this interaction seems dubious, further evaluation should be initiated.
Concerning reactions at delivery include the following:
Lack of interest in the baby, ambivalence, passive reaction.

Keeps the focus of attention on herself.
Unwillingness or refusal to hold the baby, even when offered.
Hostility directed toward father who put her "through all this."
    Inappropriate verbalizations, glances directed at the baby, with definite hostility expressed.

Disparaging remarks about the baby's sex or physical characteristics.
Disappointment over sex or other physical characteristics of the child.

Source: Gray, Cutler, Dean, Kempe, 1976. Reprinted with permission from *Child Abuse and Neglect: The Family and the Community*, copyright 1976, Ballinger Publishing Company.

her husband had been waking in the night and terrorizing the family by violent behavior.

Injuries in women resulting from family violence are often concealed or explained as accidental. The physician should be on guard for this. Marital discord is a common reason for chronic depression, especially in women. A wide variety of medical and psychological symptoms may have their roots in an abusive relationship. Often, whether a woman reveals this to her physician depends on the perceived openness of the physician to what may be viewed by the patient as a shameful secret. The investigation of depression and symptoms arising from stress should always include inquiry about family relationships.

Another aspect of conflict is the stress induced by conflicting loyalties between different family members. This may be seen, for example, in a woman who is torn between her obligations to her children and to her elderly parents, or between commitments to job and family.

When a family physician confirms or strongly suspects that a woman or her children are at risk of domestic violence, the physician must assess the immediacy of the risk and help develop an escape plan if necessary. Most communities

Table 10.4 High-risk signals in the postpartum period (on postpartum ward and in well-baby clinic)

Does the family remain disappointed over the sex of the baby?

What is the child's name?
  Who is he or she named for/after?
  Who picked the name?
  When was the name picked?
  Is the name used when talking to or about the baby?

What was/is the husband's and/or family's reaction to the new baby?
  Are they supportive?
  Are they critical?
  Do they attempt to take over and control the situation?
  Is the husband jealous of the baby's drain on the mother's time and energy?

What kind of support, other than family, is the mother receiving?

Are there sibling rivalry problems? Does the mother expect any? How does she plan to handle them? Or does she deny that a new baby will change existing family relationships?

Is the mother bothered by the baby's crying?
  How does it make her feel? Angry? Inadequate? Like crying herself?

Feedings:
  Does the mother view the baby as too demanding in his or her needs to eat?
  Does she ignore the demands?
  Is she repulsed by messiness, e.g., spitting up?
  Is she repulsed by sucking noises?

How does the mother view changing diapers?
  Is she repulsed by the messiness, smells, etc.?

Are the expectations of the child developmentally far beyond his or her capabilities?

Mother's control or lack of control over the situation:
  Does she get involved and take control over the baby's needs and what's going to happen (waiting room and during the exam interaction).
  Does she relinquish control to the doctor, nurse, etc. (undressing, holding, allowing child to express fears, etc.)?

Can the mother express that she is having fun with the baby?
  Can she view him or her as a separate individual?
  Can attention be focused on him or her and can she see something positive in that for herself?

Can she establish and maintain eye-to-eye, direct contact with the baby?

How does she talk with the baby?

Are her verbalizations about the child usually negative?

When the child cries, does she, or can she, comfort him or her?

Source: Gray, Cutler, Dean, Kempe, 1976. Reprinted with permission from *Child Abuse and Neglect: The Family and the Community*, copyright 1976, Ballinger Publishing Company.

now have shelters and supports for abused women and their children. Having this information at hand and available in the family physician's office is an essential tool in family practice.

Divorce

Divorce is an experience analogous to bereavement in its capacity to cause grief. The same feelings of anger, bitterness, guilt, and self-doubt arise, without the comfort the bereaved can derive from memories of a loving relationship. Continuing conflict over the divorce settlement or over the children serve to intensify and prolong the pain.

Children are particularly vulnerable to the effects of divorce. About one-third of children are deeply distressed by divorce and continue to be distressed for many years. Very young children (up to age 5) show regression in development: feeding and toilet problems, enuresis, sleep disturbances, and separation anxiety. In early school-aged children, distress may be concealed by denial of difficulties. At this age, however, children may harbor strong feelings of guilt derived from their fantasy of having caused the separation. Distress may be expressed in the form of school problems, somatic symptoms, enuresis, and nightmares.

Older children are often shocked and incredulous. They may be directly involved in custody battles and this is associated with later maladjustment. They suffer from conflicts of loyalty, which they may resolve by completely rejecting one parent. Adolescent children of divorced parents may have a particularly stormy adolescence and are likely to have a lower self-concept than their peers.

It is important for the family physician to identify and help the vulnerable children of divorced couples. The amount of distress in the children is proportional to the amount of conflict between parents. The Toronto Family Study (Homatidis, Johnson, Orlando, and Robson, 1986) found that vulnerable children had more school changes, fewer friends, more feelings of guilt, needed more help with schoolwork, and experienced the separation as very stressful. Other studies have shown that a good relationship with one parent, good peer relationship, academic success, and involvement in school counseling programs were associated with better adjustment.

Having identified vulnerable children, the physician can either provide counseling within the practice or ensure that the child and parents get help from an agency or school counseling service.

Younger children are often not told about an impending separation on the grounds that "they are too young to understand." This has the effect of increasing the child's anxiety and distress. The physician can help parents to understand the importance of explaining what is happening to the children.

Family physicians may in various ways become enmeshed themselves in divorce and custody proceedings. An attempt may be made by either party to enlist the physician's support in marital conflicts—a particularly difficult situation when husband and wife are both patients. On the other hand, if the physician can retain neutrality, he or she may be able to play a significant part in resolving the conflict. When divorce has become inevitable, the physician may be asked to give evidence in court, or to provide corroboration of abuse or of parenting failures. When disputes arise over visiting rights, the physician may be asked by the favored parent to certify that visits to the other parents make the child ill or anxious or that the child is being sexually abused.

Illness and Disability

Serious illness or disability has profound effects on the life of a family. The actual effect varies with the type of illness and the family member involved: a mentally or physically handicapped child; an adolescent with paraplegia, diabetes, or schizophrenia; a mother with multiple sclerosis; a father with cancer or alcoholism. The common factor in all these situations is the need for the other family members to adjust to the changed situation and to adopt new roles. With these adaptive changes come new risks to other members of the family, which may in turn affect the member who is sick or disabled. The harm caused by these changes is potentially preventable if members of the family can be helped to gain enough insight to avoid the risks.

Counseling for families of patients with schizophrenia is a good example of what can be done to help families care for patients with chronic illness. Several studies have shown big reductions in relapse rates when families are either counseled in their own homes or invited to attend group sessions with other families (Leff, 1989). Themes running through the group sessions are education about schizophrenia, teaching about problem solving, improving communication, and dealing with expressed emotion. Patients with schizophrenia are very vulnerable to criticism, hostility, and overinvolvement. Relatives may criticize patients for their apathy and lack of initiative, not realizing that these are manifestations of the illness. Family members can learn to control their negative emotions and to be more tolerant.

Although in the published studies therapy has been carried out by psychiatric teams, the methods could be adapted to family practice. The family physician or a counselor in the practice team could offer a series of sessions to a family in their home, or to members of several families at the practice center. In a less formal way, the physician could provide counseling during routine contacts with family members. The family doctor may be the only person who can reach those relatives who do not attend group sessions and who are likely to be in greatest need of help.

So much attention may be focused on a handicapped child or adolescent that the needs of a spouse or of siblings are not met. The strain of caring for a sick person may go unnoticed both by the physician and by other family members as they concentrate their attention on the sick member. Other members of the family may hide their illnesses or their despair until it becomes too late to help them. Medalie (1975) has stressed the need to be alert for the "hidden patient."

Case 10.5
An elderly woman with congestive heart failure was cared for during her long terminal illness by her husband. I saw him in the course of many home visits and although

he always looked pale I (IRMcW) never suspected anything amiss. Soon after the woman died, her husband came to see me complaining of severe fatigue. He had prostatic obstruction, renal failure, and uremia with secondary anemia, all of which had been present for the duration of his wife's illness.

The question "And how are *you* doing?" can be sufficient to allow another family member to express his or her feelings. People from families with a member who is chronically sick have higher rates of illness themselves than people from families without chronic sickness.

Terminal illness is a particularly stressful time for families, whether the sick person is at home or in the hospital. As well as grieving over the suffering, and physically exhausted by the demands on them, children or grandchildren may be disturbed by conflicts over sharing the burden of care, or by the resurgence of old conflicts that have remained dormant for years.

Case 10.6
The daughter of an elderly couple—a single woman—was dying of cancer in a palliative care unit. Despite vigorous efforts by the palliative care team, her pain remained uncontrolled and her suffering was intense. In the last few days of her life, her mother was admitted to the coronary care unit in another hospital with chest pain. After several days of observation, she was discharged home but continued to complain of pain and was very agitated. The family doctor, who was not involved in the care of the daughter, reassured her about the pain and prescribed a sedative. When her agitation continued, other members of the family became impatient with her, and one of her other children left and returned home. On the same day she died suddenly at home.

One could not imagine a clearer example of death from a broken heart. A "broken heart syndrome" (stress cardiomyopathy, myocardial stunning, takotsubo cardiomyopathy) has been described by Wittstein et al. (2005) and evidence for a physiological linkage through a strong neurohormonal surge found. This syndrome should be considered when patients present with symptoms of a myocardial infarction following strong emotional stress such as death of a loved one. In retrospect, her care might have been different if the palliative care team, coronary care team, and family doctor had recognized her as a highly vulnerable person. The risk of cardiac arrest might have been anticipated. Her intense suffering was inevitable, but an urgently convened family conference might have helped the family to respond by increasing their support.

Communication problems are common, even in well-functioning families. According to Stedeford (1981), a psychiatrist who has done much work with the families of the dying, poor communication causes more suffering to dying patients and their families than any other problem except unrelieved pain. Married couples, even when very close to each other, may find it very difficult to talk to each other when one becomes terminally ill. Information may be withheld from key members of the family. A dependent child, for example, may not be told that his parent is dying. He may therefore feel, for the rest of his life, that he has been deprived of precious moments with his mother or father. A spouse may try to conceal the diagnosis from the patient, thus imposing intolerable strains on their relationship.

The adaptation of a family to a sick member may itself become a problem when it comes to rehabilitation. The spouses of alcoholics may become so used to their adaptive role that they find it difficult to relinquish control if their spouse recovers. A spouse may be drawn into facilitating alcohol abuse. Parents of a handicapped child may be so overprotective that the child is denied the opportunity to become independent. The sick role of an adult member may be reinforced so strongly by the family that rehabilitation becomes impossible.

Bereavement

The loss of a loved one is the greatest emotional trauma a person can experience. As we have seen, the loss has profound effects on both mind and body, making the bereaved person especially vulnerable to physical illness as well as to mental breakdown. However well prepared the person may be, the effect is one of devastation, isolation, and loss of purpose. Dr. Samuel Johnson described his own feelings after his wife's death in these words: "I have ever since seemed to myself broken off from mankind; a kind of solitary wanderer in the wild of life, without any direction or fixed point of view: a gloomy gazer on a world to which I have little relation."

Feelings of anger and guilt are common, and these are sometimes projected toward the physician ("If only he had diagnosed it sooner"). Friends can make the problem worse by trying to avoid discussion of feelings or even avoiding the bereaved person for fear of not knowing what to say.

Somatic symptoms are common: loss of appetite, loss of weight, diarrhea, and pain. The illness may be so severe as to suggest a life-threatening disease. There is a pitfall here for the unwary physician. If intensive investigations are set in motion without allowing the patient to express his or her grief, the result may be mental breakdown and suicide. It is sometimes forgotten, too, that other types of loss can cause grief—loss of a pregnancy, loss of health, of job, or of valued possessions, even death of a family pet. Loss of a parent presents unique challenges as it tends to bring to the forefront many, often previously repressed, issues in a person's life. The death of a child can widen any small cracks in a marital relationship and without assistance, separation and divorce are common outcomes.

Family physicians encounter grief in many forms. In caring for a dying patient they may be able to prevent some of the things that trouble the bereaved. They can reduce the dying person's pain and suffering to a minimum, protecting him or her from traumatic and disturbing investigations and therapies that cannot serve any useful purpose. They can ensure that the death is prepared for, so that there is no last minute rush to the hospital by ambulance. They can assure the family that the patient is not suffering, tell them how well they are caring for the patient, and ensure that distant family members come in time to see the patient. They can be aware of family members who may find it difficult to express their needs, such as school-aged children.

After bereavement, they can ensure that the family is offered support in bearing the grief, either from themselves or from some other person. When bereaved persons become ill, they can remember that person's vulnerability and encourage the expression of feelings. Physicians too, experience emotional reactions to the death of a patient, even if anticipated and planned for. These emotions may run the gamut from guilt, to shame and personal loss. It behooves practitioners to be aware of these reactions and have in place a method of coping with them.

Poverty

Even in the wealthiest countries, the poor have higher rates of illness and early death. The differences in death rates between social classes are not removed by having a national health service with free access to medical care. In Britain, for example, after more than 60 years of the National Health Service, there are still large differences between rich and poor. Some of these differences are no doubt due to environmental factors. Tudor Hart (1971) in Britain and Ford (1976) in the United States have shown that the poorest areas of the country also have the poorest health services.[2] Even though economic barriers may have been removed, there are other less visible barriers between the poor and the health services: difficulties with transport, long waits in clinics, lack of knowledge of services, communication problems, and the sheer weight of problems a family has to bear, of which illness is only one. Large income differentials between the wealthiest and the poorest in society have been found to be an independent factor in determining population health (Daniels, Kennedy, and Kawachi, 2000). Many of these problems can be eased by family physicians who help poorer families to use the health and social services and mobilize extra support for them. Shi, Starfield and colleagues have found that access to primary care can mitigate the negative effect of large income differentials on health (Shi, Starfield, and Kawachi, 1999). Nevertheless, medical care has a limited role as a factor in social inequalities in health[3] (Marmot, Bobak, and Smith, 1995).

Thirty-six women staying in shelters or transitional housing were invited to form focus groups at five locations to discuss their health concerns. The groups, conducted by Susan Woolhouse MD, explored the women's experiences and interactions with family physicians. Two dominant themes emerged. Power imbalances within patient–physician relationships could make women feel demeaned, marginalized, and unimportant, creating a reluctance to consult about their health. Women who described close and trusting relationships with their family physicians experienced support and collaboration, with continuity of care being of paramount importance (Woolhouse, Brown, and Lent, 2004).

A study in Scotland has compared affluent areas of the country with poor areas. More than 3,000 patients were surveyed and data collected on demographic and socioeconomic factors, health variables and factors related to quality of care. Patients in the most deprived areas had more long-term illness, more multimorbidity, and more psychological problems. Patients in the more deprived areas had more problems to be discussed, but shorter time with their doctors than patients in affluent areas. General practitioners' stress was higher than in affluent areas (Mercer and Watt, 2007).

In poorer countries, poverty is a major reason for ill health through malnutrition, overcrowding, contaminated water, and ignorance of hygiene. Some of these problems may be so basic that the physician's most important task is to work with the community to raise standards of public health. In these conditions, however, a family approach to health is even more necessary. Teaching mothers about nutrition and about the management of infant diarrhea, for example, can improve child health and reduce infant mortality.

Uprooting

Migration of various kinds is one of the most traumatic experiences a family can undergo. The trauma varies with the type of migration, from the forced movement of refugees, to the "upwardly mobile" movement of a family on its way up the social scale. The trauma also varies with the cultural and language change involved in the move. Migration affects different members of a family in different ways. To an ambitious person, the move may be a challenge, to the spouse an alienating experience. A woman who moved to my (IRMcW) practice with her husband from another part of the country said she felt like "a snail without a shell." Younger children may be unaffected, older children disturbed by breaks in friendships and school careers. Migration is associated with an increase in illness rates and with an increase in utilization of health services.

Unemployment

Loss of job, with its resulting loss of income, loss of self-respect, and loss of social status is traumatic both for the individual and for the family. When the loss of job is associated with failure of a business or a family farm, the effect is even greater. Unemployment is reported to be associated with higher illness and death rates.

How Family Doctors Work with Families

We know very little about how family physicians work with families as groups. Very little research has addressed this question. Apart from Huygen's book and some case studies, the literature on the subject has been mainly concerned with theory development. One thing we know is that family physicians rarely function as family therapists. Almost certainly family physicians do help families in their own way, by providing information and support at times of vulnerability, and by helping family members toward self-knowledge. Only long-term descriptive studies will tell us how this is done and how effective the help is.

Although a family physician may not be able to act as family therapist in his or her own practice, he or she can help selected families by referring them for family therapy. Many families, however, are resistant to family therapy, lacking even the recognition that they have a problem. Family physicians still have to work with these families as best they can.

The Family Conference

We do not know how often family physicians see whole family groups together. Encounters with parent–child and husband–wife pairs are probably frequent in most practices. Encounters with larger groups may occur naturally at times of crisis and during home visits, but these can rarely be as effective as a specially arranged family conference.

A family conference is especially helpful when a life-threatening or disabling disease has been diagnosed, when difficult treatment or placement choices have to be made, and when a family member is terminally ill (Schmidt, 1983). Who attends the conference will vary with circumstances. Usually it will include the patient and all close family members who are locally available. Besides the family physician, it may include other members of the health-care team: a nurse, social worker, or consultant, who is involved in the patient's care.

The conference can deal with both cognitive and affective issues. Providing information to the whole family together can minimize the risk of misinformation, especially if questions are invited and responded to with care.[4]

The conference can provide an opportunity for family members to express feelings that they have found difficult to express before. With good listening skills, the physician may pick up cues to family conflicts or to a family member who is especially vulnerable. This may, for example, be a member who sits silent throughout the conference, or one who does not attend at all, even though he or she is readily available.

Case 10.6
An elderly woman who was dying of liver cancer was being cared for at home by her widowed daughter, who was also working full time as a librarian. Two teenaged granddaughters also lived in the home. The patient also had another daughter living nearby. The patient wanted to die at home and the whole family supported her in this. The burden of care, however, was falling mainly on the daughter, who was beginning to show signs of exhaustion. The rest of the family seemed unaware of this, and she had been unable to express her feelings to them.

At a family conference held in the home, the patient, her two daughters, and two granddaughters were present. The family physician, attending nurse, and a volunteer from a hospice organization were also present. The patient's daughter was able to express her feelings of exhaustion and despair and the other members of the family understood for the first time how close to breakdown she was. Arrangements were made to provide her with relief and support. The physician and nurse answered questions about the patient's symptoms and clarified the arrangements for getting help in case of crises. The patient was able to remain at home until her death.

Precepts of Family Care

The following precepts summarize the content of this chapter. We regard them as the basic responsibilities of a family physician to the families of his or her patients.

1. Look out for vulnerable families and give them extra support.
2. Provide good information at times of serious illness. Ask, "Have you any questions?"
3. "Be there" at times of crisis: serious illness, terminal illness, and bereavement.
4. Take the initiative at times when you may be needed—on discharge from the hospital, for example. Do not assume people will know when to call you for advice or assistance.
5. Look out for vulnerable family members, the "hidden patient."
6. Look out for patients who are family scapegoats or presenting symptoms of a family problem.
7. Avoid being drawn into taking sides in family conflicts.
8. Offer a family conference at critical times.

The Universal Importance of the Family

The family is important in all parts of the world. The principles set out in this chapter are as important—if not more important—in poverty-stricken parts of the world as they are in affluent countries. Dr. Cicely Williams, a pediatrician who spent her life working in Africa, and who was the first person to describe kwashiorkor, was emphatic about the need to involve the family if child health was to be improved. In her Blackfan Lecture (1973) at Boston Children's Hospital she said "the conditions that mostly damage children are gastroenteritis, respiratory diseases, dyspepsia, worms and maternal inadequacy.... Malnutrition and 'failure to thrive' are of course due to numerous causes, not only to insufficient food."

The public health services can improve the macroenvironment by instituting water supply, refuse disposal, pest control, food hygiene, and so forth. But it is the microenvironment in the home and its surroundings that are most important to the child. These are controlled by the parents and depend on their values and their diligence.

Whether in rich or poor countries, "developed" or "developing," the health of individuals is influenced by family life, and families are affected by the illnesses and misfortunes of their members.

References

American Academy of Pediatrics. 2003. Report of the Task Force on the Family. *Pediatrics* 111(6):1541–1571.

Baker SP, O'Neill B, Ginsburg MJ, Li G. 1992. *The Injury Fact Book*, 2nd edn. New York: Oxford University Press.

Batty GD, Morton SMR, Campbell D, Clark H et al. 2004. The Aberdeen Children of the 1950's cohort study: Background, methods and follow-up information on a new resource for the study of life course and intergenerational influences on health. *Paediatric and Perinatal Epidemiology* 18: 221–239.

Brennan M. 1974. Personal communication.

Community Childhood Hunger Identification Project. 1991. *A Survey of Hunger in the U.S.* Washington, DC: Food Research and Action Center.

Daniels N, Kennedy B, Kawachi I. 2000. *Is Inequality Bad For our Health?* Boston, MA: Beacon Press.

Day T. 1995. *The Health Related Costs of Violence against Women in Canada, The Tip of the Iceberg.* London, Ontario: Centre for Research on Violence against Women and Children.

DeNavas-Walt C, Proctor BD, Lee CH. 2006. Income, Poverty and Health Insurance Coverage in the United States: 2005. U.S. Census Bureau, August.

Dingle JH, Badger GF, Jordan WS. 1964. *Illness in the Home–A Study of 25,000 Illnesses in a Group of Cleveland Families.* Cleveland, OH: Western Reserve University Press.

Doherty WJ, Baird MA, eds. 1987. *Family Centered Medical Care: A Clinical Casebook.* New York: Guilford Press.

Duvall EM. 1977. *Family Development*, 5th edn. Philadelphia, PA: Lippincott.

Ford AB. 1976. *Urban Health in America.* New York: Oxford University Press.

Gray JD, Cutler C, Dean J, Kempe CH. 1976. Perinatal assessment of a mother–baby interaction. In: Kempe CH, Helfer RE, eds., *Child Abuse and Neglect: The Family in the Community.* Cambridge: Ballinger.

Haggerty RJ, Roghmann KH, Pless IB. 1975. *Child Health and the Community.* New York: John Wiley.

Hart JT. 1971. The inverse care law. *Lancet* 696:405.

Heise, L., Pitanguy, J., Germain, A. 1994 Violence against women: The hidden health burden. World Bank Discussion Papers. Washington D.C.

Hinkle LE. 1974. The effect of exposure to culture change and changes in interpersonal relationships in health. In: Dohrenwerd BP, Dohrenwerd BS, eds. *Stressful Life Events: Their Nature and Effects.* New York: John Wiley.

Homatidis G, Johnson L. Orlando F, Robson B. 1986. *The Toronto Family Study.* Toronto: Toronto Board of Education Publications.

Huygen FJA. 1982. *Family Medicine: The Medical Life History of Families.* New York: Brunner/Mazel.

Klaus AS, Kennell JH. 1976. *Maternal–infant Bonding.* St. Louis, MO: C.V. Mosby.

Kraus AS, Lilienfeld AM. 1959. Some epidemiologic aspects of the high mortality rate in the young widowed group. *Journal of Chronic Disease* 10:296.

Leff J. 1989. Family factors in schizophrenia. *Psychiatric Annals* 19(10):542.

Marmot M, Bobak M, Smith GD. 1995. Explanations for social inequalities in health. In: Amick BC III, Levine S, Tarlow AR, Walsh DC, eds., *Society & Health.* New York: Oxford University Press.

Maughan B, McCarthy G. 1997. Childhood adversities and psychosocial disorders. *British Medical Bulletin* 53:156.

McCain, M and Mustard, F. (1999). *The Early Years Study: Reversing the Real Brain Drain.* Ontario, The Canadian Institute for Advanced Research, and The Founders' Network.

McEwen BS, Seeman T. 1999. Protective and damaging effects of mediators of stress: Elaborating and testing the oncepts of allostasis and allostatic load. *Annals of New York Academy of Sciences* 89630–89647.

Medalie JH. 1975. The hidden patient. Lecture at Quail Hollow Conference. November. Case Western Reserve School of Medicine.

Medalie JH, Goldbourt U. 1976. Angina pectoris among 10,000 men.Psychosocial and other risk factors as evidenced by a multivariate analysis of a 5-year medicine study. *American Journal of Medicine* 60:910.

Mercer SW, Watt GC. 2007. The inverse care law: Clinical primary care encounters in deprived and affluent areas of Scotland. *Annals of Family Medicine* 5(6):503–510.

Meyer RJ, Haggerty RH. 1962. Streptococcal infections in families, factors altering individual susceptibility. *Pediatrics* 29:539.

Miller FJW, Court WKM, Walton WS, Knox EG. 1960. *Growing up in Newcastle upon Tyne*. London: Oxford University Press.

Mistry R. 2002. *Family Matters*. Toronto: McClelland and Stewart.

National Alliance to End Homelessness. *Homelessness Counts*. January 10, 2007.

Nesser WB. 1975. Fragmentation of black families and stroke susceptibility. In: Kaplan BH, Cassel JC, eds., *Family and Health: An Epidemiological Approach*. Chapel Hill, NC: University of North Carolina Press.

Pless IB, Satterwhite BB. 1973. A measure of family functioning and its application. *Social Science and Medicine* 7:613.

Ramsey CN, Abell TD, Baker LC. 1986. The relationship between family functioning, life events, family structure, and the outcome of pregnancy. *Journal of Family Practice* 22:521.

Ransom DC, Vandervoort HC. 1973. The development of family medicine: Problematic trends. *Journal of the American Medical Association* 225:1098.

Roland A. 1988. *In Search of the Self in India and Japan*. Princeton, NJ: Princeton University Press.

Schmidt DD. 1983. When is it helpful to convene the family? *Journal of Family Practice* 16:967.

Schor EL, Menaghan EG. 1995. Family pathways to child health. In: Amick BC III, Levine S, Tarlow AR, Walsh DC, eds., *Society and Health*. New York: Oxford University Press.

Seeman TE, Crimmins E, Huag M-H et al. 2004. Cumulative biological risk and socioeconomic differences in mortality: MacArthur studies of successful aging.*Social Science and Medicine* 58:1985–1997.

Shi L, Starfield, Kennedy B, Kawachi I. 1999. Income inequality, primary care, and health indicators. *Journal of Family Practice* 48(4):275–284.

Smith K, Joshi H. 2002. The Millennium Cohort Study. *Population Trends* (Spring):30–34.

Stedeford A. 1981. Couples facing death: Unsatisfactory communication. *British Medical Journal* 183:1098.

U.S. Census Bureau 2006. http://pubdb3.census.gov/macro/032006/pov/toc.htmWadsworth MEJ, Kuh DJL. 1997. Childhood influences on adult health: A review of recent work from the British 1946 national birth cohort study, the MRC National Survey of Health and Development. *Paediatric and Perinatal Epidemiology* 11:2–20.

Williams CD. 1973. Health services in the home. *Pediatrics* 52:773.

Wittstein IS, Thiemann DR, Lima JAC, et al. 2005. Neurohormonal features of myocardial stunning due to emotional stress. *New England Journal of Medicine* 352:539–548.

Woolhouse S, Brown JB, Lent B. 2004. Women marginalized by poverty and violence: How patient–physician relationships can help. *Canadian Family Physician* 50:1388–1394.

Notes

1. I am indebted to Dr. Michael Brennan for these observations.

2. The Inverse Square Law, published by Tudor Hart in 1971, states that areas with greatest need for medical care tend to be provided with fewer resources. For a first-hand account of practice among the inner city poor, see David Hilfiker's *Not All of Us Are Saints: A Doctor's Journey with the Poor.* New York: Ballantine Books, 1994.

3. For a discussion of social inequalities in health see Marmot, Bobak, Smith (1995). Poverty does not account for the social class gradient in mortality and morbidity rates. These decrease with every step upward in social status from lowest to highest. The difference between the two highest levels clearly cannot be attributed to poverty. Moreover, the differences are found in most of the major causes of illness and death. There is no simple explanation for the relationship between social class and health. Social class is related to many factors with known relationships to health: early life experience, education, material conditions, health behavior, negative emotions arising from lack of control over one's life, and amount of social support. In this regard, it seems significant that differences between countries in the social class gradient are related more to differences in the distribution of wealth than differences in overall wealth.

4. For an excellent guide, see Conducting a Family Conference, chapter 6 in *Family-Oriented Primary Care* by Susan McDaniel, Thomas Campbell, and David Seaburn. New York: Springer-Verlag, 1990.

Part II

Clinical Problems

The following five clinical chapters are intended to illustrate the principles delineated in Part I of the book. They do not intend to cover the whole field of clinical family medicine.

11

Acute Sore Throat

Upper respiratory infection is the most common diagnosis made in general practice, and sore throat is one of the most common presenting symptoms. Seventy years ago, a discussion of acute sore throat would have centered on the clinical and bacteriological diagnosis of diphtheria and its differentiation from streptococcal infection. The uncommon acute epiglottitis is now the main life-threatening type of throat infection encountered by family physicians. Diphtheria is likely to be encountered only in communities where social disorganization has reduced rates of primary immunization.

With the virtual eradication of diphtheria and the coming of penicillin, attention shifted to the diagnosis of streptococcal sore throat. Penicillin provided for the first time a means of preventing both the suppurative complications of sore throat and the nonsuppurative (principally rheumatic fever; acute glomerulonephritis does not appear to be preventable by treatment of streptococcal infection). At the time when penicillin was introduced, rheumatic fever was a common and serious health problem. In Toronto in 1949, the annual incidence in children was 0.33%. Even after penicillin became available, rheumatic fever remained common. In my (IRMcW) first 10 years in general practice (1954–1963), I saw 15 new cases of acute and subacute rheumatic fever. Most were mild. The course of the illness was 3 months or less in all but one. Clinical evidence of carditis was present in seven patients, but was severe only in two. One patient was left with a valvular lesion. Two patients developed chorea. All patients except four were ambulant when first seen and in six the course of the illness was subacute throughout.

In the past 20 years, the decline in incidence has been dramatic. In school-aged children in the United States it has declined by more than 90%. The annual incidence of rheumatic fever in most parts of North America is now between one and two cases per million population. Even in affluent countries there remain some high-risk communities, notably those with a high proportion of aboriginal people.

In societies with low living standards, rheumatic fever remains common and serious. In the 1982, the incidence in the Caribbean islands of Martinique and Guadeloupe was 19.6 and 17.4 per 100,000 inhabitants under 20, respectively. After the introduction of a 10-year educational program targeting the public and health-care workers, including general practitioners, there was a progressive decline in the incidence rate. By 1992, the frequency had fallen by 78% in Martinique and 74% in Guadeloupe (Bach et al., 1996). The highest reported rates of acute rheu-matic fever are documented in aboriginal children in northern Australia where a conservative estimate places it at 245 to 351 per 100,000 population. In New Zealand, Pacific Islander children have rates of 80 to 100 per 100,000. By con-trast, the non-indigenous population of New Zealand have incidence rates of less than 10 per 100,000 (Carapetis, McDonald, and Wilson, 2005).

We cannot assume that rheumatic fever will not emerge again as a serious health problem in affluent communities. Several outbreaks have recently been reported in the United States (Kaplan and Hill, 1987) and have recurred in cer-tain areas such as Utah and elsewhere (Veasy et al., 2004). We still do not know why the incidence has declined so dramatically in the past 20 years in so many areas. Four explanations deserve attention: a rise in living standards, an increase in herd immunity, the use of penicillin, and a change in the streptococcus. The first two reasons are supported by the continuing high incidence of rheumatic fever in conditions of poverty, overcrowding, and malnutrition. On the other hand, the incidence in affluent societies continued to decline after living standards had ceased to change significantly. If the penicillin treatment of streptococcal sore throats was the reason, we would have expected to see a steep decline after the introduction of penicillin rather than a gradual decline over a period of 30 years. Also, we know that many cases of rheumatic fever either had no history of sore throat or had one so mild that no doctor was consulted.

Although the issue is still controversial, there is a strong body of evidence supporting the existence of rheumatogenic and nonrheumatogenic group A strep-tococci. The existence of nephritogenic serotypes is well established. Although rheumatic fever has declined so steeply, there has been no corresponding decline in the incidence of streptococcal sore throat. The decline, moreover, has been steeper than one would expect from a change in herd immunity. It is possible, therefore, that recent outbreaks of rheumatic fever have been caused by the reemergence of rheumatogenic strains of streptococci and that further outbreaks will occur. At the time of periodic outbreaks of acute rheumatic fever, there have been reports of an increased number of mucoid strains of *Streptococcus pyo-genes*, predominantly M-type 18 (Veasy et al., 2004). Eventually, we may see a vaccine against rheumatogenic strains for people with genetic markers indicating susceptibility to rheumatic fever. For the present, the best means of prevention is the detection and treatment of streptococcal infection.

A Strategy for the Management of Acute Sore Throats

When rheumatic fever was still common, the American Heart Association rec-ommended that throat cultures should be done on all patients with sore throat and that those with positive cultures should have intramuscular benzathine penicillin G to maintain therapeutic blood levels for 10 days. With the decline in incidence, these recommendations have been modified. Oral penicillin is now recommended, and less stress is placed on posttreatment throat cultures and cultures of family contacts.

The main decisions facing the family physician seeing a patient with sore throat are whether to prescribe penicillin and whether to do a rapid latex-agglutination test or throat culture. Developing a strategy illustrates some of the principles described in Chapter 8. With the decline in rheumatic fever, the emphasis has shifted away from the prevention of this disease to the reduction of unnecessary prescribing of antibiotics. Evidence from Britain (Howie and Foggo, 1985) indicates that 80% of patients attending with sore throats receive penicillin. The reported prevalence of positive throat cultures for streptococci in patients attending with sore throat is between 7% and 30% (Hillner and Centor, 1987). The problem for family physicians in communities with low rates of rheumatic fever is how to attain the objectives of therapy for streptococcal sore throat at reasonable cost while reducing to a minimum the unnecessary prescription of antibiotics. Avoidance of overtreatment is important, not only for economic reasons and for prevention of allergic reactions, but also because it can result in the growth of penicillinase-producing organisms. In a national survey done in the United States between 1989 and 1999 (Linder, Randall, and Stafford, 2001) it was found that more than half of adults presenting with sore throat to community primary care physicians received an antibiotic. Further there was documented a shift from penicillin and erythromycin to more expensive nonrecommended antibiotics such as the fluoroquinolones.

The objectives of treatment for streptococcal infection in these communities are now primarily to shorten the illness, to prevent septic complications, and to prevent rheumatic fever in those at special risk. The following facts are important to remember when developing a strategy.

In a systematic review of the literature Del Mar and colleagues (Cochrane Review, 2006) found that antibiotics used to treat sore throat had their greatest effect at day 3 when they reduced soreness and fever by 50%. However, the overall number needed to treat to prevent one sore throat at day 3 was just under six. Treatment can, therefore, increase comfort, reduce the period of infectivity, and return patients quickly to school or work.

Clinical assessment can substantially alter the probability of streptococcal infection in patients with sore throat. The clinical cluster of sore throat, temperature 38°C or above, enlarged and tender tonsillar lymph nodes, pharyngeal exudate, and absence of cough has a positive predictive value of at least 25% and a negative predictive value of 95%. The predictive value of clinical assessment is lower in children (Forsyth, 1975).

Because predictive value varies with prevalence, we would expect the predictive value to vary with the prevalence of streptococcal infection in patients with sore throat. This is indeed the case. The positive predictive value of the clinical cluster has varied from 26% to 62% with prevalence rates of 5% to 20% (Centor, Meier, and Dalton, 1986).

In other words, it is possible, by clinical assessment alone, to separate patients with sore throat into groups with a very high probability of being not streptococcal and a moderately high probability of being streptococcal. Between these is an intermediate group in which the probability of streptococcal infection is between 5% and 30%. The "gold standard" for the diagnosis of streptococcal infection in these estimates is a positive throat culture.

A positive throat culture does not distinguish between infection with streptococcus and the carrier state. Confirmation of infection requires a rise in the anti-streptolysin O (ASO) titer. Because this is not applicable in clinical practice, there is no certain way of distinguishing between infection and the carrier state. The prevalence of the carrier state varies between populations and from time to time in the same population. There is some evidence that it is lower under epidemic conditions. Studies in different communities have shown a rate of between 2% and 10%, with higher rates in children than in adults. Contrary to a widespread assumption, a low colony count in culture does not indicate the carrier state (Kellogg and Manzella, 1986).

The carrier state is a problem for several reasons. When associated with an upper respiratory illness it leads to unnecessary antibiotic treatment. When streptococci are found in symptomless persons, it is impossible to know, without showing a rising ASO titer, whether the person is a carrier or has subclinical infection. We also know that a subclinical infection can be followed by rheumatic fever.

A single throat swab has 90% sensitivity for streptococcal infection, when two swabs are used as the gold standard. In other words, there are 10% false negatives. The false negatives result from faulty technique in taking or processing the swab (Kellogg and Manzella, 1986). Improved sensitivity necessitates proper technique in obtaining the swab. Vigorous swabbing of the both tonsils or tonsillar fossae and the posterior pharynx, while avoiding contact with the tongue or buccal mucosa is necessary.

Our knowledge of the risk of rheumatic fever, and of the preventive effects of penicillin, is based on studies done when the incidence of rheumatic fever was much greater than it is now. The attack rate in young males in epidemic conditions was 3% in untreated patients and 0.3% in those who received penicillin. The attack rate in untreated children under endemic conditions was two out of 311 patients with rises in ASO titer (0.64%). Although the prevention of rheumatic fever by oral penicillin has never been demonstrated by a controlled trial, it is known that oral penicillin for 10 days can eradicate streptococci from the throat.

Pooling the data from several studies, Tompkins, Burnes, and Cable (1977) estimated the risk of serious allergic reactions to be 0.64% of patients treated with intramuscular penicillin and 0.025% of patients receiving oral penicillin. They estimated the risk of mild reactions to be 0.3% with intramuscular penicillin and 0.52% with oral. Serious reactions were defined as moderate to severe anaphylaxis or serum sickness, usually requiring hospitalization. These figures assume that penicillin will not be given to patients known to be allergic to it. Fatal reactions to penicillin are very rare in adults and rarer in children. There were no deaths in 315,000 US Navy recruits given intramuscular penicillin and one in 94,655 patients treated in US venereal disease clinics between 1954 and 1969.

Specificity of these tests is in the 90% to 95% range, but sensitivity can vary between 60% and 95% with some as low as 31%. Because of the high specificity and generally lower sensitivity, a positive test is useful in the diagnosis of strep pharyngitis, but a negative test does not rule it out. Some guidelines therefore recommend doing a throat culture if the rapid test is negative (Bisno, Gwaltney, Kaplan, and Schwartz, 2002). However, sensitivity has varied with the rigor of the method used for culture. It is still not clear that the latex-agglutination test is as sensitive as culture of a single throat swab (Kellogg and Manzella, 1986; *Lancet*, 1986). The great advantage of the test over culture is its rapidity. The answer is available within 1 hour, so that a decision about treatment can be made while the patient is in the office.

Using cost-effectiveness as their criterion, Tompkins, Burnes, and Cable (1977) recommended the following strategy: if the prevalence rate of streptococcal infection is 30% or more, give antibiotics without culture; if the prevalence rate is 5% or less, do not give antibiotic; if the rate is between 5% and 30%, culture and give antibiotic to those who are positive. We believe this advice still holds good, not only in economic terms, but in terms of benefit to the patient. The latex-agglutination test is now an alternative to culture for the intermediate group.

After using decision analysis for comparing different strategies for managing throat infections, De Neef (1986) observed that the optimal strategy depends on the physician's main objective, whether it is to prevent rheumatic fever, reduce the severity of symptoms, or to minimize the unnecessary use of antibiotics.

If a rapid test is available, why not use it for all patients? Let us look first at the effect of using the test on an adult patient with a sore throat but no enlarged, tender cervical glands, no exudate, and a temperature less than 38°C, when the prevalence rate of streptococcal infection in patients with sore throat is 20%. The pretest probability of streptococcal infection in this patient is 3% (Centor, Meier, and Dalton, 1986). Table 11.1 shows the effect of the test if its sensitivity is 90% and specificity is 96%. (In Tables 11.1, 11.2, and 11.3, the category of streptococcal infection includes those who are carriers. There is no way of distinguishing these at the time of diagnosis.) If the test is negative, as it will be in 934 out of 1000 patients, the effect is negligible—a 2% difference in predictive value. If the test is positive, the predictive value increased by 38%. But does this justify doing the test? Twenty-seven people harboring streptococci will receive treatment, who would otherwise have been untreated. On the other hand, 39 false positives will be treated unnecessarily. Because the infections are clinically mild, the benefit in symptom reduction will be very small. The risk of rheumatic fever will be extremely low.

Let us now look at the effect of using the test in a patient with temperature above 38°C, pharyngeal exudate, enlarged and tender cervical glands, and no

Table 11.1 Predictive value of streptococcal antigen test for streptococcal infection when prevalence rate is 3%

		Streptococcal Infection		
		Yes		No
Streptococcal	Positive	27	a b	39
Antigen Test	Negative	3	c d	931
		30		970

Pretest probability = 3%
Sensitivity = 90%
Specificity = 96%
Posttest probability with positive test = $\dfrac{a}{a+b} = 41\%$

Posttest probability with negative test = $100\% - \dfrac{d}{c+d} = 100\% - \dfrac{931}{934} = 1\%$

Change from pretest probability with positive test = +38%
Change from pretest probability with negative test = −2%

Table 11.2 Predictive value of streptococcal antigen test for streptococcal infection when prevalence rate is 60%

		Streptococcal Infection		
		Yes		No
Streptococcal	Positive	540	a b	16
Antigen Test	Negative	60	c d	384
		600		400

Pretest probability = 60%
Sensitivity = 90%
Specificity = 96%
Posttest probability with positive test = $\dfrac{a}{a+b} = \dfrac{540}{556} = 97\%$

Posttest probability with negative test = $100\% - \dfrac{d}{c+d} = 100\% - \dfrac{384}{444} = 16\%$

Change from pretest probability with positive test = 37%
Change from pretest probability with negative test = 44%

cough (Table 11.2). The pretest probability in this patient at a prevalence rate of 20% is about 60% (Centor, Meier, and Dalton, 1986). As one would expect from a pretest probability at this level, the test has a major effect. A positive test increases the pretest probability by 37%, and a negative test decreases it by 44%. Again, does this justify using the test? About one-third of the patients (384 out of 1,000)

Table 11.3 Predictive value of streptococcal antigen test for streptococcal infection when prevalence rate is 18%

		Streptococcal Infection			
		Yes		No	
Streptococcal Antigen Test	Positive	162 *a*	*b*	33	
	Negative	*c* 18	*d*	787	
		180		820	

Pretest probability $= 18\%$
Sensitivity $= 90\%$
Specificity $= 96\%$
Posttest probability with positive test $= \dfrac{a}{a+b} = \dfrac{162}{195} = 83\%$

Posttest probability with negative test $= 100\% - \dfrac{d}{c+d} = 100\% - \dfrac{787}{805} = 2\%$

Change from pretest probability with positive test $= 65\%$
Change from pretest probability with negative test $= 16\%$

are saved from having unnecessary penicillin. On the other hand, 60 false negatives out of every 1,000 patients are deprived of penicillin and, since they are clinically severe infections, they will also be deprived of the benefits of symptom relief and shortening of the illness.

With an intermediate clinical picture and a prevalence rate of 20%, the pretest probability is 18% (Centor, Meier, and Dalton, 1986). A positive test increases the pretest probability by 65%, and a negative test decreases it by 16% (Table 11.3). Out of 1,000 patients, 787 are saved from unnecessary penicillin if the policy without testing was to prescribe penicillin for all. If the policy without testing was not to prescribe, then 162 patients out of 1,000 benefit by having penicillin for moderately severe clinical infections.

On the basis of the above evidence, we believe the following strategy is appropriate in our present state of knowledge:

1. For adults with sore throat but no exudate, no enlarged and tender cervical glands, and temperature less than 38°C, and for patients with sore throat with no glands or exudate as part of an influenza-like illness: no agglutination test or throat culture, no penicillin.
2. For adults with sore throat, no cough, enlarged and tender cervical glands, exudate, and temperature above 38°C: prescribe penicillin (or appropriate substitute if allergic to penicillin) but do not do agglutination test or throat culture.
3. For adults with a clinical picture between the above categories, do agglutination test or throat culture and prescribe penicillin or appropriate substitute if positive.

Management of Acute Sore Throats in Children

For children with acute sore throat, Dippel, Touw-Otten, and Habbema (1992) used decision analysis to evaluate five strategies:

1. Symptomatic treatment.
2. Direct treatment with penicillin.
3. Agglutination test: if positive, treatment with penicillin.
4. Culture: if positive, treatment with penicillin.
5. Culture: start treatment immediately with oral penicillin; stop treatment if culture is negative

Outcomes were expressed in terms of quality—adjusted life—days lost. The probability of carrier state and compliance were both taken into account in the analysis. The probability that acute sore throat is streptococcal is higher in children than in adults.

In the analysis, the most favorable outcome followed strategy number 3 for patients with at least a 40% probability of having a streptococcal infection. As an illustration, a child with acute sore throat, fever (38.5°C), pain on swallowing, no cough or rhinitis, red throat and tonsillar exudate, and large tender cervical lymph nodes has a 60% probability of streptococcal infection. This strategy assumes a low incidence of rheumatic fever. If the incidence of rheumatic fever is high, the penicillin should be given intramuscularly; if it is low, oral penicillin is recommended.

Family physicians often come under pressure to prescribe antibiotics for mild or moderate throat infections against their better judgment. The reasons are often understandable—important meetings, weddings, examinations, holidays. Throat culture is of little help because of the delay in getting the result. Now that rapid tests are available, the physician can demonstrate to the patient whose test results are negative, before he or she leaves the consulting room, that an antibiotic is not indicated.

For patients who are not allergic to penicillin, in communities where rheumatic fever is not prevalent, oral penicillin V for 10 days is the treatment of choice. One of the most common prescribing errors is the use of amoxicillin for sore throat. This is not only unnecessary, but also increases the cost of treatment and exposes the patient to the risks of additional side effects, especially if the sore throat is due to mononucleosis.

For those who are allergic to penicillin, erythromycin estolate is the treatment of choice. In communities where rheumatic fever is a high risk, or in patients who are at special risk because of a past attack of rheumatic fever or a family history of the disease, or when compliance may be poor, intramuscular injections of penicillin are preferable. When oral penicillin is prescribed, the reasons for giving a 10-day course, and the importance of completing it, should be explained to the patient or to the parent. Under existing conditions in most Western countries, the swabbing of family contacts is not usually necessary. Where rheumatic fever is prevalent, swabbing is indicated, with treatment of those found to be positive. A family physician with responsibilities for community health can also approach the prevention of rheumatic fever through the routine swabbing of schoolchildren.

Family Aspects of Streptococcal Infection

Streptococcal infection spreads within families. The risk of spread within the family is increased when there is overcrowding in the household, especially when sleeping accommodation is shared. In their study of 1,000 families in Newcastle-upon-Tyne, Miller,Court, Walton, and Knox (1960) described 20 "streptococcal families," in whom streptococcal infections recurred in different members of the family over periods of months or years.

Meyer and Haggerty (1962) studied streptococcal infection over a 1-year period in 16 families, comprising 100 persons. Throat cultures were done on all family members every 3 weeks, with additional cultures at times of acute illness. ASO titers were measured in all subjects every 4 months. The families were interviewed periodically, and each one kept a diary recording illnesses, therapy, and life events. A rating scale was used to measure levels of chronic family stress.

There were no significant differences in illness rates associated with the acquisition of group A as compared to non–group A streptococci, or with the various types of group A streptococci. There was also no relationship between likelihood of illness and number of colonies on the agar plate. There was no way of knowing, however, whether the organisms isolated were causally related to the illnesses. Only 28% of beta-hemolytic streptococcal acquisitions, detected by throat culture, were followed by increases in ASO titer. Acquisition rates were highest in school-aged children, second highest in 2- to 5-year-olds, adults next, and lowest in children under 2 years.

There were striking relationships between stressful life events and the occurrence of streptococcal infection. Thirty-five percent of the 56 illnesses associated with beta-hemolytic streptococci were preceded by acute stress. Nineteen percent of beta-streptococcal acquisitions without illness were preceded by acute stress, and 10% of non-streptococcal respiratory infections. The types of stressful event recorded were loss of a family member, serious illness in a family member, father's loss of job, divorce in a near relative, a birth in the family, and stressful events outside the family, such as witnessing violence. Stressful events were four times more frequent in the 2 weeks before all three types of infection than in the 2 weeks after. The number of streptococcal acquisitions, the number of illnesses associated with beta streptococci, the number of prolonged carriers, and the number with ASO titer responses all increased with increasing scores of chronic stress.

Acute Epiglottitis

Although rare, acute epiglottitis is an important condition for family physicians because of the possibility of rapidly worsening airway obstruction. Since the introduction of Haemophilus influenza type b vaccine, the annual incidence in American children has declined from 3.5 cases per 100,000 population in 1980 to 0.6 per 100,000 in 1990. During the same period, the annual incidence is adults remained relatively stable, with a mean incidence of 1.8 cases per 100,000 (Frantz and Rasgon, 1993).

The key features are severe sore throat and pain on swallowing. Drooling of saliva, stridor, and sitting erect are signs of impending respiratory obstruction and should lead to emergency admission to the hospital. In children, inflammation is usually confined to the epiglottis. The swollen epiglottis may be seen on examination of the throat. In adults, the inflammation often affects the pharynx, uvula, and base of the tongue (Frantz, Rasgon, and Quesenberry, 1994).

Infectious Mononucleosis

Infectious mononucleosis (IM) usually presents to the family physician as an acute sore throat. The emergence of the disease illustrates how the pattern of illness in a population changes with social conditions, and how disease categories evolve with changes in medical knowledge. Before 1920, there were many reports of a febrile illness with generalized glandular enlargement, known as glandular fever. Lymphocytosis was reported in some of these patients, but no specific blood picture was described. In 1920, Sprunt and Evans described a series of cases with generalized glandular enlargement and specific hematological findings: a relative and absolute lymphocytosis and atypical mononuclear cells. They called this disease infectious mononucleosis. From this time, the clinical picture and mononucleosis were required criteria for the diagnosis.

In 1932, Paul and Bunnell discovered that sheep erythrocytes were agglutinated by the sera of patients with IM. This heterophil–antibody reaction became the basis of the Paul–Bunnell test and its later refinements. Although the Paul–Bunnell test was often positive in the presence of the clinical and hematological picture, it could be positive in the absence of illness, and it could be negative with the clinical picture. It therefore became customary to divide patients into "heterophil–antibody-positive" and "heterophil-negative" IM.

Between 1964 and 1968 it emerged that heterophil-positive IM was associated with seroconversion to the recently discovered Epstein–Barr virus (EBV) (Epstein, Achong, and Barr, 1964). Further studies showed that many young adults had antibodies to the EBV without having had IM. The presence of EBV antibodies is not necessarily therefore an indication of recent infection. One antibody, however— the VCA-IgM antibody—appears during the acute phase of the infection and disappears shortly after reaching maximal levels. Because this antibody is detectable in 97% of patients with clinical IM, it can be used as a diagnostic test.

The question of what criteria are used for the gold standard in diagnosis becomes important when one is establishing the sensitivity, specificity, and predictive value of a diagnostic test. If the heterophil–antibody test is being evaluated, it cannot itself be used as the gold standard for the diagnosis. Until the discovery of the EBV, only the clinical and hematological picture could be used as the ultimate criterion for IM. Because these were themselves uncertain criteria, it was difficult to establish the predictive value of the heterophil–antibody tests, or any other test, with precision. Some studies did not even state what their gold standard for the diagnosis was. With the discovery of the EBV, we have reached a new stage in the evolution of IM as an illness category. It can now be defined as an EBV infection associated with clinical and hematological features. These features, together with VCA-IgM antibodies, are the ultimate criteria for diagnosis and the gold standard against which the heterophil–antibody test is measured. Because EBV antibody tests are not suitable for routine use, this enables us to use the heterophil–antibody test as a substitute, with precise knowledge of its value.

Children living under poor or crowded conditions undergo seroconversion to EBV in the first 3 years of life, usually without an illness. Under better and less crowded conditions, seroconversion is delayed until later in life—usually adolescence and young adulthood—and then may be associated with the clinical syndrome of IM. IM has emerged, therefore, as a disease in affluent societies with low population densities. Within these societies, it affects the more affluent members. This is why it is especially common in college students, half of whom enter college before seroconversion to EBV.

Epidemiology
The incidence of IM in any population depends on its standard of living and age distribution. The incidence of IM in the general population of Europe and North America is about 1 per 1,000 per year. More than 85% of patients with IM are between the ages of 15 and 30. Among college students the annual incidence is between 10 and 20 per 1,000. A family physician's experience of IM will depend very much on the economic status and age distribution of the practice. The average family physician in Europe, North America, and Australasia will see about two cases per year; a physician who cares for a large student population may see 10 times as many.

Clinical Presentation
Sore throat occurs in 85% of patients and is the most common presenting symptom. The great majority of patients with undifferentiated sore throat do not require clinical examination beyond the head and neck, or any blood tests. The question for the family physician, therefore, is how to select out those patients with a high probability of IM for further investigation. I have found the most useful screening test to be palpation of the posterior cervical glands. These are enlarged in 90% of patients in the first week of the illness and are rarely enlarged in other forms of pharyngitis. Their presence is therefore a very sensitive screening test for IM. If the posterior cervical glands are enlarged, the search strategy will include palpation of axillary and inguinal glands and of the spleen. The spleen is palpable in about 50% of cases, but the peak sensitivity is not reached until the second week.

Other early cues to a diagnosis of IM are a period of malaise before the onset of the sore throat, a discrepancy between the severity of the malaise and the mild appearance of the throat, and increasing redness and exudate in the throat in a patient who is taking penicillin.

The appearance of the throat is indistinguishable from that of streptococcal sore throat. About half the cases have a gray-white exudate, which may become very extensive and may resemble the membrane of diphtheria. The throat infection may be mild or severe. In some cases, there is pharyngeal edema extensive enough to cause respiratory obstruction. Fever is usually present, but may be intermittent, so is not always found when the patient is first seen. The liver is often affected in IM and jaundice is present in 5% to 10% of cases. A patient presenting with sore throat and jaundice should suggest IM.

The degree of glandular enlargement varies greatly. Sometimes the cervical gland enlargement is great enough to produce a bull-necked appearance. Occasionally, an enlarged gland is the patient's presenting complaint.

Investigation

Patients suspected clinically of having IM should have a white cell count and differential, and a test for heterophil antibodies if atypical lymphocytes are less than 40% of the total white cells (see following text). In the first week, some abnormality in the white cell count is usually present. The characteristic finding is a relative and absolute lymphocytosis, often associated with a polymorphonuclear leukopenia. Atypical lymphocytes are a defining feature of IM and distinguish it from other illnesses producing a lymphocytosis. By the second week, lymphocytes may form as much as 60% of the total white cells; for a diagnosis of IM, atypical lymphocytes should be at least 20% of the total white cells. Toxoplasmosis, viral hepatitis, rubella, adenovirus, herpes and cytomegalovirus infections, and influenza B are also associated with lymphocytosis, but with lower levels of atypical lymphocytes.

A number of heterophile–antibody tests are available. In the original Paul–Bunnell test as modified by Davidsohn and Walker (1935), the antibody is measured by its effect in agglutinating sheep red blood cells. The antibody is removed by absorption with bovine erythrocytes but not by absorption with guinea pig tissue. The test is quantitative, the results being expressed as the highest titer in which agglutination occurs. Rapid, nonquantitative tests such as the monospot are based on the agglutination of red cells on a slide after absorption with guinea pig or bovine red cells. Horse red cells are used in the monospot test because the antibody has proved to have higher agglutination activity against these than against sheep cells.

In a prospective study of IM in West Point cadets, Evans, Niderman, Cenabre, West, and Richards (1975) measured the sensitivity and specificity of three heterophil–antibody tests and a test for antibody to EBV IgM, using as their gold standard the clinical and hematological picture, appearance of antibody to EBV, and positivity of at least one heterophil–antibody test. A titer of 1/40 was used as the criterion of positivity. The results illustrate the changes in sensitivity with the evolution of the illness. During the first week, 85.7% of sera were positive by the horse red cell test, 69.2% by the beef red cell, and 68.8% by the sheep red cell test. In the second week, the sensitivities were 100.0%, 85.7%, and 80%, respectively, and in the third week, 100.0%, 100.0%, and 80.0% respectively. Thus, even the most sensitive test, attaining 100% sensitivity in the second week, was only 85% sensitive during the first week of the illness, at the stage when many patients first present to the family physician.

The sensitivity of tests for heterophil antibody also varies with age. They are less sensitive in children and older patients with IM.

Evans, Niderman, Cenabre, West, and Richards (1975) established the specificity of the heterophil-antibody tests by testing the sera of healthy EBV-negative cadets who later developed IM. The beef hemolysin test was positive in no sera, the horse cell test in 6.7%, and the sheep cell test in 12%, giving specificities of 100%, 93.3%, and 88.0%, respectively.

The horse red cell test is therefore the best test for the family physician, provided the result is assessed along with the clinical and hematological picture. If negative, it should be repeated if the patient is not recovering by the third week. In practice, quantitative results are not necessary. Rapid slide tests provide positive/negative results with equivalent sensitivity.

The West Point study showed that the horse cell test was still positive in 73% of patients 1 year after the illness, the sheep red cell test positive in 25% at 1 year. No sera were positive with the beef hemolysin test at 6 months. A persisting positive test can be a source of confusion if found in a patient who was not seen in the acute stage of IM. It may lead to some other illness being erroneously diagnosed as IM. Confusion may also be caused by the reappearance of heterophil antibodies in the course of some other illness—usually respiratory —months or years after the attack of IM (the so-called anamnestic reaction).

By reserving the white cell count and antibody test for patients with sore throat who have a high pretest probability of IM, family physicians are greatly increasing the predictive value of the tests. Is it necessary to test for heterophil–antibody if the clinical picture is typical and if more than 20% of white cells are atypical lymphocytes? Ho-Yen (1983) argues that it is not necessary if atypical lymphocytes are 40% or more of the total, for he found that 98 out of 100 consecutive patients with greater than 40% atypical lymphocytes were serologically positive for IM. If we apply the principles in Chapter 8, the heterophil–antibody test is certainly not going to be useful when the pretest probability of IM is 98%. When the percentage of atypical lymphocytes is between 20 and 40, the probability of IM is 69%, of toxoplasmosis 5%, and of cytomegalovirus 2%; 24% remain undiagnosed. The value of the heterophil–antibody test is increased accordingly. The process of diagnosis is illustrated in Figure 11.1. Is the distinction between IM and these other infections clinically important? We think it is, because their natural history is different. Toxoplasmosis, for example, is a mild illness, but has a longer average duration than IM, and glandular enlargement may continue for months.

Streptococcal throat infection may coexist with IM. How often this occurs is not known. The frequency of positive cultures varies widely in different reports and there is no clear evidence that it is different from the frequency in the general population. My own practice has been to do a throat culture if the throat infection is more than mild and to prescribe antibiotic for those who are positive. Ampicillin

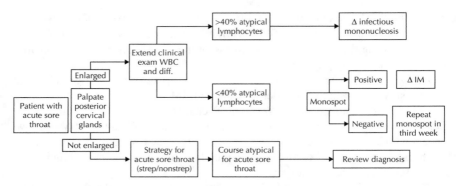

Figure 11.1 Search strategy for infectious mononucleosis in patients with acute sore throat.

or amoxicillin should not be used because of the frequency with which it produces skin rashes in patients with IM.

Management

Infectious mononucleosis is usually a mild illness with a duration of less than 4 weeks. Serious complications occur only in 1% of patients, but a larger number have severe symptoms that can give rise to anxiety. The question for the family physician in these more severe cases is whether or not to admit the patient to the hospital. In my own experience, the condition most often requiring admission is extensive swelling or exudate in the throat.

In the hospital, the throat can have frequent attention, and, if respiratory obstruction occurs, it can be detected and treated before it becomes dangerous. Respiratory obstruction is an uncommon but serious complication of IM. A patient who develops dyspnea or stridor requires urgent admission to the hospital.

One of my (IRMcW) patients requiring admission to the hospital and surgical consultation was a young woman with severe abdominal pain. Abdominal pain raises the question of ruptured spleen, so it should always be taken seriously. Ruptured spleen is a rare complication but has a high mortality rate unless detected early. In those wishing to return to athletic activities, contact sports must be avoided until resolution of splenomegaly. Clinical judgment may require imaging techniques such as ultrasound to confirm complete resolution.

References

Bach JF, Chalons S, Forier E, Elana G, Jouanelle J, Kayemba D et al. 1996. 10-year educational programme aimed at rheumatic fever in two French Caribbean islands. *Lancet* 347:644.

Bisno AL, Gerber MA, Gwaltney JM, Kaplan EL, Schwartz RH. 2002. Practice guidelines for the diagnosis and management of group a streptococcal pharyngitis. *Clinical Infectious Diseases* 35:113–125.

Carapetis JR, McDonald M, Wilson NJ. 2005. Acute rheumatic fever. *Lancet* 366(9480):155–168.

Centor RM, Meier FA, Dalton HP. 1986. Throat cultures and rapid tests for diagnosis of Group A streptococcal pharyngitis. *Annals of Internal Medicine* 105:892.

Davidsohn I, Walker PH. 1935. Nature of heterophilic antibodies in infectious mononucleosis. *American Journal of Clinical Pathology* 5:455.

De Neef P. 1986. Comparison of tests for streptococcal pharnygitis. *Journal of Family Practice* 23:551.

Dippel DWJ, Touw-Otten F, Habbema JDF. 1992. Management of children with acute pharyngitis: A decision analysis. *Journal of Family Practice* 34(3):149.

Epstein MA, Achong BG, Barr YM. 1964. Virus particles in cultured lymphoblasts from Burkitt's lymphoma. *Lancet* 1:702.

Evans AS, Niderman JC, Cenabre LC, West B, Richards VA. 1975. A prospective evaluation of heterophile and Epstein-Barr virus-specific IgM antibody tests in clinical and subclinical infectious mononucleosis: Specificity and sensitivity of the tests and persistence of antibody. *Journal of Infectious Diseases* 132:246.

Forsyth RA. 1975. Selective utilization of clinical diagnosis in treatment of pharyngitis. *Journal of Family Practice* 2(3):174.

Frantz TD, Rasgon BM. 1993. Acute epiglottitis: Changing epidemiologic patterns. *Otolaryngology—Head and Neck Surgery* 109:457.

Frantz TD, Rasgon BM, Quesenberry CP. 1994. Acute epiglottitis in adults: Analysis of 129 cases. *Journal of the American Medical Association* 272(17):1358.

Hillner BE, Centor RM. 1987. What a difference a day makes: A decision analysis of adult streptococcal pharyngitis. *Journal of General Internal Medicine* 2:244.

Howie JGR, Foggo BA. 1985. Antibodies, sore throats, and rheumatic fever. *Journal of the Royal College of General Practice* 35:223.

Ho-Yen DO. 1983. Is the serological diagnosis of infectious mononucleosis always necessary? *British Medical Journal* 287:1187.

Kaplan EL, Hill HR. 1987. Return of rheumatic fever: Consequences, implications, and needs. *Journal of Pediatrics* 111:244.

Kellogg JA, Manzella JP. 1986. Detection of group A streptococci in the laboratory or physician's office. *Journal of the American Medical Association* 255:2638.

Lancet Editorial. 1986. Rapid detection of beta hemolytic streptococci. *Lancet* 1:247.

Meyer RJ, Haggerty RJ. 1962. Streptococcal infection in families. *Pediatrics* 29:539.

Miller FJW, Court WDM, Walton WS, Knox EG. 1960. *Growing up in Newcastle upon Tyne.* London: Oxford University Press.

Paul JR, Bunnell WW. 1932. The presence of heterophile antibodies in infectious mononucleosis. *American Journal of Medical Science* 183:80.

Sprunt TP, Evans FA. 1920. Mononuclear leucocytosis in reaction to acute infections ("infectious mononucleosis"). *Bulletin of the Johns Hopkins Hospital* 31:410.

Tompkins RK, Burnes DC, Cable WE. 1977. An analysis of the cost-effectiveness of pharyngitis management and acute rheumatic fever prevention. *Annals of Internal Medicine* 86:481.

Veasy LG, Tani LY, Daly JA, Korgnski K, Miner L, Bale J et al. 2004. Temporal association of the appearance of mucoid strains of Streptococcus pyogenes with a continuing high incidence of rheumatic fever in Utah. *Pediatrics* 113:e168–e172.

12

Headache

Headache is among the 12 most common presenting complaints in family practice in industrialized societies. It is also one of the most common reasons for patients to use alternative therapies. In approximately 20% of patients, the headaches are secondary to an organic disease process. The large majority of secondary headaches are caused by relatively benign conditions such as sinusitis (Table 12.1). A very small proportion are caused by life-threatening conditions that are rare in family practice, such as cranial tumor and other brain lesions, cranial arteritis, and subarachnoid hemorrhage. These present us with a challenge, because we have to respond to those cues that distinguish these patients from the large majority with primary headache. Patients with primary headache present another kind of challenge. About 16% become chronic sufferers and there is good reason to believe that the initial assessment and management may be a factor in preventing long-term disability (Headache Study Group, 1986).

Classification of Headaches

In 2004, the International Headache Society published a second edition of its widely used classification system (ICHD II, 2004). As in the first edition, migraine headaches are broadly divided into those with and those without aura. Tension-type headaches (TTH) may or may not have pericranial tenderness. The system is designed as a taxonomy of headaches, not of patients. Many patients have more than one type of headache and should receive a different diagnosis for each headache. The old term "combined headache" has been abandoned. Because individual episodes may be aborted by treatment, or poorly remembered, there is no need to attempt diagnosis of every headache. The most typical episodes without treatment should be described.

Table 12.1 Final diagnosis in 265 patients presenting to family physicians with a new complaint of headache

	Number of Patients	Percentage
Cluster headache	5	1.9
Classical migraine (def.)	8	3.0
Classical migraine (poss.)	5	1.9
Common migraine (def.)	6	2.3
Common migraine (poss.)	59	22.2
Muscle contraction (def.)	45	17.0
Muscle contraction (poss.)	81	30.5
Acute sinusitis	16	6.0
Posttraumatic headache	8	3.0
Cervical spine headache	4	1.5
Temporal arteritis	1	.4
Drug-induced headache	5	1.9
Birth control pill	7	2.6
Ocular headache	4	1.5
Meningitis	1	.4
Fever	2	.8
Viral rhinitis	3	1.1
Allergic rhinitis	1	.4
Wine intolerance	1	.4
Vascular abnormalities	1	.4
Intracranial lesion	1	.4
Possible demyelinating disorder	1	.4
Totals	265	100.0

Def., definite; poss., possible.

From Headache Study Group, 1986.

The IHS Classification is still controversial. Like the former system (Ad Hoc Committee, 1962), it does not rest on empirical evidence from experimental or descriptive biology. A pathological basis has been demonstrated for only two of the main categories: migraine with aura and cluster headache. The distinction between migraine without aura and TTH is still one of degree; TTHs are more variable in duration, more constant, less severe, more often bilateral, and less often associated with nausea. There is still, therefore, a case to be made for regarding recurring benign headaches as a continuum until the evidence justifies two discrete categories (Marcus, 1992). This was the position taken in the first edition. The IHS response to this is that the system should be regarded as evolving, not written in stone. They justify retaining the category distinctions on the grounds that it will increase the precision of clinical research.

The new IHS categories are organized in a four-level hierarchy. For example, the first-level category, "tension-type" headache, is divided at the second level into episodic and chronic forms. This is justified by the differences in management between the two forms. At the third level, patients with TTHs are divided into those with and those without disorder of the pericranial muscles. The fourth level is used to indicate the pathogenic factors, such as anxiety, depression, and oromandibular dysfunction. It is suggested that in general practice, diagnosis will be made at the first level, whereas other levels will be needed for research purposes (ICHD II, 2004). Although this may be generally correct, it should not be taken as a rule of diagnosis in general practice. The degree of precision required depends on the context. Concern about the cause of their headaches is a major reason for patients to consult a family physician (Headache Study Group, 1986). A diagnosis at the first level may be sufficient for these patients. The key to a successful consultation is often an understanding of the meaning of the headaches for the patient and a diagnosis sufficient for reassurance that no serious disease is present. The provision of reassurance may explain why many patients seen with headaches do not return for a second visit (Becker et al., 1988). On the other hand, many patients with TTHs are anxious and depressed, so that diagnosis at the fourth level is required. And management of a complex illness such as recurrent headaches requires diagnosis at many levels.

Migraine

Cerebral blood flow in the posterior part of the cerebral hemisphere is reduced at the onset of a migraine with aura. This hypoperfusion lasts during the aura and into the headache phase, sometimes persisting longer than the headache. Hypoperfusion is followed by hyperperfusion. These findings are not sufficient to support the theory that the migraine aura is caused by constriction and dilatation of cerebral arteries. Recent findings suggest that the process is one of spreading cortical depression, a wave of neuronal depolarization that spreads across the cortex, followed by a period of relative silence, then a return of neuronal activity. Although this may explain the aura of migraine, it does not explain the pain. This may be the result of interactions between neurotransmitters released by the sensory and sympathetic nerve endings in the intracranial arteries. In contrast, migraine without aura shows no changes of spreading cortical depression although there may be blood flow changes in the brainstem. Nevertheless, migraine without aura responds to triptans which are highly specific for 5-HT receptors suggesting some commonality with migraine with aura.

Serotonin has long been known to be involved in the pathogenesis of migraine. Plasma serotonin is increased early in the attack and decreased in the later stages. Serotonin acts on many different neuroreceptors in blood vessels, inducing either vasodilatation or vasoconstriction, depending on the locally dominant receptor. Sumatriptan binds to serotonin 1D receptors in the intracranial vasculature, thus blocking release of a neuropeptide involved in the interactions believed to produce the pain (Hoffert, 1994; Olesen, 1994). Ergotamine, methysergide, and sumatriptan all act on 5-HT receptors, but sumatriptan is the first antimigraine drug to have receptor selective properties (Moskowitz and Cutrer, 1993). In spite of the elucidation of the mechanism of migraine headaches, migraine should not be seen as "caused" by a single factor, even though a final common pathway for the headaches can be identified. The causal web is complex and multifactorial, and the balance of factors varies from one patient to another. In a recent review of the biology of migraine, a leading authority concludes that "it is now time for physicians to acknowledge that migraine is a neurobiologic, not a psychogenic disorder" (Olesen, 1994)—a view that exemplifies the either/or thinking that pervades much of modern medicine. For family physicians, migraine is more likely to be viewed as a coupling of biological and behavioral processes in a complex, nonlinear relationship.

Any explanation of migraine must account for a condition of great complexity and diversity. The aura may include visual and other sensory hallucinations, mood changes, intense emotions, and disorders of consciousness. At the height of an attack there is severe headache, together with nausea, vomiting, and other vegetative symptoms. The attack may be preceded by a variety of prodromal symptoms, including emotional states. The finding of a mechanism for one of the manifestations of migraine does not mean that the "cause" of migraine has been found. The mechanism, for example, may explain the headache of migraine but does not explain why the mechanism was activated in the first place. Even the discovery of a successful therapeutic agent does not depend on elucidation of the cause of migraine, for it may act on a final common pathway for the symptoms of migraine without affecting the underlying process leading to the pathway. Moskowitz and Cutrer (1993) suggest that sumatriptan may work in this way. If this is so, a favorable response to the drug is not necessarily diagnostic of migraine, because other types of headache may have a similar final common pathway. Because clinical practice is concerned primarily with the relief or prevention of suffering, a successful remedy may render the further elucidation of causal explanation less urgent. A new pragmatic taxonomy may emerge, based on response to treatment rather than pathophysiology. With headache in general, and migraine in particular, the complexity of the processes involved make it unlikely that any single system of classification, or any one form of therapy will be sufficient. The ability to abort an attack is not the same thing as being able to prevent recurrences. Attacks of migraine can be triggered by numerous external factors as well as by physiological and emotional states. A patient's response to attacks may be such as to reinforce the tendency to recurrence. There are, therefore, many possible therapeutic approaches to migraine, and the development of a successful drug should not lead to a neglect of other approaches.

In some patients, migraine headaches become chronic, persistent, and disabling. Of these, Sacks (1985) writes: "The most severely afflicted patients defeated my therapeutic endeavors until I started to enquire minutely and persistently into their emotional lives. It now became apparent to me that many migraine attacks were drenched in emotional significance, and could not be usefully considered...unless their emotional antecedents and effects were exposed in detail." Two forms of association between the emotions and bodily states have been postulated. Emotions have their involuntary physiological concomitants, and chronic emotional tension may be expected to have its physiological counterpart in vegetative symptoms. The emotional tensions, however, are often repressed, so that the patient's state is experienced as one of chronic pain. The second type of association is the one described by Freud as conversion. In this reaction, somatic symptoms become a substitute for repressed emotion. The association between the symptoms and the emotion is symbolic, not physiological. The substitution takes place usually in the voluntary motor and sensory systems. The location and distribution of the dysfunction (e.g., paralysis or analgesia) is the patient's image of the body, not the anatomical structure of the nervous system. The distinction is by no means clear-cut. A vegetative symptom may become, by a process of learning and conditioning, a symbolic substitute for repressed emotion. The chronic migraine state may therefore be the physiological concomitant of repressed emotion and become the symbolic substitute for the emotion, with all the uses to which the substitution can be put: avoidance, regression, self-punishment, and so on. "In migraine, the symptoms are fixed and bounded by physiological connections; but its symptoms can constitute...a bodily alphabet or protolanguage, which may secondarily and subsequently be used as a symbolic language" (Sacks, 1992).

Assessment of the Patient with Headache

The interview and history are by far the most important parts of the assessment. It is very important to allow the patient to express feelings and fears and to ascertain his or her expectations of treatment and perception of the cause of the headache.

The important data to be obtained from the history are length of headache history, frequency of headaches, mode of onset, duration, site of headache, severity, description of pain, precipitating factors, warning symptoms, accompanying symptoms, relieving factors and coping strategies, history of trauma, current medications, and family history of headaches. If time is limited, anxiety to obtain all the data should not be allowed to reduce the opportunity for the patient to express himself or herself. If necessary, the full picture can be obtained over two or more visits.

Grouping a number of headache patients together in one category is an abstraction from a much larger picture. In each patient, the symptom of headache has to be considered in the larger context of the whole person. The family physician's knowledge of the context may come from a number of sources but most probably from previous knowledge of the patient and the family and from the patient's records. Any deficiencies in this knowledge will need to be made up for during the initial visits. It is important to know about current problems in the patient's life, previous illness patterns, and self-medication. A history of pain syndromes or a tendency to symptom formation is particularly important.

At the completion of the interview and history, the physician should already have ascertained, with a high probability of being correct, whether the headaches are primary or secondary and, if primary, whether they fall into the categories of migraine with aura or cluster headache. Texts on headache sometimes say that a full neurological examination should be done on every patient. For the primary physician this is poor advice. In most patients, a full neurological examination would be redundant and would only reduce the time available for listening to the patient. Apart from certain routines, the physical examination—its kind and extent—will be determined by the physician's hypothesis after completing the interview and history. A hypothesis of sinusitis will direct the physician's attention to the nose and sinuses; a headache of recent and sudden onset to the body temperature and a test for neck rigidity; a history of neurological symptoms to the appropriate neurological examination; and malaise accompanying the headaches to a search for infection. On the other hand, a patient with tight-band headache who breaks down and cries may have little or no physical examination at all.

Besides a directed search, the physician should also have certain routines that are done for all patients or all patients in certain categories. The selection of routines is discussed in Chapter 8. These are not necessarily done on all patients; one or all may be omitted. The important thing is that the physician has to justify their omission to himself or herself. The routines headache patients may include pulse, blood pressure, fundi, selected cranial nerves, neck movements, palpation of neck and scalp, and, in patients over50 years, sedimentation rate. Hypertension seldom presents with headache; many patients, however, expect to have their blood pressure taken, and their visit provides an opportunity to detect hypertension unrelated to the headaches.

The Diagnosis of Headache

This section deals with the distinction between the main headache categories. The family physician's main tasks are to distinguish primary from secondary headache and, within these categories, to identify certain disorders with a specific etiology, specific therapy, or a threat to life.

Migraine with Aura

The distinguishing features of migraine with aura are recurrent headaches preceded or accompanied by focal neurological disturbances and also accompanied by nausea and/or vomiting. The headache is usually described as throbbing and severe and may be unilateral or bilateral. The frequency of the headaches varies greatly from one patient to another and in the same patient at different times. The most common neurological disturbances are visual. Typically, the patient first notices a small area of scintillation and blurring in the field of vision. This gradually enlarges into a ring of zig-zag lines, shaped like the fortifications of an ancient castle. Hence the term fortification spectrum. The enlarging ring is followed by a crescent of blindness—the scotoma—which is followed in turn by restoration of vision. The whole sequence takes 15 to 20 minutes to pass over the visual field. Typically, the headache begins as the aura wanes. Some patients may experience flashing lights, scotomata, or hemianopia. Others may have transient neurological disturbances of other kinds—paresthesia, vertigo, or aphasia, for example. The tongue, hands, and feet are areas of predilection for paresthesia. These begin peripherally and spread centripetally. The rate of spread is very much slower than in the aura of epilepsy—an important distinguishing feature. In contrast to the crescendo of migraine—transient ischemic attacks (TIAs) are maximal at onset, after which they recede. The anatomical distribution of a TIA corresponds to the distribution of the artery involved.

Attacks of migraine—with or without aura—may be preceded by premonitory or prodromal symptoms such as restlessness, insomnia, emotional arousal, mood changes, thirst, water retention, and gastrointestinal disturbances. After the attack, there may be a period of cognitive disturbance during which it is unwise for the patient to be doing work that involves judgment and decision making. The prodromal symptoms can warn the patient to prepare for an attack. On the other hand, they may have a disturbing effect on the family.

Migraine with aura usually begins in childhood or early adult life. Onset after the age of 50 is rare. The pattern of attacks varies greatly between patients and in the same patient at different periods of life. Some patients may have only occasional attacks throughout life. Some may have occasional attacks at one time of life, frequent attacks at another. Others may have the full syndrome at one time of life and transient neurological symptoms without headaches at another. In childhood, the manifestation of migraine may be recurrent vomiting attacks (the periodic syndrome). In some patients, the pain may be felt in one side of the face—the so-called facial migraine.

In certain rare variants of the migraine syndrome, the headaches are accompanied and followed by motor neurological deficits such as hemiplegia or ophthalmoplegia. These motor phenomena require further pursuit.

Migraine without Aura
The attacks are distinguished from migraine with aura chiefly by the absence of preceding neurological symptoms. The most common symptoms accompanying the headache are nausea, vomiting, photophobia, phonophobia, and general sensory excitability. Other symptoms include dizziness, drowsiness, abdominal pain, diarrhea, and nasal stuffiness.

If nausea is the only symptom accompanying the headache, differentiation from TTH may be difficult, especially if the headache is not typical of migraine. The Headache Study Group found that only six patients out of 65 classified as having common migraine were considered "definite" after 1 year of follow-up. Very frequent migraine (>15 days per month for at least 3 months) is called chronic migraine provided there is no medication overuse. Typically, chronic migraine evolves from migraine without aura.

Cluster Headache (Migrainous Neuralgia)
The salient features of cluster headache are its periodicity, its great severity, and its preponderance in males. The syndrome is periodic in two senses. Bouts of headaches, lasting from 2 to 12 weeks, alternate with pain-free intervals of several months to several years. Within each bout, headaches occur one or more times a day, often with great regularity. The headache is almost always unilateral and centered around the eye and is so severe that the sufferer cannot keep still. It is usually accompanied by lacrimation from the eye on the affected side. The conjunctiva is often injected in this eye, and there may be some drooping of the upper eyelid and miosis. If the patient is seen between headaches, these signs are of course absent. The male-to-female ratio in cluster headache is about 6 to 1. Most patients are between the ages of 20 and 40.

Tension-type Headache and Recurrent Nonspecific Headache

The IHS (ICHD II) continues to include TTH, episodic and chronic, in its classification system. The headache is defined by the features that distinguish it from migraine: moderate severity, bilateral distribution, longer duration, and absence of nausea and photophobia. The chronic form is distinguished from the episodic by the persistence of headaches for longer than 6 months. In addition, both episodic and chronic TTH are subdivided into those with and without pericranial tenderness elicited by manual palpation.

This classification and nomenclature remains controversial. The physiological basis for these headaches has not been established, and in practice it is often difficult to make a clear distinction between common migraine and "tension-type" headaches. This difficulty is reflected in the discussions within the classification subcommittee of the International Headache Society(ICHD II, 2004, p. 32). The issue can be further complicated as TTH can occur in migraineurs making treatment decisions even more difficult.

After reviewing all the available clinical data in 265 new patients with headache, using the 1962 classification, the Headache Study Group (1986) was unable to classify 50% of the patients with any degree of certainty. Thirty percent were classified as having "possible muscle contraction headache" and 22% as "possible common migraine." For these reasons, such patients were described in the first edition of this book as having recurrent nonspecific headache (RNSH). Anxiety was associated with the headaches in about 60% of these patients and depression in about 25%. In many patients with RNSH, the headaches are related to transient situational anxiety and reactive depression. In some, the anxiety is focused on the cause of the headache. Of 1,331 patients attending primary care physicians with new headache, 1,131 (85%) did not return for a second visit within the 14-month study period (Becker et al., 1988). This suggests that in the great majority of patients with headache seen by family physicians, the condition is self-limiting or responds to measures such as reassurance and counseling. The following consultation is a good example of this type of headache.

Patient: I thought I'd better get a checkup. I just don't feel 100%. I've had really bad headaches for about a week (putting hand on right forehead). I've got constant headache: along here (draws finger across forehead) and down here (down each side of nose). When I bend my head over it hurts (bending her head over). My whole head feels like it's being squashed (squeezing head between hands). I don't know—I take Tylenol, but it doesn't seem to make much difference.

Doctor: Uh huh.

Patient: It's really very sore here (rubs nose). The back of my head here hurts, the top hurts (hand on crown). Hurts sort of everywhere you know. I don't know whether it's a cold.

Doctor: Have you had this before?

Patient: Like what do you mean?

Doctor: This collection of symptoms?

Patient: Last year I had sinus trouble: so blocked I couldn't even blow my nose. I've only got a slight dribble from my nose now. Doesn't seem as if I need to blow my nose all the time. Maybe a cough or a sneeze.

Doctor: Uh huh (nods).

Patient: ... apart from that, nothing really. I've got this really bad headache (right hand on forehead).

Doctor: Are you a headachy person generally?

Patient: Not really, no ... I get headaches from time to time. Seems like my whole head's throbbing—not all the time: some of the time.

Doctor: You mentioned that you feel a bit low too, apart from the headache.

Patient: I had a car accident a couple of months ago now. I had a month when I had this flu-type thing, and a bad bronchitis-type thing as well. It took me ages to shake, and ever since then I just haven't felt right. I just sort of—I don't know—I feel really lethargic. I just don't feel 100%.

Doctor: What sort of treatments did you have during the course of that illness. A lot?

Patient: First of all I had an antibiotic because he (the doctor she consulted near her home because she did not have a car) said it was a chest infection. And then he put me on ventolin because I got asthma as well. And then he sort of he thought it would get better.

I was sort of coughing all night. It was awful—I couldn't shake it. Its the worst thing I've ever had (pause). My Dad died in March. I was—I don't know. A lot of people said to me "you're stressed"—plus the car accident. I don't know—it's the worst illness of my life, really. If all I've got is a cold, it should be getting better by now. Its not. I thought I'd better get checked out.

Doctor: Yes, sure.

Patient: You can't keep taking Tylenol all the time.

Doctor: A lot's happened to you.

Patient: I feel really weak. I cough every now and then even now.

Doctor: When did you have the original bout?

Patient: Oh, at the end of May it started—hung on till the middle of June.

Doctor: Do you feel you got over it completely at any stage?

Patient: No. I don't feel I've ever got over it and I feel really weak—cough every now and then still. I feel lightheaded all the time. I don't have any energy—feel weak and tired all the time.

Doctor: Are you sleeping all right?

Patient: No.

Doctor: Not sleeping? What's keeping you awake?

Patient: I don't know—ever since my Dad died—I don't know. Plus, another thing too— my husband moved out in March. Ever since he moved out, I haven't really ... you know.

Doctor: You've had a lot, haven't you.

Patient: I don't know. I've been trying to cope on my own. I haven't really felt well for a long time. That's why I don't sleep properly.

Doctor: How are you coping?

Patient: Oh, well—you know. I'm going red now (puts hands to her face, looks upset). I can feel it. I can't get used to sleeping on my own, and that's why I don't sleep properly. But since my Dad died, that's another thing—that was really shocking— I never really slept very well—even worse after that.

Doctor: His death was unexpected, was it?

Patient: (Describes father's sudden death at home, then gives a long sigh) I don't know what's wrong with me, whether it's stress—you know.

Doctor: Do you feel anxious and stressed?

Patient: I had an anxiety attack on the Saturday night—after the funeral. I thought I was going to die then. I couldn't breathe. It's awful. It came on suddenly, my heart was beating fast. My mother was with me—she thought I was going to die, too. I went to the local doctor. He told me to go home and behave myself and stop being stupid.

Doctor: How did you feel about that?

Patient: I felt awful. I felt there was something seriously wrong with me. He said, "Go for a jog if you feel like that." I told him, "How can I jog—I can't breathe." So he put me on these Valium tablets. Then three weeks later I had this car accident because I went to sleep at the wheel. So I haven't taken anything since. But since then I've been taking yoga classes—learning to relax.

Doctor: That's good. Do you feel it's helping?

Patient: I feel it's starting to. Now when I feel anxious I start to do the deep breathing. I can visualize the tranquility.

Doctor: Do you do it each day?

Patient: I try to do it at least once a day.

Doctor: Excellent. That's a very constructive thing to do.

Patient: I really enjoy it. I used to do it. Especially after the car accident. I knew how it happened. It was Good Friday. I was really upset at Mums—just the memories, I suppose. Got to me and I was crying. So I took a tablet in the afternoon because I felt really anxious. I was driving home.

Doctor: You were lucky.

You've told me about the tiredness and lethargy and headaches. Is there anything else you can tell me about how you are feeling?

Patient: About how I'm feeling? (describes how she has been irritable and "on edge.")

At a follow-up visit, doctor and patient explored her feelings of anger, guilt, and sadness. Once the connection was made between her emotional state and the headaches, she had the requisite skills to deal with it herself. An antihistamine was prescribed because there was an element of sinus inflammation complicating the headache.

In some patients, intermittent headaches evolve over a period of years to a chronic state of daily headaches. By this stage, patients are often depressed, sleep poorly, and make frequent use of analgesics. The natural history and pathophysiology of the chronic condition is not well understood. One concept is that intermittent common migraine is transformed over a period of 8 to 10 years to daily chronic headaches of the tension type (Saper, 1990).

Besides the clinical history and description of the headaches, it is important in TTH to answer certain questions. First, what is the patient's perception of the problem? What does he or she think the headaches are caused by? What prompted the patient to consult a doctor? It is common for patients to have fears about the cause of the headaches, especially about cerebral tumor. Second, is the patient depressed or suffering from chronic or recurrent anxiety, with or without depression? It is especially important to explore feelings, life experiences, and interpersonal relationships. There may be no clear relationship between times of anxiety and the times of headaches. Patients may say that the headaches occur even when they are most relaxed. Has the patient noticed any triggering factors or relieving factors? Even if these have not been noticed by the time of the first consultation, keeping a headache diary may bring them to the patient's attention. What medication is the patient taking? If the patient is new to the practice, he or she may have been receiving prescriptions for tranquilizers or narcotics.

Medication-Overuse Headache
This is an important diagnostic category in family practice, though the frequency is unknown. Without careful a careful history, patients may be diagnosed erroneously as chronic migraine or frequent TTH. What distinguishes medication-overuse headache is the use of migraine drugs and/or analgesics on a frequent and regular basis. In this way, episodic TTH may evolve into a chronic state. Generally use of ergotamine, or triptans or opioid analgesics for more than 10 days per month, and of more than 15 days for simple analgesics is required to merit this diagnosis. It is very important to make this diagnosis as patients in this category rarely respond to preventative medications.

The Diagnosis of Patients with Subarachnoid Hemorrhage
or Intracranial Mass
Subarachnoid hemorrhage (SAH), subdural hematoma (SDH), and intracranial tumor (ICT) are rare in family practice. An American study of 58 practices reported an annual incidence rate per 100,000 patients of 1.9 for SAH, 4.1 for SDH, and 6.1 for ICT (Becker et al., 1993b). The figure for SAH is lower than that reported in a general practice study from the Netherlands: 4.2 per 100,000 per year (Linn et al., 1994).

The incidence of intracranial lesions in patients presenting to family physicians with new headache is about 0.4% (Headache Study Group, 1986; Becker et al., 1988). Even in neurological practice, the incidence of intracranial lesions in headache patients with a normal neurological examination is only 2.4% (Frishberg, 1994).

Subarachnoid hemorrhage has a mortality rate of 50%, and it is estimated that 36% of patients die before they reach the hospital. It has been estimated that 40% to 60% of patients have warning signs caused by small leaks several days or weeks before the main hemorrhage. These estimates, however, are based on retrospective studies. In a recent prospective study in general practice only two of 37 reported patients with SAH had previous episodes of headache (Linn et al., 1994). A SAH causes severe headache of sudden onset, often with vomiting, prostration, syncope, nuchal rigidity, and loss of consciousness. Patients with this type of headache have a high likelihood of serious neurological disorder. Of 148 general practice patients with this kind of headache reported by Linn et al. (1994), 37 had SAH, nine had intracerebral hematomas, four had meningitis or encephalitis, and one each had SDH, giant aneurysm without bleeding, bleeding into a tumor, cerebral infarct, and intraventricular bleeding. Thirty-four patients were not investigated, and in 59 the investigations were negative. None of these 93 patients had developed a serious neurological disorder after 1 year of follow-up. The same investigators had reported in an earlier study that a large proportion of patients with sudden severe headache and negative investigations subsequently develop migraine (Wijdicks, Kerkhoff, and van Gijn, 1988).

Patients with sudden, severe headache plus other evidence of SAH should be admitted immediately to a hospital with a neurosurgical unit. For those with sudden severe headache alone, the evidence indicates that an urgent CT scan or MRI should be done. Because the CT scan is negative in about 6% of patients with SAH (Becker et al., 1993a; Linn et al., 1994), a lumbar puncture should be done in patients with strong clinical evidence of SAH and negative imaging studies. Because MRI has a sensitivity of more than 90% in picking up soft tissue lesions, it is likely that it will eventually be the investigation of choice if available.

The indications for CT scan in the early detection of intracranial mass are less clear-cut. Patients who present with headache plus neurological abnormalities, symptoms of raised intracranial pressure, or seizure pose no difficulty, because all will be either investigated or referred to a neurologist. About half of patients with ICT, SAH, or SDH who present with headache have additional signs or symptoms (Becker et al., 1993b). Those with typical migraine or episodic TTHs do not need further investigation unless this is indicated on other grounds, such as the patient's anxiety. A CT scan should be considered in patients with persistent, worsening headaches of recent origin, even if there are no neurological signs or symptoms, and in patients whose headaches have changed in frequency or intensity. CT scans with contrast medium give a higher yield of abnormalities. In one study (Becker et al., 1993a), family physicians ordered CT scans for 3% of patients presenting with headache. In half of these, an ICT was suspected because of the above clinical presentation. Of 293 CT scan reports reviewed, 14 indicated that an ICT, SAH, or an SDH was present. Two of these were found to be false positives. Forty-four (15%) of the reports noted incidental findings of little clinical significance. The rest (83%) were negative. Thus, the true positives were heavily outnumbered by false positives and incidental findings, some of which (e.g., cerebral atrophy) had the potential for causing long-term anxiety. Fifty-nine (17%) of the CT scans were ordered because of patients' expectations or medicolegal concerns.

In the present state of knowledge, therefore, clear indications for further investigation, and clear evidence of benefit, exist only for patients with sudden severe headache and headache with additional signs and symptoms. In the remainder, good clinical judgment must be the guide in selecting those few for whom the benefits of further investigation are likely to outweigh the risks.

Cranial (Temporal) Arteritis

Headache is a common presenting symptom in this inflammatory condition of the cranial arteries. Cranial arteritis is a general disorder of elderly people, closely related to polymyalgia rheumatica. In fact, these two conditions are probably variants of the same pathological process. Because the disorder is a generalized one, the headaches usually occur with symptoms such as malaise, sweating, myalgia, and arthralgia. In some patients, the headache may be overshadowed by other more florid symptoms such as high fever, vomiting, vertigo, visual disturbances, and other neurological symptoms. The disease is virtually unknown under the age of 50.

The importance of this condition is that if diagnosis is delayed, involvement of the intracranial arteries can cause blindness and cerebrovascular accidents.

The response to steroids is dramatic, although the treatment does not completely remove the risk of serious complications. The results are so satisfactory, however, that the early diagnosis of cranial arteritis is important preventive medicine. Because the disease is uncommon in general practice, this poses a challenge to the family physician. Hence the need for awareness and for routine ESRs in older patients with headaches or joint and muscle pains.

Examination may reveal tenderness and thickening of the affected scalp arteries. This sign, however, is not 100% sensitive and cannot be relied on for ruling out cranial arteritis (see sensitivity, Chapter 8). The most sensitive test is the ESR, which is nearly always above 50 mm per hour and usually much higher. The diagnosis is based on the clinical findings and ESR, with appropriate tests to rule out other causes of a very high sedimentation rate, such as myelomatosis, systemic lupus erythematosus, carcinomatosis, and pernicious anemia. Treatment should be started with prednisone as soon as the diagnosis has been made. The dramatic response to steroids is an additional confirmation of the diagnosis. Biopsy of the temporal artery may be done, but the test is not very sensitive, and a negative test is of little value. Treatment should not be withheld while a patient is waiting for a biopsy.

Sinusitis
In the Headache Study Group (1986) data, 6% of patients with new headache presenting to family physicians were diagnosed as having acute sinusitis, according to rigorous criteria that included X-ray confirmation for maxillary sinusitis.

Morbidity studies record an incidence of 21 to 25 episodes per 1,000 listed patients per year, usually based on a clinical diagnosis without X-ray or ultrasound. A study using ultrasound as confirmation reported an incidence of 14.1 episodes per 1,000 patients per year (van Duijn, Brouwer, and Lamberts, 1992). Not surprisingly, sinusitis tends to be overdiagnosed when only clinical criteria are used. In cases where ultrasonography was negative, the clinical diagnosis was upper respiratory infection, rhinitis, headache, or "other." The sensitivities and specificities of ultrasonography are 89 percent and 95 percent, respectively, for maxillary sinusitis and 90 percent and 75% to 95% for frontal sinusitis (van Duijn, Brouwer, and Lamberts, 1992). Of the symptoms and signs recorded, five were independently related to a positive ultrasound: onset of symptoms with a common cold, purulent rhinorrhea, pain on bending, unilateral maxillary pain, and pain in the teeth. Given this cluster of symptoms, the diagnosis can be made on clinical grounds and treatment with amoxicillin initiated. According to van Duijn, Brouwer, and Lamberts (1992), 55% to 65% of the doctors' clinical diagnoses were correct. Only 5% of cases were missed.

In the study by van Duijn et al. (1992), the start and end point of the episodes were not clear-cut, nor was the border between sinusitis and nose complaints or facial pain.

Van Buchem et al. (1995) found that sinusitis (confirmed by X-ray, ultrasound, and antral puncture) cannot be predicted by history or clinical examination. Relying on clinical diagnosis alone means that large numbers of patients may be receiving antibiotics unnecessarily. Family physicians are probably basing their decisions to prescribe an antibiotic on severity of symptoms rather than diagnostic label, as Howie (1973) found with respiratory infection. Whether or not this is justified must await clinical trials of antibiotic treatment.

Posttraumatic Headache
Headache following injury presents two kinds of problems for the family physician: deciding whether the headache is a result of intracranial hemorrhage and identifying the different contributory factors in patients with continuing headaches that persist long after the injury. Headache is the most frequent symptom following mild head injury. Dizziness, fatigue, nausea, weakness, depression, insomnia, and cognitive impairment are also reported. Many patients with cognitive symptoms do not report them unless specifically asked about them (Packard, 1994). Most patients improve gradually in the first six months after the injury, but in 15% to 30% the condition becomes chronic. Headache persisting longer than 6 months despite treatment, with no tendency to improve, is a predictor of chronicity. The belief that posttraumatic headache is a form of compensation neurosis is not supported by the evidence (Packard, 1994).

Persistent headaches for long periods after the injury may have a number of components: vascular, muscle-contraction, and localized headache at the site of injury. Injuries to the cervical spine may be followed by persistent neck pain. The psychological element is often important. The accident may have been traumatic mentally as well as physically, leaving depression, guilt, and a sense of grievance. The long process of litigation and compensation are often important factors.

Management depends on which of the above components are most prominent. Listening to the patient and understanding fears and feelings is important. Questions of compensation should be settled as soon as appropriate. Local treatment, such as infiltration with local anesthetic, ice packs or heat, physiotherapy, or acupuncture may be helpful where there is localized pain and tenderness. For generalized headaches, some of the strategies described for chronic TTH are appropriate.

For patients with headache immediately after head injury, assessment and observation are necessary. The patient may already have been observed for a period of time either in the emergency department or as an inpatient. The assessment includes examination of the fundi, pupils, and cranial nerves and observation of the patient's state of consciousness, especially any suggestion of drowsiness. If there are no neurological signs and no altered state of consciousness, and if the headache is not severe, the patient can be allowed to go home and be observed or report progress at appropriate intervals. If the patient is alone, he or she should be asked to report progress. If family members are present, they should be asked to report any change in level of consciousness or any new symptom such as vomiting. If the headache is persisting, and especially if it is getting worse, the patient should be reexamined at frequent intervals for new neurological signs. If circumstances at home make frequent observation impossible, admission or readmission to the hospital may be necessary.

Trigeminal Neuralgia

The pain of trigeminal neuralgia is so characteristic that it does not usually present difficulties of diagnosis. The patient is usually elderly. The pain is felt in the distribution of one of the branches of the trigeminal nerve. It is described as very severe, shock-like, and of short duration although recurring frequently. Usually, the patient has identified trigger zones that produce the pain when touched. The patient may have found it necessary to avoid washing or shaving this area or stimulating it by chewing or biting. Examination of the cranial nerves is usually negative.

The pain usually responds to carbamazepine. The dose is individualized to the patient. A dose of 200 mg three times daily is usually sufficient to control the pain. If it is, then it may be reduced gradually after a few weeks to a maintenance dose or until it can be discontinued altogether. If carbamazepine does not control the pain, diphenylhydantoin may be added. Gabapentin may be tried as well. If pain is intractable, stereotaxic surgery to the Gasserian ganglion removes the pain, but in some patients the sensory aftereffects are almost as troublesome as the pain.

Therapy

Treatment of Migraine Attacks

It is important to initiate any antimigraine drug as early as possible in the attack. In mild cases of migraine with or without aura, early use of aspirin, ibuprofen, or other NSAID may abort or diminish the severity of the attack.

The effectiveness of sumatriptan for attacks of migraine with or without aura, and for cluster headaches, has been demonstrated in placebo-controlled trials and in studies comparing it with combinations of ergotamine and caffeine, and aspirin and metoclopramide (Tfelt-Hansen, 1993; Plosker and McTavish, 1994). Subcutaneous sumatriptan in a dose of 6 mg aborts migraine attacks within two hours in more than 80% of patients. Taken orally, 100 mg is effective in 60% to 70% of patients. The subcutaneous route should therefore be used in patients who do not respond to oral sumatriptan. In about one-third of patients, the headache recurs in 4 to 5 hours, but responds in most patients to a second dose of sumatriptan (Cady, Rubino, Crummett, and Littlejohn, 1994). The maximal recommended dose during a 24-hour period is 300 mg orally and 12 mg subcutaneously. Although there is no conclusive evidence of a link between myocardial ischemia and sumatriptan, a few cases with a temporal association have been reported, and 3% to 5% of patients report chest tightness after sumatriptan. In the present state of knowledge, therefore, sumatriptan is contraindicated in patients with a history of ischemic heart disease or uncontrolled hypertension (Tfelt-Hansen, 1993; Plosker and McTavish, 1994); it should not be used together with ergot preparations or selective serotonin reuptake inhibitors (SSRI). The combination of a triptan and SSRI may lead to the serotonin syndrome. Sumatriptan can also be administered intranasally.

Sumatriptan is also effective in the treatment of cluster headaches. Because these reach maximum intensity very rapidly, the subcutaneous route is preferable.

Controlled trials to date have been carried out only among patients who have migraine as defined by the International Headache Society (Olesen, 1990), so the effectiveness of sumatriptan for other types of headache is not known. No trials have yet been reported with patients drawn entirely from general practice.

Ergotamine tartrate is an alternative to sumatriptan, given in a dose of 2 mg by mouth or rectum early in the attack, to a maximum of 6 mg in one day and 12 mg in one week. Dihydro-ergotamine-45 is superior to ergotamine tartrate in having fewer side effects and less rebound potential. Neither drug should be given in pregnancy or when ischemic heart disease or uncontrolled hypertension is present. Dihydro-ergotamine-45 is given intranasally or parenterally.

Prophylaxis of Migraine Attacks

IHS guidelines (1993) recommend that migraine-abortive drugs not be used more than six times a month. Patients who use excessive amounts of migraine-abortive drugs may experience rebound headaches that then become chronic. Prophylactic treatment to reduce the frequency of headaches is indicated in patients with frequent (more than two or three migraines a month) severe attacks. Beta-adrenergic blocking agents (especially propranolol) and calcium channel blockers are commonly used, although the evidence for efficacy of the latter class of drugs is not strong. Tricyclic antidepressants can be effective in reducing attacks. Nonsteroidal anti-inflammatory drugs can be used prophylactically as well as abortively and are particularly useful for menstrual migraine (Baumel, 1994). Anticonvulsants such as valproic acid or divalporex are effective prophylactic agents for migraine, as well. Because of its serious side effects (retroperitoneal and cardiac fibrosis), methysergide is rarely used. It should be used only for medium-term therapy of up to 4 months, and only if the benefits are thought to outweigh the risks.

Chronic Headache

The first aim of the family physician is to prevent the chronic state by dealing effectively with the early stages of a headache problem. The Headache Study Group found that the strongest predictor of a good outcome at 1 year was the patients' statement after the first visit that they had been able to discuss their headaches and associated problems fully with the doctor. Nevertheless, some patients will develop chronic headaches, and some will have them when they come to the practice as new patients.

Six important principles should be remembered if the management of chronic headache is to be successful:

1. The original reason for the headaches is not necessarily the same as the reason that makes them chronic. Headaches that began as responses to stress may eventually become autonomous symptoms, perpetuated by a combination of physiological mechanisms and inappropriate cognitive and emotional responses to pain. This is why the search for problems in the patient's life at

this stage may be unhelpful. On the other hand, chronic headaches may be the correlate of repressed emotional tension or conflict. By a process of conditioning, they may also have become a response to factors that are a substitute for the original stimulus.

2. Complete removal of the headaches is not a realistic objective of therapy. Success should be measured by patients' ability to function, their assessment of the severity and frequency of the headaches, their use of medication, and the extent to which the pain ceases to dominate their lives.

3. The patient should become an active participant in the treatment. Success depends on the insight the patient gains into the factors that contribute to the continuation of the headaches and on their capacity to control them.

4. Unresolved family tensions may be among the initial causes of the patient's problem and the reasons for its chronic state. Family relationships should be assessed and family members involved in the therapeutic program.

5. Overmedication is a common feature of chronic headache. A detailed drug history should be taken and the elimination of ergotamine and analgesic dependency is an important objective of treatment.

6. Treatment must be individualized. A successful coping strategy for one patient may make the headaches worse for another patient. For one patient, relaxation may relieve the headaches; for another, keeping busy and active may give relief.

In the course of the assessment, the physician should gain insight into the patient's thoughts and feelings about the headaches, including any specific fears about their cause. Armed with this information, the physician can then proceed to explain the physiological changes that lead to headache, providing reassurance where necessary, dealing with specific fears and misconceptions, and describing how thoughts and emotions can increase susceptibility to headaches.

The next step is a headache diary. The patient records over a period of several weeks the severity, site, and duration of headaches, as well as noting thoughts and feelings and recording precipitating factors and coping strategies. The severity can be quantified on a five-point scale and the site indicated on a diagram of the head. The diary serves two purposes: it increases the patient's self-understanding (a necessary precondition of self-control) and it gives the physician a basis for the design of a therapeutic strategy.

In the next phase, the physician, building on this knowledge, teaches the patient strategies for controlling the headaches. These may include relaxation, attention focusing, imagery, and thought management. Alternatively, the patient may be referred to a headache clinic or clinical psychologist for this therapy, or for biofeedback.

Opioids in Chronic Headache
Opioids are often prescribed for patients with chronic headache, usually the drugs of lower potency such as codeine, oxycodone, and propoxyphene. Even though some patients find that only these drugs will give them relief from pain, and

take them for years without ill effects or escalation of dose, their use remains controversial.

Reservations about the use of opioids are based on three grounds: lack of knowledge about the pathophysiology of headache, fear of drug dependency and addiction, and the risk of adverse side effects. Opioids are most effective for nociceptive pain—that is, pain arising from organic disease such as cancer. They are less effective for neurogenic pain such as trigeminal neuralgia, and pain of uncertain origin, especially when behavioral factors are prominent. Although a sterile inflammatory reaction appears to be a factor in migraine headache, chronic headache is often of uncertain origin. On the other hand, severe chronic headache is a feature of some chronic diseases (e.g., systemic lupus erythematosus) and opioids are the drug of choice.

Although opioids are addictive for some patients, recent studies have shown that when they are prescribed for chronic noncancer pain in patients with no history of drug abuse, the risk of addiction or escalation of dose is very small (Ziegler, 1994). The main adverse effect of milder opiates is constipation. This requires prophylactic management with stool softeners, with added Senokot when necessary, but is not a reason for withholding the drug. The adverse effects of mild analgesics, such as aspirin and acetaminophen, are potentially more serious. Long-term use of aspirin has been one of the most common causes of nephropathy, and acetaminophen in large doses is hepatotoxic.

Another reason for concern is the contribution of daily intake of drugs to the perpetuation of headaches. The evidence indicates, however, that ergotamine and analgesics, rather than opioids, are the factors in drug-induced headache (Ziegler, 1994).

The decision about prescribing opioids should be based on the individual features of each patient, including type of headache, evidence of relief from opioids, emotional stability, ability to function, and availability of alternatives.

References

Ad Hoc Committee on Classification of Headache. 1962. A classification of headache. *Journal of the American Medical Association* 179:717.

Baumel B. 1994. Migraine: A pharmacologic review with newer options and delivery modalities. *Neurology* 44(Suppl 3):S13.

Becker LA, Iverson DC, Reed FM, Calonge N, Miller RS, Freeman WL. 1988. Patients with new headache in primary care: a report from ASPN. *Journal of Family Practice* 27(1):41.

Becker LA, Green LA, Beaufait D, Kirk J, Froom J, Freeman WL. 1993a. Use of CT scans for the investigation of headache: A report from ASPN, Part 1. *Journal of Family Practice* 37(2):129.

Becker LA, Green LA, Beaufait D, Kirk J, Froom J, Freeman WL. 1993b. Detection of intracranial tumours, subarachnoid hemorrhages, or subdural hematomas in primary care patients: A report from ASPN, Part 2. *Journal of Family Practice* 37(2):135.

Cady AK, Rubino J, Crummett D, Littlejohn TW. 1994. Oral sumatriptan in the treatment of recurrent headache. *Archives of Family Medicine* 3:766.

Frishberg BM. 1994. The utility of neuroimaging in the evaluation of headache in patients with normal neurologic examinations. *Neurology* 44:1191.

Headache Classification Subcommittee of the International Headache Society. 2004. The International Classification of Headache Disorders 2nd Edition. *Cephalalgia*. 24, Supplement 1 (ICHD II).

Headache Study Group of The University of Western Ontario. 1986. Predictors of outcome in headache patients presenting to family physicians: A one year prospective study. *Headache* 26:285.

Hoffert MJ. 1994. Treatment of migraine: A new era. *American Family Physician* 49(3):633.

Howie JGR. 1973. A new look at respiratory illness in general practice: A reclassification of respiratory illness based on antibiotic prescribing. *Journal of the Royal College of General Practitioners* 23:895.

Linn FHH, Wijdicks FM, van der Graff Y, Weerdesteyn-van Vliet AC. Bartelds AIM, van Gijn J. 1994. Prospective study of sentinel headache in aneurysmal subarachnoid haemorrhage. *Lancet* 344:590.

Marcus DA. 1992. Migraine and tension-type headaches: the questionable validity of current classification systems. *Clinical Journal of Pain* 8(1):28.

Moskowitz MA, Cutrer FM. 1993. Sumatriptan: A receptor-targeted treatment for migraine. *Annual Review of Medicine* 44:145.

Olesen J. 1990. The classification and diagnosis of headache disorders. *Headache* 8(4):793.

Olesen J. 1994. Understanding the biologic basis of migraine. Editorial. *New England Journal of Medicine* 331(25):1713.

Packard RC. 1994. Posttraumatic headache. *Seminars in Neurology* 14(1):40.

Plosker GL, McTavish D. 1994. Sumatriptan: A reappraisal of its pharmacology and therapeutic efficacy in the acute treatment of migraine and cluster headache. *Drugs* 47(4):622.

Sacks OW. 1985. *Migraine.* Berkeley, CA: University of California Press.

Saper JR. 1990. Daily chronic headache. *Headache* 8(4):891.

Tfelt-Hansen P. 1993. Sumatriptan for the treatment of migraine attacks—a review of controlled clinical trials. *Cephalalgia* 13:238.

van Buchem I, Peeters M, Beaumont J, Knotternus JA. 1995. Acute maxillary sinusitis in general practice: the relation between clinical picture and objective findings. *European Journal of General Practice* 1:155van Duijn HP, Brouwer HJ, Lamberts H. 1992. Use of symptoms and signs to diagnose maxillary sinusitis in general practice: Comparison with ultrasonography. *British Medical Journal* 305:684.

Wijdicks EFM, Kerkhoff H, van Gijn J. 1988. Long-term follow-up of 71 patients with thunderclap headache mimicking subarachnoid haemorrhage. *Lancet* 2:68.

Ziegler DK. 1994. Opiate and opioid use in patients with refractory headache. *Cephalalgia* 14:5.

13

Fatigue

Tiredness, lack of energy, fatigue, or lassitude is the seventh most common presenting complaint in general practice. Of patients presenting with a new leading complaint of fatigue, half or more receive a diagnosis of depression or anxiety state, or both (Kroenke, Wood, Mangelsdorff, Meier, and Powell, 1988). In about one-third, an organic disease is diagnosed. Of these, the most common is an acute infection, followed by cardiovascular and endocrine diseases. Infectious mononucleosis and viral hepatitis commonly present with fatigue. Endocrine and metabolic conditions associated with fatigue are early pregnancy, menopause, diabetes mellitus, hypothyroidism, and hypokalemia. In the ensuing decades, a more recent, practice-based study in the Netherlands (Okkes, Oskam, and Lamberts, 2002) followed 5,915 patients who presented with general weakness and tiredness, for a period of 10 years. At the end of that time, 37.5% were not further diagnosed, 25.6% had an organic diagnosis (chiefly infectious diseases), and 10% had a psychological diagnosis. Since depressive illness has increased in that time period, the marked decline in the proportion of patients who present with fatigue and who are ultimately diagnosed with depressive illness may suggest that it has become more acceptable for depressed patients to explicitly identify their experience as being psychological in nature.

For a long time, fatigue has been associated in physicians' minds with anemia. Studies in the general population and in general practice, however, have shown that patients with hemoglobin levels down to 8 g per 100 mL do not suffer from fatigue any more frequently than people with normal levels (Knotternus, Knipschild, Van Wersch, and Sijstermanns, 1986).

Iatrogenic fatigue may be produced by one of the many drugs that can cause fatigue. Among the most common are birth control pills, antihypertensives, diuretics, tranquilizers, and steroids.

The remaining patients do not receive a specific diagnosis. In some of these the fatigue is related to aspects of the patient's way of life, such as insufficient sleep, overwork, poverty, or too little exercise. Women with young children, especially if they are single parents, are especially vulnerable (Valdini, Steinhardt, and Jaffe, 1987; Pelosi et al., 1990). Daytime somnolence may be an indication of sleep apnea.

Little is known about the natural history of fatigue. A prospective study showed that 67% of patients presenting with fatigue as chief complaint improved over 1 year. They had much higher medical care utilization rates than control subjects, however, and substantial limitations in function (Nelson et al., 1987). Another prospective study of patients presenting with fatigue of more than 1 month duration, excluding those with major medical illness, showed that only 28% had improved in 1 year. Older patients and those with greater functional impairment were less likely to improve. The fatigued patients as a whole had much greater functional impairment (as measured by the Sickness Impact Profile) than matched controls (Kroenke, Wood, Mangelsdorff, Meier, and Powell, 1988).

Assessment of Patients Presenting with Fatigue

The first part of the assessment includes listening to the patient's account of the symptoms, trying to understand their meaning for the patient, and following up any cues to their cause. It is important to explore what the patient means by tiredness or lack of energy. There are qualitative differences between the tiredness of depression, organic disease, and overactivity, which can only be identified by an exploratory dialogue. Most patients presenting with fatigue have other symptoms, and these may provide cues to the diagnosis. Pregnancy, medication-related fatigue, and obvious organic disease such as HIV infection and congestive cardiac failure should be readily identified at this stage. If the diagnosis is not apparent, then conditional probabilities will depend to some extent on the age and sex of the patient and on the length of history. The shorter the history, the more probable is a diagnosis of acute infection. Acute infection is also more probable in younger patients than in the elderly. Depression and anxiety are diagnosed on positive evidence, not by exclusion. In the great majority of patients, clinical assessment over the course of one or two visits will enable one to make a very probable diagnosis, which can then be tested by observation over time or response to therapy. In many patients, no tests are necessary at this stage. If they are indicated, it is usually to confirm some specific infection such as mononucleosis, hepatitis, or pyelitis or to rule out organic disease (see *Case 13.1*).

In a small number of patients, the fatigue will continue and none of the initial hypotheses will be verified. At this stage other hypotheses must be considered, this ranking order again depending on the age and sex of the patient. In older patients, an occult infection or malignancy must be considered. If a repeat physical examination is negative, screening tests such as blood count, ESR, stool occult blood, urine microscopy, and chest X-ray may help to change the probabilities. But further tests after the initial investigation are seldom helpful in patients with persistent fatigue (Sugarman and Berg, 1984; Valdini, Steinhardt, and Feldman, 1989).

Because of the importance of early diagnosis, it is important to think of subacute bacterial endocarditis in elderly patients with fatigue of recent onset. Fever is usually present but may be intermittent and therefore will not be detected unless regular readings are taken. A heart murmur is usually heard, but no other signs can be expected in the early stages of the illness. Once the diagnosis is considered, confirmation by blood culture is not usually difficult. The most common error is not thinking of the hypothesis.

Hypothyroidism and diabetes should be considered, especially in older patients. Even though anemia is not considered a common cause of fatigue, the early stages of pernicious anemia should be remembered in older patients, and a mild anemia may be the cue in older patients to a gastrointestinal malignancy.

Even after intensive observation and investigation, there will remain a few patients in whom the cause of the fatigue is not apparent. Sometimes depression will be missed at first assessment, and it is advisable to repeat the assessment, perhaps using an assessment scale, when the fatigue persists. If the psychological assessment is still negative, however, one should not assume that the problem is psychogenic just because all tests for organic disease are negative. Sufferers from chronic fatigue syndrome are not helped by physicians who imply that their troubles are all psychogenic (see p. 303).

Depression

Substantial numbers of patients presenting with fatigue to family physicians are suffering from anxiety states, or depression, or both. Depression is very common in Europe and North America, probably in all parts of the world. In some cultures, however (e.g., Chinese and Indian), there is no equivalent for the English word depression. The state described by the word is more likely to be expressed in terms of bodily disease.

In describing his own illness, William Styron (1990) registered

a strong protest against the word "depression." It may be that the scientist generally held responsible for its currency in modern times, a Johns Hopkins Medical School faculty member justly venerated—the Swiss-born psychiatrist Adolf Meyer—had a tin ear for the rhythms of English and therefore was unaware of the semantic damage he had inflicted by offering "depression" as a descriptive noun for such a dreadful and raging disease. Nonetheless, for over seventy-five years the word has slithered innocuously through the language like a slug, leaving little trace of its intrinsic malevolence and preventing, by its very insipidity, a general awareness of the horrible intensity of the disease when out of control.

The older English term melancholia seems a more fitting one than its successor. In Europe and North America, about 20% of females and 10% of males have a major depression at some time in their lives. Depression is one of the most common diagnoses in family practice, ranking from fourth to twelfth in frequency in different studies.

British studies indicate that general practitioners treat about four new episodes of depression per month. About 40% of depressed patients in general practice have a coexisting organic illness. According to Watts (1984), the prevalence of chronic depression (duration of 3 years or more) is 4.5 per 1,000 patients in the practice.

Depression is more common in females than in males, and its prevalence increases in middle age. It is more common in the poor than in the well-to-do and is especially common in conditions of social deprivation, as in the inner cities of the Western world.

The spectrum of depression in general practice differs from that in psychiatric practice. A much larger proportion of patients in general practice have mild depression, with fewer of the classic manifestations (Sireling, Freeling, Paykel, and Rao, 1985a; Sireling, Paykel, Freeling, Rao, and Patel, 1985b). Many patients have a combination of depression and anxiety. Vegetative symptoms such as loss of weight and anorexia are much less common, and many patients are not overtly depressed. Because of this, a physician who has had psychiatric training in a department of psychiatry may have difficulty in adjusting diagnostic criteria accordingly. A British study found that depressed patients most likely to be missed by general practitioners were those who looked and behaved in a less depressed way and who did not complain of or admit to depression. They were more likely to have been depressed for more than a year and were more likely to have a coexisting organic illness (Freeling, Rao, Paykel, Sireling, and Burton, 1985).

How depression presents appears to vary in different cultures. In North America, Europe, and Australasia, where most studies have been done, fatigue is a common presenting symptom, but physiological symptoms, pain, and anxiety symptoms are also common. The fact that patients rarely complain of feeling depressed is probably a result of several causes: lack of insight into their condition, difficulty in putting their feelings into words, and assumptions about what complaints are legitimate in a medical context.

Depression is not easy to identify in a person of widely different culture from the observer. Western physicians, for example, may find it difficult to know when an Asian or African patient is depressed. The converse is also true. I have noticed that residents coming from Asia have difficulty in identifying depression in North American patients. Because many family physicians have patients from different cultures, this is an important consideration.

Family physicians and other generalists also miss depression in patients from their own culture. Studies comparing generalists' diagnoses with valid semistructured interviews have shown that the physicians identified only half of those with depression (Goldberg and Huxley, 1980; Freeling, Rao, Paykel, Sireling, and Burton, 1985). However, it is not enough to show that generalists fail to identify depression. We need to know what the consequences are. Do the patients who are not identified fare less well than those who are? Do those who are not identified have less severe depression? Is the patient's mood disorder recognized but given some other name? A doctor might recognize that a patient is depressed but consider labeling unwise. He may feel that the depression is likely to remit spontaneously, that treatment is not indicated at the time, or that the patient is unlikely to accept the diagnosis. In these studies, the doctors' recognition of depression is measured against standardized psychiatric assessments applied by mental health professionals who have no previous knowledge of the patient. The assumption that the standardized assessment is the gold standard for general practice patients may well be correct but cannot be taken for granted.

Of the patients whose depression is not recognized at the index visit, 10% are recognized at a subsequent visit, and 20% remit spontaneously. The remainder, however, remain depressed for long periods (Paykel and Priest, 1992). Depression is more likely to be missed in patients with chronic organic disease, those who have been depressed for a long time, and those who present with somatic or atypical complaints (Freeling, Rao, Paykel, Sireling, and Burton, 1985). In a large cohort study of psychological disorders in general practice (Ormel et al., 1990), doctors recognized all severe depressions and 62% of neurotic depressions. Comorbidity of depression and anxiety was common. More than half the patients with depression also manifested anxiety, and over two-thirds of those with major anxiety disorders manifested borderline depression. Psychological disorders with recent onset or exacerbation were twice as likely to be recognized, and improved at follow-up, than those with chronic disorders. Patients presenting with psychological or social reasons for encounter were 40 times more likely to be recognized than those presenting with bodily symptoms. The same observation was also made by Tylee, Freeling, Kerry, and Burns (1995). After a 14-month follow-up period, recognized patients had less psychopathology and better social functioning than those not recognized. Recognition predicted a better outcome independently of treatment.

The evidence does indicate that a number of patients with major depression are not being identified. Because these patients are likely to respond to antidepressant drugs, it is reasonable to infer that they would benefit from a diagnosis. It also appears that recognition itself, irrespective of specific treatment, may lead to a better outcome. It should also be noted that some of the key studies of depression in general practice have included only patients in the 16 to 65 age groups. The results, therefore, cannot be generalized to the elderly population. One study has shown that general practitioners identified a large majority of elderly patients with depression, although only a minority received a prescription for an antidepressive (MacDonald, 1986).

In most studies of the recognition of depression by generalists, the cases of unrecognized depression have come mainly from doctors with a low sensitivity for identifying depression. To control for doctors' sensitivity, Tylee, Freeling, and Kerry (1993) compared a patient identified as depressed with one not identified as depressed by the same doctor ($n = 36$ doctors). The association between organic illness and unrecognized depression was strongly confirmed. Patients with serious coexisting organic disease were five times more likely to have their major depression missed than those without organic disease, and those with mild organic illness three times more likely. The severity of the depression was only slightly greater in the recognized patients than in the unrecognized. More patients in the recognized group felt that their depressed mood was different from normal sadness. Tiredness was more prevalent in patients with unrecognized depression.

Physicians who are more likely to recognize depression make more eye contact with patients, are good listeners, and are less likely to interrupt patients. They are also more likely to explore psychological and social issues (Paykel and Priest, 1992). All of these are features of the patient-centered clinical method. Recognition of depression occurs more frequently in consultations that are longer, where the doctor tolerates silence, notices nonverbal behavior, and uses patients' responses in further discussion, and where patients present psychological symptoms early (Paykel and Priest, 1992). The deficiencies probably reflect a lack of awareness of the many faces of depression and inadequate training in interviewing methods.

At one end of the spectrum, depression is a devastating and potentially fatal disease; at the other, it merges with the inescapable sadness of life. Family physicians are witnesses to a great deal of sadness: the sadness of disappointment, the sadness of loss, the sadness and despair of overwhelming misfortune, and the sadness of old age and mortality. This is not a "disease" to be cured by medication or cognitive therapy. In some ways, sadness in these circumstances may be a necessary experience, because it invites reflection and self-examination, perhaps also self-forgiveness and healing. Perhaps some of the "depressions" missed by general practitioners are feelings of this kind. The need may not be for cure, but for presence, support, and a listening ear. Kay Toombs, severely disabled by multiple sclerosis, tells of a visit she paid to her physician. She said "I don't know why I've come to see you." "Yes, you do," he replied, "you came because you wanted to know that somebody gives a damn."

The issue of "missed" cases of depression should be viewed against the background of mental illness in primary care practice and in the general population. In the Netherlands (Verhaak, 1995), a population sample of 13,014 people had a 2-hour health interview, including the General Health Questionnaire (GHQ), and kept a health diary for 3 weeks. For 3 months following the interview, all the visits to their general practitioners were recorded. The general practitioner recorded the diagnosis, including for each an assessment on a five-point scale ranging from "completely somatic" to "completely psychological."[1]

Thirty-five percent of the population over the age of 15 expressed at least one psychological complaint during the interview, and a further 15% recorded such complaints in the health diary. Thirteen percent scored above the GHQ threshold for psychiatric illness (a point prevalence rate of 125/1000). Of the GHQ positives, however, only 48% consulted their general practitioner during the 3-month recording period. Women, divorced persons, and the unemployed were overrepresented in the GHQ-positive group. Of those who expressed psychological problems but were GHQ-negative, only 40% consulted their general practitioner in the 3-month period. It seems that many people with psychological problems, even identified as psychiatric cases, do not see medical care as the solution to their problem.

Two-thirds of the GHQ-positive patients who consulted their general practitioner were recognized by the doctor as having a psychological component to their illness. One-quarter of the people who expressed psychological complaints but were GHQ-negative were recognized as having a psychological component.

Of the GHQ-positive patients who consulted their general practitioner, only one-sixth expressed psychological complaints. Of all the patients who reported psychological problems in the health interview and diary, and who consulted their general practitioner, fewer than 10% presented with psychological complaints. Two-thirds of the GHQ-positive patients, and half the mentally distressed GHQ-negative patients, received a psychological diagnosis from their general practitioner. The most frequent diagnoses were anxiety, depression, and sleep disorder. Verhaak (1995) writes: "a psychiatric category system does not seem the most appropriate way of classifying mental problems encountered in primary care. The picture which emerges from general practice looks more like a rather disorganized collection of symptoms, pointing mainly to anxiety and depression, with some stress and addiction among it."

What we see here is a much more complex world than the one defined by the categories of the *Diagnostic and Statistical Manual of Mental Disorders* (DSM IV). Many people with psychological problems do not see themselves as in need of medical help. Perhaps they should; but on the other hand, perhaps they know their needs better than we do. If patients present to their doctor with psychological problems, they are likely to receive a psychological diagnosis. If they have psychological problems, but present with physical complaints, they are more likely to receive a physical diagnosis. Are general practitioners missing the true diagnosis or simply responding to patient's expressed needs in a quite appropriate way? Even when general practitioners identified a psychological problem, they seldom gave counseling or prescribed psychotropic drugs. Would patients have been better treated in this way, or was recognition itself sufficient?

The answer to these questions probably lies somewhere between the two points of view.[2] Not everybody with emotional distress has a serious psychiatric problem. Every case of sadness or anxiety does not need formal therapy. Psychiatric categories and diagnostic rating scales do not fit well with patients seen by general practitioners. On the other hand, we do fail to identify some patients who would benefit by treatment. We know that we have failed to identify depression in some patients who badly needed help.

In his book *Beyond Depression* (2004) Christopher Dowrick adds evidence to the complexity of the concept of depression in general practice. Writing from his experience in general practice and social work, from his own research, and from a wide reading in psychology, medical history, sociology, and philosophy, Dowrick draws our attention to the factors which make for the complexity. Among these are questions concerning depression as a diagnostic construct, inability of psychiatrists to agree on categorizations of mood disorders, the placebo effects, comorbidity in general practice, and the suffering of many kinds which faces family doctors day after day. While urging us to hone our skills in the detection and diagnosis of depressive disorders, and applying evidence-based treatment wherever we can, Dowrick reminds us that "in the complicated and confused world of primary care, the usefulness of the diagnosis is unclear, and our attempts to apply it may cause as many problems as we solve."

Etiology of Depression

The ways in which depression has been classified reflect the changing views about the nature of the condition. At one time, a distinction was made between endogenous and reactive depression or between psychotic and neurotic. The implication was that depression was either biological in origin or environmental—an example of the way in which monocausal and linear thinking has dominated medicine. We now know that depression does not have to be either biological or environmental—it can be both.

In an important study of depression in women, Brown and Harris (1978) have shown that social factors are important in all types of depression, including those thought to be endogenous. Brown and Harris identify three types of factors: those that make a woman more vulnerable to depression, those that precipitate a depression, and those that influence the way the depression will be clinically expressed. Women developing a depression were much more likely than those without depression to have had a traumatic life event in the 9 months before the onset. These events involved loss and disappointment, separation or threat of separation from a key figure, an unpleasant revelation about somebody close, a life-threatening illness in a close relative, and loss of employment.

The key factor is not change in itself but the meaning that the event has for the person. Also important as precipitating events were major difficulties in life, such as a poor marriage, bad housing, financial problems, or difficulties with children. A traumatic life event or a major difficulty were precipitating factors in 83% of depressions. Minor events could also precipitate depression if they served to bring home to a person the implications of a long-term loss or disappointment.

The factors that made a woman vulnerable to depression were those that tended to isolate her, reduce her supports, and lower her self-esteem. The lack of a confidant, especially the inability to confide in a spouse, was important. Having three or more children at home and not being employed outside the home were factors increasing isolation. Regarding the past, the death of the woman's mother during childhood was the most significant factor.

Whether or not a depression had severe features such as retardation of thought was related to three factors. Severe depression was more likely to be associated with past bereavements, such as the death of a parent or sibling during childhood or the death of a spouse several years previously. Less severe depression was more likely to be associated with loss by separation rather than death. Women were more likely to have a severe depression if they were older, if they had had a previous depression, and if a traumatic event occurred after the onset.

The fact that social factors are important in depression does not necessarily mean that all depressed patients have "problems." If they have current problems, these should be identified, but it is counterproductive to be incredulous when a patient and spouse insist that they are happily married and have no major stresses in their lives. After the initial stimulus of a life stressor, recurrent depressions can eventually become autonomous (see the discussion of kindling below).

About half of all patients with major depression have excessive levels of blood cortisol, suggesting a response to stress that disrupts serotonin and norepinephrine transmission. Most antidepressant drugs act on either serotonergic or noradrenergic neurotransmitter systems, or both. By blocking reuptake, they increase the availability of these neurotransmitters. These imbalances of endocrine and neurotransmitter systems may in turn reflect changes at the more basic level of gene transmission and brain structure. In affective disorders, 50% of the first episodes are associated with significant stressors, but only 36% of the second or third episodes. Animal studies indicate that an acute stressor can turn on genes for substances that initiate long-term changes in the structure of brain cells (Post, 1992). In the theory of kindling, Post postulates that the trauma of events like childhood bereavement could change the structure of the developing brain, making the person vulnerable to depression when under stress in later life. If each episode increased the vulnerability, later depressive episodes could occur with little or no environmental stimulus. This would also explain the greater severity of depression in women who had had previous episodes (see Brown and Harris, 1978). If this is so, then adequate treatment of early episodes of depression should reduce vulnerability to later attacks.

The emerging picture of depression is one of an illness in which short- and long-term changes in the central nervous system are coupled in a nonlinear relationship with life experiences and social relationships. The nonlinearity is seen in the capability of any part of the circular chain to produce change. Life events can elicit changes in brain structure, which in turn alter the response to future events. Social isolation increases depression, which in turn increases social isolation (see *Case 8.5*). Intervention at any point in the circle can be therapeutic: drug therapy, social support, cognitive therapy. Relief from depression can transform the perception of life events from negative to positive.

The fact that neurotransmitter systems are disturbed makes it unnecessary to invoke such mechanisms as somatization to explain the physical symptoms that many depressed patients present. Neurotransmitters circulate widely in the body, and one might expect such a widespread bodily disturbance to be accompanied by pain and other symptoms. Because it is so difficult to describe the anguish of depression, it is not surprising that patients complain first of bodily sensations, which they can express in words. Even a person as articulate as William Styron (1990) found his experience to be indescribable:

I was feeling in my mind *a sensation close to, but indescribably different from, actual pain.*...That the word "indescribable" should present itself is not fortuitous, since it has to be emphasized that if the pain were readily describable most of the countless sufferers from this ancient affliction would have been able to confidently depict for their friends and loved ones (even their physicians) some of the actual dimensions of their torment, and perhaps elicit a comprehension that has been generally lacking; such incomprehension has usually been due not to a failure of sympathy but to the basic inability of healthy people to imagine a form of torment so alien to everyday experience. *For myself, the pain is most closely connected to drowning or suffocation*—but even these images are off the mark. William James, who battled depression for many years, gave up the search for an adequate portrayal, implying its near-impossibility when he wrote in The Varieties of Religious Experience: *"It is a positive and active anguish, a sort of psychical neuralgia wholly unknown to normal life."*

The current way of classifying depression relies on degree of severity and association with manic symptoms, rather than on etiology. Major depression is distinguished from dysthymia by its greater severity. Bipolar depression and cyclothymia are distinguished from other depressions by the occurrence of mania or hypomania. These patients appear to be distinct genetically from those with depression alone, and to differ in prognosis and response to drugs (Michels and Marzuk, 1993). In general practice, mania or hypomania are much less common manifestations of these disorders than depression. Depression may exist without any concurrent disorder or may coexist with other physical or mental problems. Depression is often present in patients with chronic disease, including the disabilities of old age. It is very common in the advanced stages of cancer. It occurs in sufferers from schizophrenia and in people who abuse alcohol and other drugs.

Diagnosis
As well as complaints of tiredness and lack of energy, the following cues should suggest depression (Widmer and Cadoret, 1978):

1. Persistent ill-defined symptoms for which no physical basis can be found, especially dyspepsia, dizziness, bowel dysfunction, hyperventilation, and palpitation.
2. Persistent unexplained pain, especially headache, backache, and abdominal pain.
3. A recent increase in the number of attendances at the office or requests for visits; or, in the case of a mother, frequent attendances with minor problems in the children.
4. Difficulty in sleeping.
5. Symptoms of anxiety arising in a person with no previous history of psychological illness. The symptoms may be the physiological expression of anxiety—palpitations, sweating, trembling—or they may be fears about personal health or health of loved ones. Anxiety symptoms arising for the first time in middle age should be assumed to be caused by depression until proved to the contrary.
6. Incongruity between a patient's apparent physical well-being and the dire nature of his or her complaints—for example, the robust, healthy looking man who feels awful.
7. Incongruity between the severity of a patient's symptoms and the minor nature of the presenting complaint—for example, a patient with a head cold who feels exhausted.
8. Failure to recover in the expected time from an illness, operation, or injury.

One of the reasons why depression is missed in general practice is that patients are not usually overtly depressed. They are often smiling when they first enter. Those with more severe forms of depression, however, will usually strike the physician as being unhappy, and the first cue may be the feeling "this patient makes me feel depressed."

Another reason is the occurrence of depression in a member of the family other than the patient being treated at the time: the spouse of a chronically ill or dying patient, or the mother of a disturbed child. It may need a question like "And how are you doing?" to allow them to express their pain.

The most common diagnostic error we have noted in residents is the failure to ask the most sensitive and specific question of all: "Do you feel depressed, low in spirits, down in the dumps?" (It is often necessary to express the question in several ways, because some patients do not identify their feeling as depression.) Instead of asking this question, residents will often ask much less sensitive and specific questions about appetite, constipation, and weight loss, which leave them uncertain about whether or not the patient is depressed.

Once the key question has been asked, other defining attributes of depression can be sought. The following are in approximate order of sensitivity and specificity:

1. Sleep disturbance. Nearly all patients have some trouble with sleeping, either difficulty in getting to sleep, frequent waking, or early waking.
2. Loss of interest in life. Tasks and hobbies lose their interest; life loses its joy.
3. Loss of concentration. Work takes longer to complete; tasks are postponed.
4. A tendency to worry about small matters, the anxiety often going around and around in the mind like an obsession.
5. Feelings of worthlessness and failure; self-reproach about past failures and supposed defects of character.
6. Bouts of crying or wanting to cry. Patients will often cry during the interview—a strong cue to depression, especially in males.
7. Irritability. Patients are often aware of being irritable and feel guilty about the effect on spouse or children.
8. Loss of appetite, constipation. These symptoms are of less diagnostic value because they are shared with many other conditions.

If the patient admits to feeling depressed and other evidence is supportive, the diagnosis can be made on positive grounds. The diagnosis of depression is not made by exclusion. Sometimes the patient insists that he or she is not depressed, even though strong evidence points to this. If the patient is convinced that the symptoms point to some organic disease, he or she may angrily reject the suggestion that the problem is psychogenic.

Whatever the nature of the depression, social factors should be assessed in all cases. Prominent among these will be family factors, especially the marital relationship, the quality of family life, and the presence of any problems with children, parents, in-laws, or other relatives. It is important to listen to the patient's life story, both the early experiences and relationships with parents and the more recent life events, especially losses of various kinds such as bereavement, separation, loss of home, or loss of job. The purpose of the inquiry is also to assess the strength and quality of social supports, since these play an important part in recovery.

Structured questionnaires are available for the detection of depression and can be used clinically. Whether or not they are used is a matter of the physician's preference.

One of the pitfalls of diagnosis is the concurrence of depression with the early stages of organic disease. Carcinoma of the pancreas, hypothyroidism, and pernicious anemia are well known for this. To avoid this pitfall, it is advisable to screen for organic disease, especially in older patients. Physical examination will exclude gross evidence of physical disease. The ESR is a valuable screening test for occult cancer or chronic infection, and serum B12 and tests of thyroid function will be helpful in some patients.

Case 13.1

An elderly woman asked for a home visit because of extreme fatigue. There was strong evidence of depression, no localizing symptoms, and examination was negative. A tentative diagnosis of major depressive illness was made, and blood was taken for an ESR. The ESR was 80 mm in one hour, and further investigation revealed a malignant carcinoma of the stomach.

Another pitfall is the confusion of depression in the elderly with dementia caused by brain failure. Depression in the elderly may present with memory loss and confusion that are entirely reversible by treatment. A trial of antidepressive treatment is advisable before concluding that a patient's symptoms are caused by brain failure.

When depression presents with physical symptoms such as pain, it may be necessary to carry out investigations to identify or exclude organic disease. The need to do these should not delay treatment of the depression. Suicide during investigation is a risk in depressed patients. One of my (IRMcW) own patients committed suicide while awaiting a barium enema for diarrhea and weight loss. When investigations are required, it is advisable to have them done as quickly as possible, so that the patient is spared unnecessary anxiety.

Depressed patients with physical symptoms are especially at risk for spurious diagnosis. The investigation may reveal some "abnormality," which becomes the explanation of their symptoms, while their depression is overlooked—for example, osteoarthritis of the spine to explain backache, hiatus hernia to explain dyspepsia, a colonic diverticulum to explain abdominal pain.

Assessing the Suicide Risk

All depressed patients should be asked about suicidal thoughts. Even patients with mild depression may have had some suicidal thoughts. Contrary to what one might expect, asking the question does not do harm by putting ideas in the patient's mind. I find that the question "Have you felt so bad that you thought of harming yourself?" nearly always produces an unequivocal response. The risk of suicide can be gauged by the persistence of the thoughts, their specificity about detail, and the existence of actual plans.

Treatment

Whatever specific treatment is given, depressed patients have a deeply felt need for reassurance and support. A person experiencing depression for the first time finds it a very disturbing experience. According to Watts (1984), after a lifetime of observing depression in general practice, "only someone who has suffered from the illness can fully appreciate the utter devastation it inflicts.... In my view, a severe depression is the most painful malady known to man."

The patient may feel he or she is going insane. It is often an immense relief to be told that he or she is not going mad, that he or she has a very common problem, and that the great majority of depressions clear completely in a few weeks or months. It is reassuring to be told that the guilt feelings, anxieties, and joylessness are symptoms of depression and will clear when the depression lifts. It is helpful to know that one cannot be expected to alter one's mood by an act of will. The patient will often have been told by unsympathetic family members to "snap out of it" or "cheer up." The family doctor can also help by explaining to members of the family how they can help the patient.

Besides individual psychotherapy and support, everything possible should be done to mobilize social supports for the patient. This may include the involvement of spouse and other relatives, help with children, and the development of contacts outside the home. Cognitive therapy, aimed at altering depressive thought patterns, has been found to benefit depressed patients referred by general practitioners (Teasdale, Fennell, Hibbert, and Amies,1984). Because this involves 20 one-hour sessions with a clinical psychologist, it is not a form of therapy general practitioners are likely to use themselves. It is possible that a modified form could be adapted for general practice. It is likely that the support given to depressed patients by family physicians already has a cognitive element.

Besides the support provided to all depressed patients, general practitioners have three main management decisions to make: the prescription of antidepressants and other drugs, referral to a psychiatrist, and admission to the hospital. The main criterion used by family physicians in prescribing antidepressants is severity of symptoms. The effectiveness of antidepressants in psychiatric outpatients has been well established, but there have been very few trials in general practice. In view of the differences between the two patient populations, this is a serious gap in our knowledge. Because some patients respond very well to explanation and reassurance, it may be wise to wait until the second visit before starting an antidepressant, especially in those with mild depression.

Tricyclic antidepressants (TCAs) have proved effective in a placebo-controlled trial in general practice patients with major and minor depression, in a dosage of 125 to 150 mg daily (Hollyman, Freeling, Paykel, Bhat, and Sedgwick, 1988). Those with major depression showed the greatest benefit over placebo. There is no evidence that a daily dosage of 75 mg is any more effective than placebo.

The newer selective serotonin reuptake inhibitors (SSRIs) and reversible inhibitors of monoamine oxidase A (RIMAs) are equally effective. All these drugs, given in adequate dosage, can be expected to relieve depression in two-thirds of patients, and all have a latency period of 2 to 4 weeks. The SSRIs and RIMAs have the advantage of fewer side effects and a lower risk of death from overdose. They have the disadvantage of producing or exacerbating sleep disturbance. Individual features, such as suicide risk or sleep disturbance, may indicate an SSRI or a TCA, respectively. Some reports indicate that a combination of the SSRI fluoxetine and a TCA is effective. Because fluoxetine can raise blood levels of TCAs, routine serum levels of TCAs are recommended if drugs in this category are utilized (Michels and Marzuk, 1993). Most guidelines consider one of the SSRIs as first line treatment for mild to moderate depression and the practitioner, in making a choice, will want to take into consideration side effect profiles, costs and any prior experience that a patient has had with antidepressant medication.

Atypical depression is particularly responsive to monoamine oxidase inhibitors. For mild bipolar depressions, lithium alone may be sufficient; for more severe bipolar illness, an added antidepressant is usually required (Michels and Marzuk, 1993).

The two main reasons for avoidable failure of drug treatment are inadequate blood levels and lack of compliance. Low blood levels may be caused by inadequate dosage or individual variations in blood level at the same dose. If there is no response to a full course of TCA in full dosage, a blood level should be done. Side effects are a major reason for noncompliance. These should be discussed with patients at the beginning of treatment. Side effects can be reduced by starting with a lower dose and increasing to the therapeutic dose over the first 2 weeks of treatment. Another reason for noncompliance is the interval between onset of treatment and improvement of symptoms. Patients are more likely to persevere if they have been informed of the delayed effect. Elderly patients metabolize tricyclic antidepressants slowly and require lower doses. A single evening dose may also be helpful.

The choice between the two well-tried drugs imipramine and amitryptiline may be influenced by the sedative and hypnotic properties of the latter. In elderly patients, it may be advisable to use a drug with fewer anticholinergic side effects. Sleep is important for depressed patients, and a hypnotic may be needed in the initial stages of therapy to attain restful sleep. Anxiety symptoms are commonly associated with depression and, if not relieved by sympathetic listening and reassurance, may be helped by a short course of a benzodiazepine.

Once a response to an antidepressant has been obtained, treatment should be continued for 4 to 6 months at the same dose unless side effects make this dose intolerable. As many as 50% of patients suffer a relapse if treatment is terminated too soon. Many patients have difficulty in accepting the need for a long course of treatment, so finding common ground and scheduling regular follow-up visits are important. Some discontinue treatment because they fear addiction. Patients especially liable to relapse are those with severe depression, those who have had previous episodes, those with residual symptoms after treatment, and those with overwhelming life problems (Paykel and Priest, 1992).

Lifelong prophylaxis should be considered in older patients with severe depression and in any patient who has had several episodes of unipolar or bipolar depression. Long-term prophylaxis requires a strong commitment by patient and family, therefore support, regular follow-up, and good communication are necessary.

Resistant Depression

If there is no response after a full course of an antidepressant, with adequate dosage and compliance, treatment with another antidepressant should be considered, usually one from a different group. Failure to respond is also an occasion to review the diagnosis and to identify subtypes of depression that may have implications for treatment (Warneke, 1996). Postpartum depression, a past history of manic episodes or hypomania, or a positive family history suggest a bipolar disorder, in which case lithium will be indicated.

Patients with delusions or hallucinations respond poorly to antidepressants alone, so electroconvulsive therapy should be considered. Depressions with severe anxiety, phobias, or panic attacks respond better to monoamine oxidase inhibitors. Those with obsessional features respond better to SSRIs (Warneke, 1996).

Depression may be resistant when there is overwhelming grief, misfortune, physical disability, or adverse social conditions or when there is substance abuse or other self-destructive behavior.

Electroconvulsive therapy is an important alternative to drug therapy. It is very effective and has the advantage of working more rapidly than antidepressants or lithium. It is also safer than antidepressants or lithium in pregnant women and in patients with cardiac conduction disorders (Michels and Marzuk, 1993).

Resistant depression is usually an indication for consultation with or referral to a psychiatrist. Even after referral, however, the family physician still has an important supporting role for patient and family.

Only about one in five depressed patients is referred to a psychiatrist. The main indications for referral are risk of suicide, severe depression with retardation or agitation, depression with psychotic symptoms such as delusions and hallucinations, bipolar depression with prominent manic features, and failure of therapy. The main indications for admission to the hospital are high suicide risk, severe mental retardation or agitation, and social isolation.

Chronic Fatigue Syndrome/Myalgic Encephalomyelitis

In the past, this condition was called *postinfective fatigue*. Since then, some progress has been made in establishing more definitive criteria and exploring links between this syndrome, infection, and immune dysfunction. At the same time, controversy has persisted about the status of the syndrome as a physical illness. Sufferers from this devastating illness still find themselves disbelieved by their physicians as they describe their problems—an experience of rejection that has profound effects on their morale. Because there is still no effective remedy, support and understanding from the physician is a key factor in helping patients to make the major adjustments in their lives that the illness requires. Such also is the power of the physician that legitimizing the illness, and giving it a name, can increase the support and understanding the patient receives from family, friends, and colleagues. Although not a common condition, chronic fatigue syndrome/myalgic encephalomyelitis (CFS/ME) is described at some length here because it exemplifies the management of patients who are chronically ill but have no physical findings. Other examples are patients with fibomyalgia and other chronic pain syndromes.

Nomenclature and Definition
The illness is now called *chronic fatigue syndrome* (CFS) in some parts of the world and myalgic encephalomyelitis (ME) in others. Neither name is entirely satisfactory. The disadvantage of using fatigue in the definition is that fatigue is a very inadequate description of these patients' experience. Fatigue suggests excessive tiredness, whereas these patients feel ill. To the general public, it conveys the idea that sufferers from CFS have just been "overdoing it." Myalgic encephalomyelitis has the advantage of embracing two common features of the illness—muscle pains and neurological/cognitive symptoms.

Since 1988, three case definitions have appeared: one from the U.S. Centers for Disease Control and Prevention (Fukuda et al., 1994), one from Australia (Wakefield, Lloyd, and Hickie, 1990), and one from Britain (Sharpe et al., 1991). The U.S. criteria has one serious shortcoming. The major criteria did not include evidence of neuropsychological dysfunction, which is such a prominent feature of the condition. The Australian criteria include neuropsychological dysfunction as a major criterion and do not exclude depression. They also emphasize the frequently relapsing nature of the fatigue and the fact that it is exacerbated by minor exercise. All three definitions specify that the fatigue must be severe and disabling, that it must have been present for at least 6 months, and that alternative explanations for the illness must be excluded.

The main purpose of these definitions is to clarify case selection for research purposes. Using them unthinkingly as diagnostic criteria can lead to nonsensical conclusions, as when a patient was told that she could not have CFS because she had been ill for only 5 months!

Epidemiology
Chronic fatigue syndrome occurs both sporadically and as one of the sequelae of an epidemic illness marked by muscle pains and neurological symptoms. Epidemics of CFS have been reported in several countries, one of the best documented being among the staff at the Royal Free Hospital, London (Medical Staff of the Royal Free Hospital, 1957). For a time it was known as the "Royal Free disease." Although epidemics continue to be reported, most cases of CFS now appear to be sporadic. Studies in Britain, Australia, and New Zealand indicate a prevalence rate of between 0.4 and 2 per 1,000 general practice patients. An average general practice may therefore expect to have between one and four cases. All

age groups, including children, are affected, with a peak between the ages of 30 and 44. The female/male ratio is about two to one.

The Etiology of CFS

The search for causes of CFS has followed several lines of inquiry: viral studies; studies of immune function, neurophysiological research, and exploration of the relationship between CFS and depression. They will only be summarized here.

The sudden onset of CFS in many patients and the occurrence of CFS after epidemics of an acute illness strongly suggest an infective etiology. Some early outbreaks appeared related to the virus of poliomyelitis, in that they occurred at the same time as epidemics of poliomyelitis. The outbreak in Akureyrie in 1948 was followed 5 years later by an epidemic of poliomyelitis, which affected all parts of Iceland except Akureyrie. This connection has focused attention on the enteroviruses, and Gow et al. (1991) have reported enteroviral sequences in muscle biopsies of 53% of patients with the postviral fatigue syndrome.

The occurrence of persistent fatigue after infectious mononucleosis also directed attention to the Epstein-Barr virus (EBV). Some investigators claimed that EBV was the specific causal agent and suggested that the syndrome be called chronic EBV infection. Further research has shown that many patients with CFS do not have evidence of EBV infection. The evidence now suggests that there is no specific infective agent and that the illness may be activated by a number of viruses or other agents. Viruses could act in two ways: they could persist in the cells, inducing chronic immune responses while evading antiviral immune recognition; or they could trigger immune dysfunction in an immune system already weakened by some other process. Some known infections produce illnesses similar to CFS (the Ross River virus, giardiasis, Lyme disease, leishmaniasis, toxoplasmosis, and brucellosis).

Some of the illnesses suffered by veterans of the Vietnam and Gulf wars also resemble CFS, raising the possibility of environmental toxins as etiological agents. Immunization has preceded the onset of CFS in some cases. Because CFS is a diagnosis of exclusion, it is important to consider and rule out specific causal agents. The process will include a travel history, an occupational history, and a review of possible exposure to environmental toxins.

Many studies have now shown evidence of immune system dysfunction in CFS. Two common changes in immune status have been described: chronic immune activation, including elevations in circulating cytokines, particularly tumor necrosis factor; and poor immune cell function, with low natural killer cell cytotoxic activity, poor lymphocytic proliferative response to mitogens in culture, and frequent immunoglobulin deficiencies (Patarca et al., 1995). Some evidence points to different immunological categories of CFS, which could explain differences in findings among studies, arising from different cohorts of patients. Further research may reveal a relationship between immunological category of disease and severity of illness or effectiveness of therapy (Patarca et al., 1995).

Although muscle pain and weakness are prominent features of CFS, muscle biopsy and electrophysiological testing have not produced evidence of a primary disorder of muscle. It seems likely that changes in muscle are part of a generalized disease process (Wakefield, Lloyd, and Hickie, 1990).

The common occurrence of fatigue in major depression has suggested to some investigators that CFS may be a variant of depression. About half of all patients with CFS fulfill the diagnostic criteria for major depression. However, this is no greater than it is for patients with other chronic illnesses (Hickie, Lloyd, Wakefield, and Parker, 1990). The inadequacy of fatigue as a term for the malaise of CFS has already been discussed. The fatigue of CFS is qualitatively different from the fatigue of depression, as is the effect of exercise. These differences are unlikely to emerge in the answers to questionnaires, which are the sources of data for some of the studies. CFS could only be classified as a variant of depression by ignoring neurological signs and the evidence of a generalized physical disease (pyrexia, lymphadenopathy).

Even less convincing have been attempts to explain CFS in terms of hysteria or somatization. The epidemic of CFS/ME at the Royal Free Hospital in 1955 was described in the British Medical Journal (Medical Staff, 1957). As one would expect from a teaching hospital, the clinical observations were detailed and systematic, including descriptions of neurological signs and enlargement of lymph nodes. Based on these and other observations, the authors presented a reasoned argument for concluding that the outbreak was an epidemic of encephalomyelitis. Fifteen years later, two psychiatrists (McEvedy and Beard, 1970) published a paper based on a reexamination of the data, in which they argued that the outbreak was probably an epidemic of hysteria similar to previously described epidemics of hyperventilation. They did not explain how this would account for facial nerve palsies in 19% of cases, ophthalmoplegia in 43%, bulbar palsy in 7%, and enlarged tender lymph nodes in nearly all cases. A temperature range of 37 to 37.8°C in 84% of patients, they suggested, could be within normal limits. Moreover, for their hypothesis to be correct, one would have to assume that the clinicians at the Royal Free were incapable of distinguishing between the manifestations of hysteria with hyperventilation and those of a diffuse disorder of the nervous system.

It is clear that there are many things about the body's energy that we do not yet understand. Cavadini and colleagues of Zurich University has recently been studying the effects of Tumor Necrosis Factor alpha (TNF-alpha) on energy levels. TNF-alpha is a cytokine, one of the proteins which feed other body cells by signals which switch particular genes on or off in response to infection.

Birchler and his colleagues studied the effect of TNF-alpha on the biochemical system that keeps bodies in synchronicity with the sun. The effect was profound. This response to infection could well be adaptive in normal circumstances, but in other cases malfunctioning.

Louise Pollard of King's College, London injected TNF-alpha in patients with rheumatoid arthritis, a condition often accompanied by severe fatigue, with a protein that binds to TNF-alpha, thus reducing its concentration. The patients felt less fatigued. It remains to be seen whether reducing the cytokine level will help patients with acute onset CFS and also those with the insidious form.

If it does, we should ask what gives rise to the malfunction in the immune system. Broom (2007) considers the views of Ichikawa, Yasuo and Shigenori of Japan. Yasuo might say that the body "remembers" after the stimulus subsides, but the symptoms can recur if similar circumstances arise.

Broom (2007) also describes people who are predisposed: "hard working, excessively responsible, high-performing, and greatly appreciated for their contributions to society. They are often people who want to please, are afraid of conflict, and out of touch with their own negative feelings, let alone able to express them directly."

The Clinical Picture

Two accounts by patients—one a surgeon, the other a general practitioner—convey the personal suffering engendered by this disease.

The surgeon, Thomas English, writes (1991)[3]

You catch "a cold" and thereafter the quality of your life is indelibly altered. You can't think clearly...sometimes it's all you can do to read the newspaper or to follow the plot of a television program. Jet lag without end. You inch along the fog-shrouded precipice of patient care, where once you walked with confidence. Myalgias wander about your body with no apparent pattern. Symptoms come and go, wax and wane. What is true today may be partially true tomorrow or totally false next week. You know that sounds flaky, but, damm it it's happening to you.

You are exhausted, yet you can sleep only two or three hours a night. You were a jogger who ran three miles regularly; now a walk around the block depletes your stamina. Strenuous exercise precipitates relapses that last weeks. There is nothing in your experience in medical school, residency, or practice with its grueling hours and sleep deprivation that even approaches the fatigue you feel with this illness. "Fatigue" is the most pathetically inadequate term.

Iron-man determination to be tough is self-destructive: you merely become Sinking Sisyphus. Perhaps you take a few weeks off; rest helps. Though you improve, you are still light years from your former self.

By now you are literally disabled, but the bills still roll in. Will you qualify for disability if your physicians determine that your only problem is "too much stress"? Maybe you will be lucky enough to find a doctor who can properly diagnose and treat you, and maybe you have disability insurance with a competent company that has informed consultants. Maybe.

I have talked with scores of fellow patients who went to our profession for help, but who came away humiliated, angry, and afraid. Their bodies told them they were physically ill, but the psychospeculation of their physicians was only frightening and infuriating—not reassuring. It told them their doctors had little understanding of the real problem. Many patients had depleted themselves financially, dragging in vain through expensive series of tests and consultants as their lives crumbled around them. They had lost careers, homes, families, in addition to the loss of stamina and cognitive skills. There is nothing that you hold dear that this illness cannot take from you. Nothing.

I have been very lucky. After being ill for a year and a half, I began painfully slow improvement. Despite repeated setbacks, I have progressed to the point where I am no longer continually miserable. My career, however, is but a faint memory. There is little demand for absentminded surgeons, even if I had the stamina. Too, I harbour the lingering fear that I might transmit my illness to a patient. The satisfactions of the operating room are a thing of the past. So I wait. I hope. I pray.

My activities are narrowly circumscribed. I can read again, but I avoid difficult material. I can handle light exercise, but the backpacking that was my previous delight is evanescent fantasy. I swallow my pills, follow my diet. (Treatment is palliative and based on trial-and-error application of anecdotal evidence, but it helps most patients. I enjoy passable existence, not a miasma of misery. I lack the strength to wait years for controlled studies; life is short, science is slow.) I try to educate other patients and "convert" other physicians. Sometimes I succeed.

I have survived because of caring friends and fellow patients and because of a few committed physicians who kept their minds open. They truly listened. They thought long and hard. Many were and still are ridiculed for taking CFS seriously.

The onset is either abrupt, following an acute influenza-like illness or throat infection, or gradual. Instead of the usual recovery from acute illness, "life is indelibly altered" as Thomas English puts it. Within a few days, the patient experiences a change from health and vitality to a bewildering and alarming succession of symptoms. In some patients the onset is gradual, with no clear-cut transition from health to illness. The most common symptoms are muscle and joint pains, extreme weakness and exhaustion, and cognitive disturbances such as memory loss, confusion, and clumsiness. The weakness and exhaustion are made worse by even minor exertion, and the deterioration is prolonged out of all proportion to the amount of exertion. Rest is not restorative. The sensation is not only one of weakness and exhaustion but of feeling ill.

The illness is notable for its great variety of symptoms: paresthesia, vertigo, tinnitus, sweating, shivering, anorexia, nausea, diarrhea, sore throat, headache, intolerance to alcohol, skin rashes. One of the most disturbing features is its unpredictability. The course in most cases is one of partial remissions followed by sudden unpredictable relapses. The unpredictability of the relapses engenders a feeling of insecurity, and this is heightened by the tendency of new symptoms to appear at any stage of the illness. To be plunged into this state is frightening, the sense of losing control profoundly disturbing. Depression is common, as it is in other chronic diseases. It is also possible that the mood disturbances may be a direct effect of neurological dysfunction.

Physical examination of the patient discloses little in the way of signs. Low-grade fever, red throat, and lymphadenopathy are the most frequent findings. With the exception of tests of immune function, laboratory tests are negative. There is no specific test for CFS.

The general practitioner writes[4]

Before my illness I was very fit, playing tennis twice a week and enjoying my general practice in Sydney.

A few weeks after my chest infection resolved, I developed palpitations and shortness of breath at rest. Fearing a viral cardiomyopathy, I consulted a cardiologist who found my heart to be normal. Within a few days I developed fasciculation in several muscle groups. A hastily arranged visit to a neurologist, and a prolonged electromyography (EMG) and examination, revealed normal nerve, neuromuscular junction and muscle function. However, to walk 20 m was a major ordeal

After 6 weeks of enforced rest, I returned part-time to work. Consulting for 2 hours a day left me exhausted, and I was forced to examine patients while sitting in a chair on wheels. Rising from a sitting position was extremely difficult and tiring. I rearranged my consulting room and bought thick plastic mats to cover the carpet so that I could slide along in the chair. I sat to examine patients on the couch. I could not even hold my stethoscope against the patient's back for more than a few seconds before muscle fatigue set in. My legs felt as if they had tight elastic bands around them, and any short walk was followed by the predictable muscle twitches.

I persevered with my practice, but my quality of life was extremely poor. A few hours work in the surgery each day necessitated complete rest for the remainder of the day. This ensured I could manage the following day.

The battery of routine blood tests proved normal, but in reality I was a semi-invalid. I have to be seated to throw a few balls to my son. Watching television made me giddy and the noise and movement of children made me feel so ill that I had to prevent any children coming to play with my boys.

Four months into my illness, I was referred to a specialist with an interest in the chronic fatigue syndrome. He commented that my history was classic and ordered further tests, including T4 and T8 lymphocytes and cell-mediated skin tests.

I was relieved when these tests came back abnormal as I was starting to question myself (as everyone with this illness does when they are told that all the basic tests are normal!).

Another 8 weeks of complete rest did not improve my health. I was desperate. My specialist offered me intravenous gamma globulin, which I gratefully accepted. (At this stage I would have tried anything.)

To my surprise, routine observations on my admission to hospital revealed I had a fever of 38.2°C. After four of the ten bottles of gamma globulin had been administered, my temperature returned to normal and I have not felt "fuzzy" since. One can only understand this type of sensation when one has experienced it.

I am delighted to report that I have continued to make slow progress since my infusion and, 16 months after becoming ill, I feel about 90 percent normal. I can even manage a limited number of house calls. I still need to rest every lunch hour and require 9 to 10 hours of sleep every night.

Patients' Experience of CFS

Patients describe intense feelings of uncertainty and estrangement. Uncertainties arise from the random and unpredictable nature of the symptoms, many of which are bizarre. The uncertainty is made worse by the lack of any explanation for the symptoms. Patients feel estranged from their world because of their inability to fulfill their social responsibilities and also from their bodies, over which they have lost all sense of being in control (Woodward, Broom, and Legge, 1995). The severity of the illness kindles fears of diseases such as cancer and AIDS.

A common response to the illness is to try to carry on as usual with work, household duties, care of children, and social life. With CFS, this is the opposite of what needs to be done. The result is often a downward spiral of self-doubt, deteriorating health, and increasingly desperate attempts to maintain usual activities. Patients who were able to alter their responses learned how to monitor what was happening to their bodies and to pace their lives accordingly (Woodward, 1993).

Receiving a diagnosis was a crucial turning point for many people. The diagnosis provided a framework for understanding what was happening to them—it "organized" their illness so that it ceased to be a nameless threat. It also legitimized their illness: they no longer had to justify their inability to "pull their weight" or to maintain their credibility by trying to carry on as usual (Woodward, Broom, and Legge, 1995).

Sixteen of the 50 people received a diagnosis, or affirmation that they were ill, at an early stage of their illness. Most of these felt they had consistently been treated with respect by their doctors. This affirmation enhanced their self-confidence and in most cases, gave their illness legitimacy in the eyes of family, friends, and colleagues.

For the remainder, the quest for meaning—for some acknowledgment of their suffering and explanation of their illness—was lengthy, distressing, and demoralizing. The attitude of their doctors was often skeptical and dismissive. Sometimes the people they depended on for support —spouses, parents, and friends—refused to believe that they were sick. The experience of rejection seems to be common to a large proportion of patients with CFS. The feeling that they are being held responsible for their illness gives them a sense of betrayal and may lead to a breakdown in the doctor–patient relationship.[5]

Treatment of CFS
In the absence of specific remedies, the physician must use the time-honored therapeutic methods that can apply to any chronic illness. Long before the days of effective drugs, wise physicians had ways of strengthening a patient's own healing powers. A key element in the process is enabling the patient to make some sense of the experience—providing the sense of coherence that Antonovsky (1987) describes as so essential to coping with illness. As already noted, an early diagnosis and naming of the illness are an important beginning. Legitimizing the patient's illness lifts the weight of self-doubt from his or her shoulders and helps to mobilize the support from family and friends. In some cases, it may be helpful for the doctor to meet with family members.

The confidence engendered by this approach will help the patient to eschew desperate attempts to continue with normal activities. Rest is essential, and the doctor will have to mobilize the support needed for child care, housekeeping, and absence from work. Patients have to learn how to monitor their bodies and adjust their lives accordingly. Exercise is helpful but has to be scaled to the body's capacity for it. Inappropriate exercise can lead to prolonged relapses.

As in any chronic illness, a balanced and nutritious diet is important. Some patients may wish to try special diets and these may or may not be helpful. If too rigorous, the diet and its preparation may add to the stresses of the illness. Monitoring the symptoms will help the patient to identify factors that trigger relapses or exacerbate their symptoms. At some point, patients may wish to try alternative therapies and the doctor can both support their wishes and offer advice about risks and benefits (see Chapter 21).

Denz-Penhey and Murdoch (1993) formed a group of CFS patients who met weekly for 9 months to develop a service delivery framework and models of care that would be acceptable to them. Their concern was to provide information useful to family practitioners and others caring for patients with CFS. Four clusters of tasks for the doctor were described:

1. Acknowledgment of the multiple symptoms, recognition of the patient's suffering, and a diagnosis. The group would have found it helpful to know more about the process of coming to a diagnosis.
2. More help with symptom control. To be told each time that "it's just CFS" was not enough. If the treatment involved lifestyle changes, such as rest, this should actually be prescribed by the doctor to make it acceptable to family and colleagues.
3. Avoid rigid adherence to the "disease model" and the dualistic distinction between physical and psychological illness.
4. Prevention of relapses by encouraging patients to watch for warning signals.

In addition to these tasks for the doctor, the group expressed a need for individual or group counseling to help them deal with the many problems of living experienced by sufferers from a serious chronic illness.

One of the authors of the study, a family physician with extensive experience of CFS, was surprised to learn from it how much he did not know about the expectations of patients—so difficult is it to be patient-centered.

References

Antonovsky A. 1987. *Unravelling the Mystery of Health*. San Francisco, CA: Jossey Bass.

Broom B. 2007. Meaning-full Disease: How personal experience and meanings cause and maintain physical illness. Karnac Books Ltd. London.

Brown GW, Harris TO. 1978. *Social Origins of Depression: A Study of Psychiatric Disorder in Women*. New York: Free Press.

Denz-Penhey H, Murdoch JC. 1993. Service delivery for people with chronic fatigue syndrome: A pilot action research study. *Family Practice* 10(1):14.

Dowrick Christopher. 2004. *Beyond Depression: A New Approach to Understanding and Management*. Oxford: Oxford University Press.

Cavadini G, Petrzilla S, Kohler P, Jud C, Tobler I, Birchler T, Fontana A. 2007. TNF alpha suppresses the expression of clock genes by interfering with E-box-mediated transcription. *Proceedings of the National Academy of Sciences* 104(31):12843–12848.

English, TL. 1991. Skeptical of skeptics. *Journal of the American Medical Association* 265(8):964.

Freeling P, Rao BM, Paykel ES, Sireling LI, Burton RH. 1985. Unrecognised depression in general practice. *British Medical Journal* 290:1880.

Fukuda K, Straus SE, Sharpe MC, Dobbins JG, Komaroff A 1994. The chronic fatigue syndrome: a comprehensive approach to its definition and study. *Annals of Internal Medicine* 121(12):953–959.

Goldberg D, Huxley P. 1980. *Mental Illness in the Community: The Pathway to Psychiatric Care*. London: Tavistock Publications.

Goldberg D, Huxley P. 1992. *Common Mental Disorders. A Bio-social Model*. London, New York: Tavistock/Routledge.

Gow JW, Behan WM, Clements GB, Woodall C, Riding M, Behan PO. 1991. Enteroviral RNA sequences detected by polymerase chain reaction in muscle of patients with postviral fatigue syndrome. *British Medical Journal* 302(6778):692.

Hickie I, Lloyd A, Wakefield D, Parker G. 1990. The psychiatric status of patients with the chronic fatigue syndrome. *British Journal of Psychiatry* 156:534.

Hollyman JA, Freeling P, Paykel ES, Bhat A, Sedgwick P. 1988. Double-blind placebo-controlled trial of amitriptyline among depressed patients in general practice. *Journal of the Royal College of General Practitioners* 38:393.

Knotternus JA, Knipschild PG, Van Wersch JWJ, Sijstermanns AHJ. 1986. Unexplained fatigue and hemoglobin: A primary care study. *Canadian Family Physician* 32:1601.

Kroenke K, Wood DR, Mangelsdorff AD, Meier NJ, Powell JB. 1988. Chronic fatigue in primary care. *Journal of the American Medical Assocation* 260(7):929.

MacDonald AJD. 1986. Do general practitioners "miss" depression in elderly patients? *British Medical Journal* 292:1365.

McEvedy CP, Beard AW. 1970. Royal Free epidemic of 1955: A reconsideration. *British Medical Journal* 1:7.

Medical Staff of the Royal Free Hospital. 1957. An outbreak of encephalomyelitis in the Royal Free Hospital Group, London, in 1955. *British Medical Journal* 19(2):895.

Michels R, Marzuk PM. 1993. Progress in psychiatry: Mood disorders. *New England Journal of Medicine* 329(9):628.

Murtagh J. 1992. *Cautionary Tales. Authentic Case Histories from Medical Practice.* Sydney: McGraw Hill.

Nelson E, Kirk J, McHugo G, Douglass R, Ohler J, Wasson J, et al. 1987. Chief complaint fatigue: A longitudinal study from the patient's perspective. *Family Practice Research Journal* 6(4):175.

Okkes IM, Oskam SK, Lamberts H. 2002. The probability of specific diagnoses for patients presenting with common symptoms to Dutch family physicians. *Journal of Family Practice* 51:31–36.

Ormel J, Van Den Brink W, Koeter MWJ, Giel R, Van Der Meer K, Van de Willige G,et al. 1990. Recognition, management and outcome of psychological disorders in primary care: A naturalistic follow-up study. *Psychological Medicine* 20:90.

Patarca R, Klimas NG, Garcia MN, Walters MJ, Dombroski D, Pons H, et al. 1995. Overregulated expression of soluble immune mediator receptors in a subset of patients with chronic fatigue syndrome. *Journal of Chronic Fatigue Syndrome* 1(1):81.

Paykel ES, Priest RG. 1992. Recognition and management of depression in general practice: Consensus statement. *British Medical Journal* 305:1198.

Pelosi DA, McDonald E, Stephens D, Ledger D, Rathbone R, Mann A. 1990. Tired, weak, or in need of rest: Fatigue among general practice attenders. *British Medical Journal* 301(6762):1199.

Post RM. 1992. Transduction of psychosocial stress into the neurobiology of recurrent affective disorder. *American Journal of Psychiatry* 149(8):999.

Sharpe M, Archard L, Banatvala J, Borysiewicz L, Clare A, David A. 1991. Followup of patients presenting with fatigue to an infectious diseases clinic. *Journal of the Royal Society of Medicine* 84:118.

Sireling LI, Freeling P, Paykel ES, Rao BM. 1985a. Depression in general practice: Clinical features and comparison with outpatients. *British Journal of Psychiatry* 147:119.

Sireling LI, Paykel ES, Freeling P, Rao BM, Patel SP. 1985b. Depression in general practice: Case thresholds and diagnosis. *British Journal of Psychiatry* 147:113.

Styron W. 1990. *Darkness Visible: A Memoir of Madness.* New York: Vintage Books.

Sugarman JR, Berg AO. 1984. Evaluation of fatigue in a family practice. *Journal of Family Practice* 19:643.

Teasdale JD, Fennell MJV, Hibbert GA, Amies PL. 1984. Cognitive therapy for major depressive disorder in primary care. *British Journal of Psychiatry* 144:400.

Tylee AT, Freeling P, Kerry S. 1993. Why do general practitioners recognize major depression in one woman patient yet miss it in another? *British Journal of General Practice* 43:327.

Tylee AT, Freeling P, Kerry S, Burns T. 1995. How does the content of consultations affect the recognition of depression by general practitioners? *British Journal of General Practice* 45:575.

Valdini AF, Steinhardt SI, Feldman E. 1989. Usefulness of a standardized battery of laboratory tests in investigating chronic fatigue in adults. *Family Practice* 6:286.

Valdini AF, Steinhardt SI, Jaffe AS. 1987. Demographic correlates of fatigue in a university family health centre. *Family Practice* 4(2):103.

Verhaak PFM. 1995. *Mental Disorder in the Community and in General Practice.* Aldershot, UK: Avebury, Ashgate Publishing Ltd.

Wakefield D, Lloyd A, Hickie I. 1990. The chronic fatigue syndrome. *Modern Medicine* July:16.

Warneke L. 1996. Management of resistant depression. *Canadian Family Physician* 42:1973.

Watts CAH. 1984. Depressive disorders in the community: The scene in Great Britain, 1965. *Journal of Clinical Psychiatry* 45:70.

Widmer RB, Cadoret RJ. 1978. Depression in primary care: Changes in pattern of patient visits and complaints during a developing depression. *Journal of Family Practice* 7:293.

Woodward RV. 1993. It's so strange when you stay sick: The challenge of chronic fatigue syndrome. PhD. thesis. Australian National University, Canberra.

Woodward RV, Broom D, Legge D. 1995. Diagnosis in chronic illness: Disabling or enabling. The case of chronic fatigue syndrome. *Journal of Royal Society of Medicine* 88:179/94A:1

Notes

1. The four levels of analysis in Verhaak's study correspond to four of the five levels originally described by Goldberg and Huxley (1980): mental illness in the general population, in patients consulting primary care doctors, in patients diagnosed as mentally ill by primary care doctors, and in patients referred to psychiatrists. Goldberg and Huxley add a fifth level: admission to a psychiatric institution. At each level, there is a filter that ideally should select those patients who are in need of the next level of care.

2. Verhaak's book includes an extensive discussion of these issues, as does that by Goldberg and Huxley (1992).

3. From the *Journal of American Medical Association* 1991. Copyright 1991, American Medical Association. Reproduced with permission.

4. From Murtagh J. 1992. *Cautionary Tales. Authentic Case Histories from Medical Practice.* Sydney: McGraw Hill. Reproduced with permission.

5. See also Broom DH and and Woodward RV. 1996. Medicalisation reconsidered: Toward a collaborative approach to care. *Sociology of Health & Illness* 18:357.

14

Hypertension

Hypertension is the most common chronic health problem in Western societies. Uncontrolled high blood pressure is associated with an increased incidence of stroke, myocardial infarction, congestive heart failure (CHF) and renal failure, and an increased mortality from these conditions. Treatment and control of high blood pressure results in a significant lowering of the risk of these outcomes in both younger and older patients. Several factors make hypertension a particular challenge to the family physician: its high prevalence, the fact that it does not produce symptoms, and the need for individual and personal management over a long period of time. It is a challenge to the physician's practice organization, clinical judgment, and communication skills.

The Natural History of Hypertension

Blood pressure is a physiological measurement with great variability between individuals and, within the same individual, from day to day and hour to hour. The definition of a particular blood pressure level as hypertension or normal is purely arbitrary (for a discussion of the meaning of normal, see Chapter 9). When blood pressures are taken in a population, the resulting distribution is continuous and unipolar (see Figure 14.1). There is no point at which the blood pressure level suddenly becomes a risk factor. The risk of death increases progressively from the lowest levels of blood pressure to the highest (Figure 14.2). Between diastolic 70 mm Hg and 85 mm Hg, the risk of death doubles; between 70 mm Hg and 115 mm Hg, it increases eightfold. In persons who have had a myocardial infarct, however, the curve is J shaped. The risk of death from coronary disease decreases progressively with each lower level of diastolic blood pressure down to 75 to 79 mm Hg, then increases progressively with each level below the figure (D'Agostino, Belanger, and Kannel, 1991). Hypertension is usually defined as a

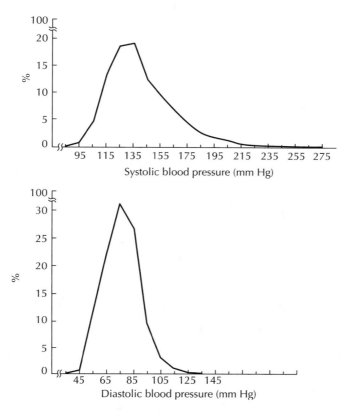

Figure 14.1 Frequency distributions of systolic and diastolic blood pressure measurements. (From Boe et al., 1957.)

sustained diastolic blood pressure above 90 mm Hg and/or a sustained systolic blood pressure above 140 mm Hg. Readings are taken in the seated position with the arm supported at heart level, legs uncrossed and three readings, two minutes apart taken. The first reading is discarded and the latter two are averaged. New automatic devices make it easy to have these readings done while the physician is attending to other patients. In cases where readings exceed 140/90, two more readings are done on the same visit and follow-up arranged to undertake search for end-organ damage. For those with readings over 160/100 a diagnosis of hypertension can be made after three visits. Patients with readings in the 140–159/90–99 range, five visits over 6 months are recommended. The most recent guidelines (Chobanian et al., 2003; Canadian Hypertension Education Program (CHEP) 2008) have identified a new category named prehypertension (120–139/80–89) which identifies people at higher risk of becoming hypertensive, especially those at the higher end of the stated range. When discussing the diagnosis with the patient, and when planning management, it is important to

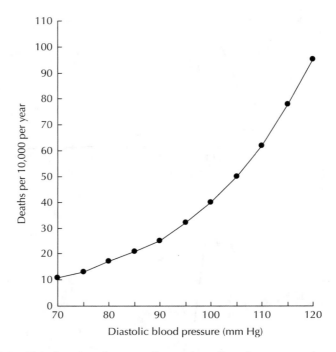

Figure 14.2 Risk function for mortality against diastolic pressure in men 35 to 44 years. (From Kannel and Gordon, 1970.)

bear in mind the arbitrary nature of this definition. Within the total category of hypertension, diastolic pressures of 90 to 104 mm Hg are usually designated as mild.

The prevalence of hypertension increases with age and varies with ethnicity (see Table 14.1). In the Framingham study (the source of much of our knowledge in the natural history of hypertension), there was an average increase of 20 mm Hg systolic and 10 mm Hg diastolic between the ages of 30 and 65. The average systolic pressure continued to rise into the eighties in women and into the seventies in men. Diastolic blood pressure peaked earlier, then declined after the age of 55 in men and 60 in women. Sixty-five percent to 75% of hypertension in the elderly was of the isolated systolic variety (Kannel, 1996). In middle-aged and elderly women, hypertension is so common that it affects a large proportion of the population. The long-term risk of developing hypertension is best conveyed by the lifetime risk statistic which is the probability of developing hypertension in the remaining years of life. This can be expressed as adjusted or unadjusted for other competing causes of death. Results of the Framingham study found that for those without hypertension at the age of 55 to 64, and who survived to 80 to 85, the lifetime risk of developing hypertension was 90% (Vasan et al., 2002) This increase would be principally in the form of systolic hypertension. The U.S.

Table 14.1 Prevalence of hypertension* among participants, by age, sex and ethnic group[†]

Factor	Ethnic group; prevalence of hypertension, % (SE)					
	White n = 6,988,494	Black n = 253,090	South Asian n = 388,930	East Asian n = 366,139	Overall n = 7,996,653	P value
Overall	20.7 (1.7)	31.5 (5.1)	30.1 (4.2)	18.5 (3.3)	21.3 (1.5)	0.02
Age, yr						
20–39	3.0 (1.3)[‡]	7.2 (4.9)[‡]	6.3 (2.4)[‡]	4.9 (3.9)[‡]	3.4 (1.2)	0.57
40–59	21.3 (2.7)	49.8 (9.0)	38.2 (6.6)	13.7 (3.2)	22.6 (2.5)	<0.001
60–79	50.2 (6.0)	62.1 (12.1)	74.9 (9.8)	61.3 (9.8)	51.6 (5.6)	
P value	<0.001	<0.001	<0.001	<0.001	<0.001	
Sex						
Female	17.9 (2.2)	36.1 (6.4)	25.9 (5.5)	21.8 (5.8)	19.0 (2.0)	0.02
Male	23.6 (2.7)	25.3 (8.6)[‡]	34.2 (5.7)	15.5 (3.4)	23.8 (2.4)	0.14
P value	0.11	0.32	0.25	0.34	0.14	

SE, standard error.
*Hypertension is defined as systolic blood pressure $\geq$ 140 mm Hg or diastolic blood pressure $\geq$ 90 mm Hg or current treatment with antihypertensive medication
[†]Data are weighted to the total adult population in Ontario (7,996,653).
[‡]Estimate with coefficient of variation > 0.33.

From Leenen, Dumais, McInnis et al., 2008.

National Health Survey showed that 15 to 20% of adults in the United States have casual blood pressures greater than 160/95 mm Hg.

A population survey in Canadian adults found a prevalence rate of 21.3% overall. Prevalence increased with age from 3.4% in those aged 20 to 39 to 51.6% in those aged 60 to 79 years (Table 14.1 from Leenen et al., 2008). In another recent population-based study using administrative data it was found that the incidence and prevalence of hypertension in the population of Ontario, Canada has risen much faster than anticipated (Tu, Chen, and Lipscombe, 2008a). Between 1995 and 2005 the age and sex adjusted prevalence had doubled from 153.1 to 244.8 per 1,000 adults. Further, there was a 25.7% increase in age and sex adjusted incidence of hypertension in the same time period.

Mild and prehypertension is much commoner than moderate and severe hypertension. In a family practice of 2,500 patients that reflects the age structure of the North American population, one can expect to find 472 patients with hypertension (Ostbye et al., 2005).

At one time the diastolic blood pressure was considered more significant as a predictor of cardiovascular disease (CVD) than the systolic. The evidence no longer supports this distinction. Even in persons with diastolic pressures of 90 mm Hg or below, the risk of CVD increases progressively with the systolic blood pressure. Combined systolic and diastolic hypertension carries only a marginally increased risk than isolated systolic hypertension (Kannel, 1996). There is evidence that some family physicians tend to pay more attention to diastolic blood pressure (DBP) in the elderly than to systolic blood pressure (SBP) (Berklowitz et al., 1998; Hyman, Pavlik, and Vallbona, 2000). Since systolic pressure increases with age, and with an aging population, the treatment of blood pressure should primarily be targeted at systolic pressure.

Hypertension and Atherogenesis

Hypertension is one of many risk factors for atherosclerotic disease, and the risk of CVD in patients with hypertension varies greatly with the number and severity of other risk factors. The assessment of coexistent risk factors is essential to the estimation of prognosis and the formulation of a plan of treatment.

Nevertheless, because the relationship between blood pressure and CVD is continuous, consistent, and independent of other risk factors, guidelines (CHEP, 2008) recommend treating all people with stage 1 or stage 2 hypertension. If other risk factors are present, the risk increases with each additional factor (see Figure 14.3).

The risk of stroke for patients with hypertension also varies with the number and severity of risk factors. The risk factors include atrial fibrillation, coronary heart disease, and cardiac failure (see Figure 14.4). The use of the Framingham risk score with published tables assists the clinician in demonstrating to the patient, the benefits of treatment.

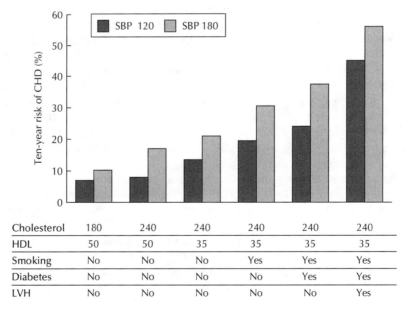

Cholesterol	180	240	240	240	240	240
HDL	50	50	35	35	35	35
Smoking	No	No	No	Yes	Yes	Yes
Diabetes	No	No	No	No	Yes	Yes
LVH	No	No	No	No	No	Yes

Figure 14.3   Ten-year risk for coronary heart disease by systolic blood pressure and presence of other risk factors. (From Chobanian et al., 2003.)

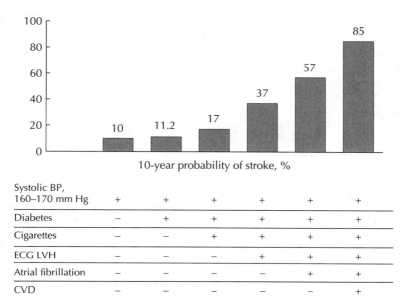

Systolic BP, 160–170 mm Hg	+	+	+	+	+	+
Diabetes	–	+	+	+	+	+
Cigarettes	–	–	+	+	+	+
ECG LVH	–	–	–	+	+	+
Atrial fibrillation	–	–	–	–	+	+
CVD	–	–	–	–	–	+

Figure 14.4 Probability of stroke in mild hypertension by intensity of associated risk factors, Framingham Study, men aged 63 to 65 years. Risk factors measured at beginning of each biennial interval. Systolic blood pressures (BPs) are casual blood pressure measurements obtained by physician. Current cigarette use was indicated as yes or no on each biennial examination. Criteria used for left ventricle hypertrophy (LVH) measured by electrocardiogram (ECG) are those of Romhilt-Estes. Cardiovascular disease (CVD) includes coronary heart disease, congestive heart failure, intermittent claudication, or stroke. Rate estimates were based on multivariate statistical modeling. (From Wolf PA, D'Agostino RB, Belanger AJ, Kannel WB. 1991. Probability of stroke: A risk profile from the Framingham study. *Stroke* 22(3):312–318. Reproduced with permission from Kannel WB 1996, *Journal of the American Medical Association* 275, 1571–1576. Copyright 1991, American Medical Association.)

Hypertension and Congestive Heart Failure

In the Framingham cohort, hypertension accounted for 39% of cases of CHF in men and 59% in women. In hypertensive patients, myocardial infarction, diabetes, left ventricular hypertrophy, and valvular disease were predictive of increased risk of CHF (Levy, Larson, Vasan, Kannel, and Ho, 1996).

Left ventricular hypertrophy (LVH) is a predictor of CHF, as well as of coronary disease, stroke, and peripheral vascular disease. The risk increases progressively with the increase in left ventricular muscle mass and with the severity of LVH by ECG criteria (Kannel, 1996). The ECG and anatomical indicators of LVH (radiography and echocardiogram) contribute independently to the risk of CHF and other sequelae. Patients who have both are at greater risk than persons with either one (Kannel, 1996). The ECG is less sensitive than the echocardiogram as a test for LVH, but economic factors make it more suitable as a routine test for patients with hypertension. Biochemical markers of heart failure such as BNP (brain naturetic protein) and a metabolite of its precursor (NT-proBNP) have been found to have high sensitivity and specificity for CHF. These tests have been mainly tested in the settings of emergency departments and cardiology outpatient clinics. Their usefulness in the setting of family practice remains uncertain, and, in any case they are not as yet widely available.

Risk Factors for Hypertension

There are populations in economically undeveloped countries that do not show the rise of blood pressure with age characteristic of people in industrialized countries. When people emigrate from undeveloped to developed societies, they change to the pattern of the new environment. In North America and Europe, population studies have not shown significant differences in blood pressure between social classes as defined by occupation, income, and education. This is not the case, however, with mortality from hypertension-related disease. In both the United States and Britain, mortality is much higher among the poor and those with lower levels of education. In the United States, African Americans have a much higher mortality from hypertension-related disease than whites. The reasons for these differences are not clear. For family physicians, however, they do signify the need for special attention to patients in lower income groups, and especially to patients of African descent.

Obesity is strongly associated with hypertension. In all age groups, the prevalence of hypertension is three times greater in the obese (20% over normal weight) than in the nonobese. The prevalence is five times higher between the ages of 20 and 44, and twice as high between the ages of 45 and 74. For every 10 kg increase in weight there is a 3 mm increase in diastolic pressure. Conversely, reduction of weight in obese hypertensive patients lowers diastolic pressure by about 5 mm Hg for each 5-kg weight loss. There is some evidence, however, that the risk of hypertension-related disease is lower in the obese.

Smoking is not a risk factor for hypertension but is strongly associated with the development of hypertension-related disease. In one MRC study of mild hypertension, which divided participants into a placebo and a treatment arm and followed them over several years(1985), morbidity and mortality rates were higher in smokers than in nonsmokers in both groups. For stroke and for all cardiovascular events, the difference between rates in smokers and nonsmokers was greater than the effect of drug treatment. For mild hypertension, therefore, smoking cessation may be the single most important management strategy.

Alcohol intake is insufficiently recognized as an etiological factor. Heavy drinkers have higher blood pressures than light drinkers or abstainers. The effect begins at about four drinks per day and is linear from eight drinks upward. The so-called type A behavior (time urgency, restlessness, ambition) also has a correlation with high blood pressure.

The contribution of salt intake to the etiology of hypertension is clear. The Intersalt study showed that the rise in hypertension observed in middle-aged urbanites is clearly linked to salt intake (Intersalt Cooperative Research Group,

1988; Elliott et al., 1996). The weight of evidence seems to support the modest reduction of dietary sodium in the general population, recommended in the U.S. Dietary Guidelines for Americans (U.S. Department of Agriculture, U.S. Department of Health and Human Services, 1995; Lenfant, 1996). Dietary sodium restriction does reduce blood pressure in hypertensive patients, the effect being greater for older people (Midgley, Mattew, Greenwood, and Logan, 1996).

High normal or Prehypertension

The increased risk of disease and death in severe and moderately severe hypertension is so great that decisions about whether to use pharmacotherapy cause little difficulty for the physician: every effort must be made to control the blood pressure. What we know of the natural history of high normal or prehypertension makes therapeutic decisions more challenging. In the first place, mild hypertension is not a high risk in the absence of other risk factors (see Figures 14.3 and 14.4). Second, a substantial number of patients with high normal blood pressure will revert to normal levels if observed over a number of years. In the British MRC trial (1985) of treatment for mild hypertension, 18% of the placebo group had readings below 90 mm Hg at the first three anniversary visits. Twenty-three percent were below 90 mm Hg at two of these visits, and 27% at one visit. Only 32% had readings above 90 mm Hg at all three visits. On the other hand, about 12% of the placebo group developed blood pressures above the mild range. At present we have no way of predicting which patients with mild hypertension will revert to normal levels without treatment, which will remain in the mild range, and which will become more severe. Patients with high normal blood pressure who are not placed on pharmacotherpy should therefore be followed at intervals.

Meta-analysis of clinical trials have shown that a reduction of DBP of 5 to 6 mm Hg resulted in a 42% reduction in strokes but only a 14% reduction in all coronary heart disease. The discrepancy between stroke and coronary disease has not been explained. Because these are relative risk reductions, their impact on an individual depends on the baseline risk without treatment. The risk of stroke in adults with a DBP from 90 mm Hg to 104 mm Hg is about 0.2% per year; for all cardiovascular events it is about 1%. Half of the people who suffer a stroke have no risk factors.

Research has shown the benefit of drug treatment for patients aged 65 to 84 with SBP of 160 mm Hg or over and a DBP of 90 mm Hg or over, either singly or combined. Rates of stroke and cardiovascular events were significantly reduced. There is insufficient evidence for or against drug treatment for hypertension in patients over the age of 84, and for patients aged 64 to 84 with SBP of 140 to 160 mm Hg (Staessen et al., 1997; Gueyffier et al., 1999; Hansson et al., 1999; Staessen et al., 2000).

Primary and Secondary Hypertension

In the general population, primary or essential hypertension—in which no specific cause is identifiable—accounts for 94% to 95% of all hypertensives. This figure

Table 14.2   Prevalence of identifiable causes of hypertension among patients with a selected clinical characteristic

Clinical Characteristics	Type of Hypertension	Prevalence (%)
Drug-resistant hypertension or increased (≥0.23 mg/dL) creatinine with ACE inhibitor	Renovascular	20
Hypertension began after the age of 60 years	Renovascular	10
Diastolic blood pressure >100 mm Hg	Renovascular	6
Hypertension began after the age of 60 years and diastolic blood pressure >110 mm Hg	Renovascular	25
Hypertension and initial serum potassium <3.4 mEg/L	Renovascular	15
Suggestive symptoms for pheochromocytoma	Pheochromocytoma	0.5
Multiple (four or more) suggestive findings for Cushing syndrome	Cushing syndrome	80–90
Hypertension and hypokalemia	Hyperaldosteronism	50

From Dosh, 2001.

is based on three studies of unselected hypertensive patients, one in an Ontario general practice (Rudnick, Sackett, Hirst, and Holmes, 1977), two in random samples in Sweden (Bergland, Anderson, and Wilhelmsen, 1976; Danielson and Dammstrom, 1981). Renal parenchymal disease was the leading cause of secondary hypertension in these populations with a frequency between 2.1% and 4.7%. Renovascular hypertension (RVH) occurred in 0.1% to 1.0%. However, since that time, improvements in diagnostic capabilities have found that primary aldosteronism (PA) (Conn's syndrome) is the most common secondary cause of hypertension (Young, 2007). Estimates of the prevalence of PA in those diagnosed with hypertension range between 5% and 11%. The prevalence of secondary causes of hypertension varies with clinical characteristics (Table 14.2). Only about 0.1% of hypertensives are surgically curable. These facts have important implications for the investigation of hypertension in general practice—to be discussed below.

Measuring the Blood Pressure

Studies have shown considerable discrepancies between blood pressure readings taken by physicians and by trained observers. Similar, though smaller, discrepancies were found between nurses and trained observers. Because the measurement of blood pressure may decide whether or not a patient is to be classified as hypertensive, even an inaccuracy of 4 mm Hg may be serious.

Inaccuracies can be traced to faults in equipment and to faults of technique. Because of concerns about the effects of mercury on human health and the environment, mercury sphygmomanometers are often replaced with aneroid or electronic monitors, which need to be regularly checked for accuracy.

However, aneroid and electronic sphygmomanometers may not be reliable. They require standardizing against a mercury sphygmomanometer twice a year, using a Y tube to connect both instruments to a cuff placed round a suitable object. Although aneroid models are convenient for the doctor's bag and sufficient for some purposes where accuracy is not as important, the mercury sphygmomanometer should be used in the office and in all cases where hypertension is suspected. Mercury sphygmomanometers require servicing if the meniscus cannot be clearly seen.

Using a standard adult cuff on an obese arm overestimates the pressure. A large adult cuff should be used whenever the mid-upper arm circumference exceeds 33 cm. If the circumference exceeds 41 cm, a thigh cuff should be used. For children—or for an arm circumference less than 24 cm—a pediatric cuff should be used.

A study in hospitals has shown that the heart rate and blood pressure of inpatients rises substantially when they are visited by a physician (Mancia et al., 1983). The average rise was 27 mm Hg systolic and 15 mm Hg diastolic and there were large individual differences. Visits by patients to a family physician whom they know are less likely to produce an alarm reaction. Our own observation has been that the blood pressure levels reported by consultants to whom we have referred patients are often much higher than the blood pressure we record when they return to see us. Even a visit to a known family doctor, however, is usually accompanied by some anxiety. It is better, therefore, to take the blood pressure after the patient has had 5 minutes to relax. Alternatively, some readings may be taken at home, either by a visiting nurse, or by the patient, using a home blood pressure monitor. There is good evidence that home and work blood pressures are better predictors of disability and cardiac enlargement than office measurements (Canadian Coalition, 1988). The arm should be well supported and bared, with no constricting clothing. The bladder part of the cuff should be placed over the brachial artery, with the lower edge of the cuff 3 cm above the elbow crease. The bag should be inflated until the pressure is above 200 mm Hg, or 30 mm above the level at which the radial pulse cannot be palpated. The bag is then deflated slowly, so that the mercury drops at no more than 2 mm per second. The systolic pressure is the point at which the sounds are first heard (Korotkoff phase I), and the diastolic is the point at which the sounds disappear completely (phase V). If the sounds persist to zero, muffling of the sounds should be used as the diastolic pressure (phase IV).

One of the most common errors is digit preference—the tendency for observers to record blood pressures ending in zero or even numbers.

Ambulatory blood pressure monitoring (ABPM) is a technology that is becoming more available and which provides valuable information about an individual's blood pressure over the course of a day. These devices when appropriately placed on the patient record blood pressure at various intervals during a 24-hour period. This is particularly helpful information in cases in which white coat hypertension is suspected, when blood pressure does not seem to respond to treatment, in cases of hypotensive episodes while on blood pressure medications and autonomic dysfunction. In those with hypertension, readings during the day are typically >135/85, and during sleep >120/75. ABPM readings correlate better than office readings with end-organ damage. ABPM is indicated in cases of fluctuating office blood pressure measurements, presence of symptoms suggestive of hypotension, or failure to achieve target blood pressure levels in spite of appropriate antihypertensive medication.

Investigation of Hypertension

Before the investigation begins, the blood pressure should be recorded often enough to ensure that a basal reading has been obtained. The measurement should be done in both arms and all subsequent readings done on the arm with the higher pressure.

The purpose of the investigation is to identify end-organ damage, to identify secondary hypertension, and to record baseline data on the cardiovascular system and risk factors for CVD. The history should include an inquiry about smoking, alcohol intake, dietary habits, level of activity, medication (especially estrogens and analgesics), family history of hypertension, and past history of renal disease. The examination should include weight and height, examination of fundi, heart, lungs and abdomen (including auscultation for carotid and abdominal bruits), a calculation of the Body Mass Index (BMI) and waist circumference, and a test of the urine for microalbuminuria. The radial and femoral pulses should be palpated simultaneously to detect coarctation of the aorta. If the dipstick test shows proteinuria, this should be confirmed with salicylsulfonic acid. Measuring urinary albumin excretion or albumin/creatinine ratio should be done annually in those with diabetes or renal disease.

For the great majority of patients, the only investigations needed are the serum creatinine (or the corresponding eGFR), blood glucose, lipid profile (including total cholesterol, LDL-C, HDL-C, and triglycerides), sodium and potassium, and an ECG for evidence of left ventricular hypertrophy. In those with diabetes, urinary albumin secretion should be assessed. The serum potassium will identify most cases of primary aldosteronism. For patients with labile hypertension, with attacks of sweating or palpitation, and with moderate or severe hypertension, 24-hour urine should be tested for catecholamines. Pheochromocytoma is a rare but important cause of secondary hypertension. In most patients with this condition, the blood pressure is very labile, and there is a history of attacks of flushing and profuse sweating. In others, the blood pressure is stable and there are few symptoms. Anesthetics can be fatal in patients coming to surgery with undiagnosed pheochromocytoma.

Detection of Renovascular Hypertension
Renal artery stenosis—caused either by atheroma or by fibroplasia—is a curable form of hypertension. It is, however, very rare in the general

population of hypertensive patients and therefore poses a difficult detection problem for the family physician. Indications for investigation for RVH include (CHEP, 2008):

Sudden onset or worsening of hypertension and age older than 55 years or younger than 30 years

The presence of an abdominal bruit

A rise in creatinine of >30% associated with use of an angiotensin-converting enzyme inhibitor or angiotensin II antagonist

Other atheroscelerotic vascular disease, particularly in patients who smoke or have dyslipidemia

Recurrent pulmonary edema associated with hypertensive surges.

In addition to the above criteria, renal investigation may be indicated because protein, blood, or pus is found in the urine, or because the serum creatinine is raised. Even in these patients, however, the potential benefit should be weighed against the risk of the procedure.

Patients should not be investigated for RVH unless they are fit for surgery. If they are not fit for surgery, the result will be of academic interest only. In the majority of patients who are well controlled with drugs, renal investigation need not be considered. There is, however, one exception to this rule. Patients with severe RVH may respond well to propranolol or ACE inhibitors, but this treatment can result in loss of renal function and renal failure.

When RVH is suspected, noninvasive investigations such as angiotensin-converting enzyme inhibitor (ACEI)-enhanced renal scan, duplex Doppler flow studies, and magnetic resonance imaging are used initially and angiography saved for identifying the renal artery anatomy if a procedure is to be done.

Other renal causes of hypertension include chronic glomerulonephritis, polycystic kidney disease, and hypertensive nephrosclerosis.

Endocrine Hypertension

Recent advances in detection suggests that primary hyperaldosteronism (PA) is much commoner than previously thought (Young, 2007). Traditional teaching was that low potassium was present in all cases of PA, but it is now recognized that potassium may be normal in some cases. Investigation for PA should be undertaken in the following situations (CHEP, 2008):

Hypertensive patients with spontaneous hypokalemia (K < than 3.5 mmol/L)

Hypertensive patients with marked diuretic-induced hypokalemia (K < than 3.0 mmol/L)

Patients with hypertension refractory to treatment with three or more drugs

Hypertensive patients found to have an incidental adrenal adenoma.

If PA is suspected on the basis of the above indications, screening should take place. This consists of measuring the aldosterone : renin ratio after the discontinuation of aldosterone antagonists, angiotensin receptor blockers, betaadrenergic antagonists, and clonidine. Other antihypertensive drugs may be continued. An aldosterone/renin activity ratio greater than 550 pmol/L/ng/ml/hr is considered positive and is an indication for further confirmatory tests (CHEP, 2008).

Pheochromocytoma is very rare, but should be suspected in the following:

Patients with paroxysmal and /or severe (BP>180/110nm Hg) sustained hypertension refractory to usual antihypertensive therapy

Patients with hypertension and multiple symptoms suggestive of catecholamine excess (e.g., headaches, palpitations, sweating panic attacks, and pallor).

Patients with hypertension triggered by beta-blockers, monoamine oxidase inhibitors, micturition, or changes in abdominal pressure

Patients with incidental discovered adrenal mass, hypertension and multiple endocrine neoplasia 2A or 2B, von Recklinghausen's neurofibromatosis, or von Hippel-Lindau disease.

Further investigations for pheochromocytoma will involve referral to a specialized centre.

Cushing's disease is estimated to have an incidence of 1 in 100,000 people. The classic symptoms (centripetal obesity, proximal muscle weakness, facial plethora, hirsutism, glucose intolerance, and easy bruisability) of Cushing's disease in a hypertensive patient should trigger the need to have a dexamethasone suppression test. The widespread use of newer imaging techniques is uncovering more unexpected adrenal masses (incidentalomas) some of which are hormonally active. It is estimated that between 5% and 20% of such tumors have autonomous hormonal activity and cause a subclinical Cushing's syndrome. The incidence of subclinical Cushing's syndrome is thought to be much higher (79/100,000) than the classical form of the disorder. Subclinical Cushing's syndrome may lack the classical signs of hypercortisolism but have a high prevalence of obesity, hypertension, and type 2 diabetes (Reincke, 2000).

Organizing the Practice for the Detection and Follow-up of Hypertension

Hypertension is the best opportunity for secondary prevention available to the family physician: the condition is common, the symptomless period long, the test simple, and the payoff—at least for moderate and severe hypertension—high.

In the 1970s, many population studies showed that about half of all people with hypertension were undetected—not aware of their condition. More recent studies suggest that this situation has changed as a result of more attention to case finding by family physicians. Surveys in Ontario have found only 6% of hypertensives unaware of their condition and a further 6% aware but not under treatment. Undetected hypertension was most frequent (27%) among males under the age of 40 (Birkett, 1987).

If the benefit of this prevention is to be felt by the whole practice, an appropriate management system must be in effect. The system to be described here is based on the following facts: 70% of a practice population consults their family physician at least once a year, and over 90% consult their family physician in a

5-year period. These visits, for all purposes, provide the opportunity for recording the blood pressure and identifying hypertension, especially in the young male population. This strategy is known as case finding and is contrasted with screening, a strategy applied to populations of ostensibly healthy individuals.

Why is a management system necessary? Is it not sufficient for the physician or nurse to record the blood pressure when the patient visits? The answer is that reliance on the physician's memory—even when he or she is interested in hypertension—is not enough. Physicians who have tried this report that it only succeeds in recording the blood pressure in about half the patients who attend.

The aim of the management system should be to record the blood pressure of all adults in the practice population at least once every 2 years. It is important that all members of the practice—physicians, nurses, and receptionists—should be committed to the system and be aware of their responsibilities to it. The first step is to identify patients who have had a blood pressure recorded by a mark on the outside of their record. One simple method is to attach a colored adhesive dot-color-coded for year. If, for example, the system is put into operation in 2004, those patients having a blood pressure recorded in this year would have, say, a black dot affixed, those in 2005 a blue dot, and so on. In 2006, those with a black dot would need another reading and the black dot would be replaced by another color. Of course there are other ways of doing this. If the same system is used for other preventive measures, such as immunization and Pap smears, color coding may be insufficient. In practices with computerized records, the year of the last recorded blood pressure can be included in the patient's printout. The computer can be programmed to notify the doctor and/or the patient when a repeat measurement is due.

The next step is to decide who has the responsibility for explaining the system to the patient and for taking the blood pressure. Often this will be a nurse or assistant. Whoever does it should be trained in the correct technique. The system will separate people into four categories at the first reading: definitely hypertensive (BP >180/104), probably hypertensive (BP 150/90 to 180/104), possibly prehypertensive (BP < 140/90), and normotensive (<120/80). Patients in the definitely hypertensive category will need immediate assessment and investigation by the physician. We know that, with blood pressures in this range, all patients will maintain pressures in the hypertension range over several weeks of observation. With those in the probably hypertensive category, we know that some will be confirmed after observation and some will revert to normal. Further readings on at least three occasions are required. This may be done either by the nurse or assistant, or by the physician. Those who are confirmed after observation should be assessed by the physician. For those in the probably normotensive category, recent guidelines recommend a recheck in 2 years. Those in the prehypertension category should be reevaluated in 1 year. Those patients who are asked to return for two further readings should be informed of the finding and the reasons for asking them to return. The practice should have a system for identifying and calling patients who do not return. Care is needed to avoid the label hypertension until it has been confirmed (Table 14.3).

Table 14.3 Recommendations for the follow-up based on initial blood pressure measurements for adults without acute end-organ damage

Initial Blood Pressure (mm Hg)[*]	Follow-up Recommended[†]
Normal	Recheck in 2 years
Prehypertension	Recheck in 1 year[‡]
Stage 1 Hypertension	Confirm within 2 months[‡]
Stage 2 Hypertension	Evaluate or refer to source of care within 1 month. For those with higher pressures (e.g., >180/110 mmHg), evaluate and treat immediately or within 1 week depending on clinical situation and complications.

[*]If systolic and diastolic categories are different, follow recommendations for shorter time follow-up (e.g., 160/86 mmHg should be evaluated or referred to source of care within 1 month).
[†]Modify the scheduling of follow-up according to reliable information about past BP measurements, other cardiovascular risk factors, or target organ disease.
[‡]Provide advice about lifestyle modifications (see Lifestyle Modifications).

From The Seventh Report of the Joint National Committee on Prevention, Detection, Evaluation, and Treatment of High Blood Pressure, 2003.

One of the chief reasons for poor control of hypertension has been the dropout of patients from continuing surveillance. Many surveys done in the 1970s showed that half of all known hypertensives were out of control and that many of these were not taking antihypertensive drugs and had ceased to attend their physicians. In the Canadian Heart Health Survey it was found that 42% of Canadian adults with hypertension were unaware of it and only 16% were treated and controlled (Joffres et al., 1997). Since that time, efforts at both detection and treatment have improved. In the Ontario population, using linked administrative data covering the decade from 1995 to 2005, it was found that the age and sex adjusted mortality among hypertensive patients declined by 15.5% (Tu et al., 2008b). The reduced mortality may be significant factor in the rise in prevalence of hypertension. It is not difficult to understand why control may be unsatisfactory. Because hypertension is symptomless, patients feel well until organ damage occurs. Unless the reason for lifelong treatment has been carefully explained to them, they may interpret their feeling of wellness as a reason for stopping treatment. Other patients may find that on medication they feel less well than they did before. It takes careful attention to their problems for control to be successfully maintained. Added to this are all our human tendencies to forget appointments, procrastinate, and deny unpleasant facts.

Patients will be less inclined to drop out from follow-up and treatment if they fully understand their condition and if they know that side effects of drugs can often be reduced or eliminated. Failure to keep an appointment may be the first indication that a patient does not have this understanding. The practice needs, therefore, a follow-up system that will identify patients who fail to make appointments or cancel an appointment they have made. The patients can then be offered another appointment and, when they do attend, their reasons for not coming can be explored by the patient-centered method. A follow-up system of this kind is made simpler by the use of electronic patient records that provide for these kinds of alerts. However, even in paper-based practices a system can be installed very simply. A Rolodex or box file can be used to file the patient's card by the month of his next appointment. When the patient attends, the card is moved forward to the month of the next appointment. At the end of each month, the remaining cards show which patients have not attended.

It is sometimes said that it is not the physician's responsibility to chase people who have decided to discontinue treatment. People have a responsibility for their own health—so the argument runs—and it is their prerogative to disregard their doctor's advice if they so wish. With all this we agree, provided the decision to discontinue treatment is a conscious decision, made after being fully informed of the facts. The problem is that the great majority of patients who drop out of treatment do not do so on the basis of a well-informed decision. If a patient fails to attend, we cannot assume that he or she has all the necessary information. If we are to fulfill our commitment to patients, it is our responsibility to see that they understand their position.

Discussions of treatment often focus exclusively on the question of drug therapy. It is also common to hear dogmatic statements such as "a diastolic pressure of 90 mm Hg or over is an indication for hypotensive drugs." For family physicians, the management issues are much broader than this. Every patient presents a different problem. It is true that for those with moderate and severe levels of hypertension, treatment with hypotensive drugs is necessary. Even in these patients, however, there may be exceptional reasons for not prescribing drugs: reasons such as severe mental illness, alcoholism, drug addiction, or the terminal stages of an unrelated disease. For patients with mild hypertension, many other factors have to be considered: age and sex, weight, habits, presence of other risk factors, and the patient's own wishes. Even if drugs are prescribed, they are only one part of the management of hypertension. Attention to diet, smoking reduction, weight reduction (for the obese), alcohol intake, exercise and way of life are equally important. In this discussion of therapy, therefore, we will begin with the general treatment of the patient and conclude with drug therapy.

General Treatment

The first principle is to provide the patient with full information about hypertension in general, and about his or her own condition in particular. No knowledge of hypertension can be assumed. The patient, in fact, may have incorrect information. It is not uncommon, for example, for patients to equate hypertension with nervous tension. The patient should be informed about the nature of hypertension, its risks, and the methods available for controlling it. The patient should have some indication of his or her own level of risk. Some caution is needed here because, as we have seen, prediction based on risk factors has a large margin of error for the individual patient. The patient will want to know, not only the risk of end-organ damage, but the likelihood that treatment will prevent it at his or her own age and level of blood pressure (see p. 195 for ways of explaining this to patients) If the question of drug therapy arises, the patient should know the risks attached to the drugs.

The following are of major importance in the regimen for patients with hypertension:

1. **Smoking reduction.** To stop smoking is the most effective thing the patient with mild hypertension can do to reduce his risk of CVD. For those with moderate and severe hypertension, smoking is a major risk factor.
2. **Salt restriction.** There is a consistent correlation between individual salt intake and blood pressure, and salt restriction can, in some hypertensive patients, eliminate the need for drugs altogether, and in others it can reduce the dose necessary to control the blood pressure. The goal for adults should be an intake of no more than 2.4 g of salt per day. This can usually be attained by advising patients to reduce the intake of high sodium foods, substituting low sodium foods, and adding no salt in cooking or at the table. High-sodium foods include bacon, ham, smoked fish, sausage, corned beef, salami, breakfast cereals, pickles, soy sauce, anchovies, tomato sauce, tomato juice, cheese, olives, canned vegetables, and soups. Low-sodium foods include rice, oatmeal, plain flour, pasta, fruit, fresh or frozen vegetables, fresh meat, poultry, and fish. The Dietary Approaches to Stop Hypertension (DASH) eating plan is rich in fruits, vegetables and low fat dairy products as well as potassium and calcium. It has reduced amounts of saturated and total fat.
3. **Weight reduction.** In patients who are overweight, weight reduction is effective in reducing blood pressure. A fall of 10 mm Hg systolic and 5 mm Hg diastolic may be expected for each 5kg weight loss. Weight reduction strategies should include education regarding diet, exercise, and behavioral intervention.
4. **Alcohol reduction.** Moderate drinking (two drinks per day for men and one for women) is not a risk factor in hypertension. Weekly intake should not exceed 14 standard drinks for men and nine for women. One standard drink consists of 1.5 ounce of spirits, or 5 ounces of wine, or 12 ounces of beer. At higher levels of intake there is a consistent and linear relationship between daily consumption and height of systolic pressure. Cessation of drinking in heavy drinkers reduces the systolic pressure by about 20 mm Hg systolic and the reduction is maintained unless drinking is resumed.
5. **Exercise.** Exercise is recommended to reduce the risk of hypertension in those who have normal blood pressure and to lower it in those diagnosed with hypertension. Moderate dynamic exercise (walking, jogging, cycling, or swimming) at least 4 to 7 days per week is beneficial for general health. This is in addition to the usual activities of daily living.
6. **Relaxation.** Similarly, the effect of relaxation is uncertain, but it is also beneficial to general health and can be safely advised. This part of the regimen is especially important for patients who feel a need to drive themselves, to the neglect of their health (the so-called type A personality).

Drug Therapy

All patients with a systolic pressure of 160 mm Hg or over and/or a diastolic pressure of 105 mm Hg or higher should have hypotensive drug therapy unless there are exceptional circumstances. The urgency of control depends on the level of blood pressure and the presence or absence of organ damage. If hypertension is associated with cerebral hemorrhage or encephalopathy, or left ventricular failure, the need for control is an emergency. If hypertension presents in the malignant phase (with papilledema or renal damage), the patient should be admitted to the hospital immediately. Higher levels of blood pressure without gross end-organ damage require early but not urgent control and do not usually call for admission to the hospital or referral to a consultant. Hypotensive medication should be started immediately, but there is no need to accelerate the treatment protocol described below. With moderate hypertension, the need for control is less pressing, and it can be delayed, if necessary, if the patient is not available for regular surveillance. One newly diagnosed patient with a diastolic pressure of 140 mm Hg was reluctantly persuaded to cancel his vacation so that he could begin treatment without delay. If his diastolic pressure had been 110 mm Hg, I (IRMcW) would have advised him to begin treatment after his vacation.

Threshold for drug therapy
There is no need to be dogmatic about instituting drug therapy for stage 1 hypertension (140–159/90–99) in the absence of target-organ damage. Lifestyle modification should be instituted and the patient closely followed. Consideration may be given for ambulatory blood pressure measurement or home measurement to assist in making the diagnosis. In those with end-organ damage, diabetes mellitus, or renal disease, institution of drug therapy is indicated as well as lifestyle modifications. Achieving a sustained drop in systolic blood pressure (SBP) of 12 mmHg over a 10-year period prevents one death in every 11 patients treated. In those with CVD or end-organ damage, the number needed to treat (NNT) over the same time period drops to nine.

The threshold for the initiation of drug treatment for young and middle-aged adults without target- organ damage recommended by authoritative groups in the United States, Canada, and Britain, and by the World Health Organization varies between 90 mm Hg and 100 mm Hg diastolic (CHEP, JNC7, BHS). In those over 50, generally speaking, SBP is more difficult to control than diastolic blood pressure (DBP). Focus of therapy should be on SBP in this age group as once control of SBP is achieved, DBP control is usually assured. With age, the prevalence of elevated SBP increases and by age 75 almost all hypertensive individuals have systolic hypertension and three-fourths have isolated systolic hypertension (ISH).

For relatively healthy patients between the ages of 60 and 80, the Canadian Hypertension Society recommends drug treatment for a systolic Blood pressure of 160 mm Hg or higher or for a diastolic pressure of 100 mm Hg or higher (CHEP, 2008). For those in poorer health and for those with lower levels of hypertension, individual judgment is recommended. There seems little justification at present for drug treatment of newly diagnosed mild hypertension in healthy persons over 60 unless there is target-organ damage. For newly diagnosed patients over the age of 80, treatment should be cautious and individualized. There is little trial evidence in this age group.

The Drug Regimen

The following recommendations are based on those found in the Canadian Hypertension Education Program (CHEP, 2008). These follow a critical examination of evidence, using criteria and a rating scale similar to those of the Canadian Task Force on the Periodic Health Examination (1994). The recommendations are graded from A to D, with A being based on significant results from a randomized control trial and D being based on expert opinion.

Initial therapy should be monotherapy with either a low-dose diuretic (e.g., hydrochlorthiazide, 25 mg. daily) (grade A) or, for those less than 60 years of age, a beta-blocker (grade B). Alternatively, ACE inhibitors, long-acting Calcium Channel Blockers (CCB) or angiotensin II antagonists (ARB) are acceptable (grade B). If the response is inadequate consider a combination of a diuretic and another drug from the list of first line options. If there is an adverse effect or a contraindication to diuretic and beta-blocker therapy, consider monotherapy with a drug from one of the other groups (grade C). If the blood pressure is still not controlled, try combinations such as low-dose diuretic with a dihydropyridine CCB (grade B) or CCB with an ACE inhibitor (grade C). Other combinations are possible, but carry a grade D recommendation. It is common for two or more drugs to be necessary to reach target levels of blood pressure and it is useful to explain to patients early in the course of therapy that this is not a reflection of failure on their part (after confirming adherence).

For those patients with other risk factors or target-organ damage, there may be indications or contraindications for certain drugs. For patients with stable angina and hypertension, beta-blockers are first choice (grade B). Long-acting CCBs are also acceptable (grade B). Most patients with hypertension and documented coronary artery disease should be on an ACE inhibitor (grade A). However, it is important not to lower DBP below 55 mm Hg as this has been associated with an increase in mortality. If maximal doses of beta-blockers fail to control blood pressure or in those in whom they are contraindicated (severe reactive airways disease, severe peripheral vascular disease, high degree AV block, sick sinus syndrome), long-acting dihydropyridine (e.g., amlodipine, felodipine, nifedipine) or nondihydropyridine (e.g., diltiazem, verapamil) calcium channel blocker should be added. Short-acting dihydropyridine calcium channel blockers should not be used as they have been shown to increase mortality.

The treatment of hypertension in patients with CHF should generally include ACE inhibitors (grade A) and beta-blockers (grade A). Loop diuretics such as furosemide control volume retention, but one must exercise caution because they can increase serum creatinine levels when used in excess and are a grade D recommendation. Aldosterone antagonists (grade B) are useful for advanced CHF or post-MI. In those who are intolerant of ACE inhibitors, ARBs may be used (grade A).

Studies have shown that beta-blockers can decrease morbidity, mortality, and CHF symptoms. Digoxin has been shown to decrease symptoms and hospitalizations, but not mortality in patients with CHF.

Chronic renal disease (CKD) is a risk factor for CVD and vice versa. In those with an estimated glomerular filtration rate (eGFR) <60mL/min there is an estimated 16% increase in CVD mortality. This risk increases to 30% in those with eGFR of <30mL/min. If microalbuminuria is present, CVD risk increases to 50%. Deterioration of renal function increases in the presence of uncontrolled SBP. In those with CKD, better outcomes have been shown to be associated with lower SBP levels (110–129), lower albumin excretion, and use of ACEI (Jafar et al., 2003). Most patients with CKD should receive ACEI (grade A) or ARB (grade D) plus a thiazide diuretic (grade D) or loop diuretic (grade D).

For hypertensive patients with three or more cardiovascular risk factors (male sex, age 55 or older, LVH, other ECG abnormalities, microroalbuminuria, smoking, family history of premature CVD, total cholesterol to HDL ratio >6), statin therapy is recommended (grade A). In addition, strong consideration should be given to instituting low-dose (81 mg) aspirin (ASA)(grade A in those older than 50 years of age).

Patients with Diabetes

These recommendations are based on those found in the Canadian Hypertension Education Program (CHEP, 2008).

Hypertension increases the mortality rate in patients with diabetes and accelerates vascular complications. In those with diabetes, target blood pressure levels are <130/80. In those individuals with diabetes and hypertension in whom target levels are not reached with lifestyle management, initial drug therapy should include an ACE inhibitor (grade A if >55 years of age) or ARB (grade A for those with LVH and older than 55), or dihydropyridine CCB (grade A for those older than 55), or thiazide diuretic (grade A for those older than 55). Because ACE inhibitors and ARB have additional renal benefits, they are to be preferred. However, if these drugs are not tolerated a cardioselective beta-blocker or nondihyropyridine CCB may be used.

In those with diabetes and albuminuria, ACE inhibitor or ARB is first choice (grade A).

Drug Therapy for Elderly Patients

Clinical trials have shown that drug treatment of hypertension is more effective in reducing cardiovascular events over a 5-year period in patients between the ages of 60 and 80 than in younger patients. When six large trials were combined, only 18 subjects needed to be treated to prevent one cardiovascular (cardiac or cerebrovascular) event (Mulrow et al., 1994). Since selection criteria exclude from trials the very frail and those who suffer from comorbidity such as dementia and chronic obstructive lung disease, the trial results do not apply to all hypertensive patients in this age group. Unless there are strong reasons of this kind for not treating, patients between the ages of 60 and 80 with a systolic blood pressure over 160 mm Hg and a diastolic blood pressure over 100 mm Hg, either singly or combined, should have antihypertensive therapy. Studies such as the SHEP study (1991), Syst-EUR (1997), Staessen et al. (1997) and meta-analysis have confirmed that there are significant benefits to treating the elderly who have identified hypertension. Benefits of treatment in those over 80 is less clear with active treatment resulting in a reduction in stroke and coronary events, but not in all cause mortality (BHS). For those with preexisting treated hypertension in this age group it is reasonable to continue treatment. For new onset hypertension over age 80, treatment decision should be guided by the presence of comorbidities. Naturally the physician needs to be very cautious in introducing medications to the elderly and the maxim "go low and go slow" is particularly pertinent.

For uncomplicated hypertension, a thiazide diuretic is the initial drug of choice (grade A). A small dose should be used initially (e.g., 12.5 mg of hydrochlorothiazide daily). A maintenance dose of 12.5 to 25 mg of hydrochlorothiazide daily is usually effective (grade B).

Beta-blockers are less effective in the elderly and should be used as second-line drugs in small doses (grade B). An ACE inhibitor should be considered as a third-choice drug, but evidence of benefit is lacking.

Principles of Drug Therapy
The following list of principles is adapted from Tudor Hart's book, *Hypertension* (1987).

1. There is a great variation among patients in their response to drugs, the combination and dosage needed, and their susceptibility to adverse effects. The correct dosage and combination have to be titrated individually for each person.
2. The object of treatment is to reduce the blood pressure to below 140/90 mm Hg, but this is not possible in all patients.
3. Doses of drugs should not be changed at intervals of less than 1 week.
4. A second drug should not be added until the maximum safe or tolerable dose of the first drug has been attained.
5. Dosage should be changed only one drug at a time.
6. All drugs except diuretics should be started and stopped gradually.

Control in difficult cases may require frequent monitoring of blood pressure. This may be done by having the patient attend the office several times during the day, or by visiting the patient at home, or a combination of both. The blood pressure may be monitored by physician, nurse, or patient. If the patient can take charge of his or her own monitoring, the physician has little left to do but review the patient's readings and check periodically for end-organ damage. Advances in monitoring methods now make it possible for patients to take regular readings as they go about their daily activities (Canadian Coalition for High Blood Pressure, Prevention and Control, 1988).

Once control is attained, the patient should be seen at regular intervals. As with all attendances for chronic problems, one should remember that the patient may have items on his or her agenda other than a check on blood pressure. Checks for end-organ disease should be carried out periodically, the frequency depending on the individual.

Adherence

Given the frequency of drug side effects, and the fact that hypertension itself is symptomless, it is not surprising that nonadherence to the medication schedule is a frequent problem. Surveys done in the 1970s revealed that 50% of hypertensive patients were dropping out of care within 1 year of starting treatment, and that 40% of those under care were not taking enough medication to attain control. Subsequent surveys have shown much improvement. Bass, McWhinney, and Donner (1986) showed that compliance and blood pressure control can be greatly improved with relatively minor changes in treatment methods.

The two main cues to nonadherence are failure to keep appointments and difficulty in attaining the goal blood pressure. If nonadherence is suspected, the patient should be asked a question such as "Many people find it difficult to take their medication. Do you ever miss taking your blood pressure pills?" Half of all nonadherent patients will admit to missing some of their medication.

The following measures are helpful in increasing adherence:

Involving the patient in his or her own care by monitoring his or her own blood pressure and entering into decisions about medication.
Asking about side effects and taking steps to eliminate them.
Reducing time in the waiting room.
Keeping the number of tablets to the minimum (e.g., not prescribing potassium unless it is necessary). Use fixed dose combinations to simplify the regimen, if the dose is the same as what the patient is already taking.
Tailoring the times of taking medications to the patient's daily routine.
Taking into account medication costs and utilizing low-cost generic medications when possible. A recent survey found that even in relatively wealthy countries (Australia, Canada, Germany, Netherlands, New Zealand, United Kingdom, United States), between 2% and 23% of people did not fill prescriptions or deliberately skipped doses because of cost (Schoen et al., 2007).
Utilizing electronic medication compliance aids.
Encouraging adherence with therapy by out of office contact (either by phone or mail), particularly over the first 3 months of therapy.

Hypertension in Children

Because there is increasing evidence that adult hypertension has its origins in childhood, the blood pressure should be taken periodically during childhood and adolescence. The optimum frequency is debatable. It is currently recommended that for children over 3 years of age, the blood pressurebe taken at least once with an appropriate sized cuff at every health episode (Fourth Report on the diagnosis, evaluation and treatment of high blood pressure in children and adolescents, 2004). As a minimum, we suggest once at entry to school, again at about the age of 12, and thereafter as for adults. Because high blood pressure in children is strongly correlated with obesity, the blood pressure should be taken more frequently in overweight children, as well as in those with a family history of hypertension or CVD. Children whose blood pressure is found to be at or above the 95th percentile based on table standardized for gender, height and weight, should also be followed more frequently.

When children with raised blood pressure are followed up, some do not persist at these levels. Those who have consistently raised blood pressure may be future adult hypertensives, but this is not certain (Ilsley and Millar, 1985).

Children with moderate or severe hypertension are more likely than adults to have secondary hypertension.

Case 14.1
When a 14-year-old girl came for a high school examination, she was found to have a blood pressure of 160/100. Physical examination was otherwise normal and there was no proteinuria. A hypertensive IVP showed a grossly hypotropic right kidney. After further investigations, the right kidney was removed. The postoperative blood pressure was 108/70.

References

Anderson KM, Wilson PWF, Odell PM, Kannel WB. 1991. Updated coronary risk profile. *Circulation* 83:357.

Bass MJ, McWhinney IR, Donner A. 1986. Do family physicians need medical assistants to detect and manage hypertension? *Canadian Medical Association Journal* 134:1247.

Bergland G, Anderson O, Wilhelmsen L. 1976. Prevalence of primary and secondary hypertension: Studies in a random population sample. *British Medical Journal* 2:554.

Berlowitz DR, Ash AS, Hickey EC et al. 1998. Inadequate management of blood presure in a hypertensive population. *New England Journal of Medicine* 39:1957–1963.

Birkett NJ. 1987. Hypertension control in Canada: How well are we doing? *Hypertension Canada* 13:4.

Boe J, Humerfelt S, Wedervang F. 1957. The blood pressure in a population. *Acta Medicus Scandinavia* (supplement 321) 157:1.

Canadian Coalition for High Blood Pressure Prevention and Control. 1988. Recommendations of self-measurement of blood pressure. *Canadian Medical Association Journal* 138:1093.

Canadian Hypertension Education Program (CHEP). 2008. http://hypertension.ca/chep/recommendations/recommendations-overview/

Canadian Hypertension Society Consensus Conference [1]. 1993. Pharmacologic treatment of essential hypertension. *Canadian Medical Association Journal* 149(5):575.

Canadian Hypertension Society Consensus Conference [2]. 1993. Hypertension in the elderly. *Canadian Medical Association Journal* 149(6):815.

Canadian Hypertension Society Consensus Conference [3]. 1993. Hypertension and diabetes. *Canadian Medical Association Journal* 149(6):821.

Canadian Task Force on the Periodic Health Examination. 1994. *The Canadian Guide to Clinical Preventive Health Care*. Ottawa: Health Canada.

Chobanian AV, Bakris GL, Black HR, et al. 2003 The Seventh Report of the Joint National Committee on Prevention, Detection, Evaluation and Treatment of High

Blood Pressure. The JNC7 Report. *Journal of the American Medical Association* 289:2560–2571.

D'Agostino RB, Belanger AJ, Kannel WB. 1991. Relation of low blood pressure to coronary heart disease in the presence of myocardial infarction. *British Medical Journal* 303:385.

Danielson M, Dammstrom B, 1981. The prevalence of secondary and curable hypertension. *Acta Medica Scandinavia* 209(6):451–455.

Dosh S, 2001. The diagnosis of essential and secondary hypertension in adults. *Journal of Family Practice* 50(8): 707.

Elliott P, Stamler J, Nichols R, Dyer AR, Stamler R, Kesteloot H, Marmot M, 1996. Intersalt revisited: further analysis of 24 hour excretion and blood pressure within and across populations. Intersalt Cooperative Research Group. *British Medical Journal* 312(7014):1249–1253.

Fourth Report on the diagnosis, evaluation and treatment of high blood pressure in children an adolescents. 2004. National High Blood Pressure Education Program Working Group on High Blood Pressure in Children and Adolescents. *Pediatrics*114:55–76.

Gueyffier F, Bulpitt C, Boissel JP, Schron E, Ekbom T, Fagard R, et al. 1999. Antihypertensive drugs in very old people: A subgroup meta-analysis of randomized controlled trials. INDANA Group. *Lancet* 353:793–796.

Hansson L, Lindholm LH, Ekbom T, Dahlof B, Lanke J, Schersten B, et al. 1999. Randomized trial of old and new antihypertensive drugs in elderly patients: Cardiovasculare mortality and morbidity the Swedish Trial in Old patients with Hypertension-2 study. *Lancet* 354:1751–1756.

Hart JT. 1987. *Hypertension*, 2nd edn. Edinburgh: Churchill Livingstone.

Hyman DJ, Pavlik VN, Vallbona C 2000. Physician role in lack of awareness and control of hypertension. *Journal of Clinical Hypertension (Greenwich)* 2:324–330.

Ilsley CD, Millar JA. 1985. Hypertension in children. *British Medical Journal* 290:1451.

Intersalt Cooperative Research Group 1988. Intersalt: an international study of electrolyte excretion and blood pressure. Results for 24 hour urinary sodium and potassium excretion. *British Medical Journal* 297(6644):319–328.

Jafar TH, Stark PC, Schmid CH, Landa M, Maschio G, D Joog PE, et al. 2003. Progression of chronic kidney disease: The role of blood pressure control, proteinuria and angiotensin-converting enzyme inhibition: a patient-level meta-analysis. *Annals of Internal Medicine* 139:244–252.

Joffres MR, Ghadarian P, Fodor JG et al. 1997. Awareness, treatment and control of hypertension in Canada. *American Journal of Hypertension* 10:1097.

Kannel WB, Gordon T. 1970. The Framingham study, sec. 26. Washington, D.C.: US Department of Health,Education and Welfare.

Kannel WB. 1996. Blood pressure as a cardiovascular risk factor: Prevention and treatment. *Journal of the American Medical Association* 275:1571.

Leenen FHH, Dumais J, McInnis NH, Turton P, Stratychuk L, Nemeth K, Lum-Kwong MM, Fodor G. 2008. Results of the Ontario Survey on the Prevalence and Control of Hypertension.*Canadian Medical Association Journal* 178(11):1441–1449.

Lenfant C. 1996. High blood pressure: Some answers, new questions, continuing challenges. Editorial. *Journal of the American Medical Association* 275:1604.

Levy D, Larson MG, Vasan RS, Kannel WB, Ho KKL. 1996. The progression from hypertension to congestive heart failure. *Journal of the American Medical Association* 275(20):1557.

Mancia G, Grassi G, Pomidossi C et al. 1983. Effects of blood pressure measurement by the doctor on patients' blood pressure and heart rate. *Lancet* 2:695.

Midgley JP, Mattew AG, Greenwood CM, Logan AG. 1996. Effect of reduced dietary sodium on blood pressure: A meta-analysis of randomized controlled trials. *Journal of the American Medical Association* 275(20):1590.

Mulrow CD, Cornell JA, Herrera CR, Abdulmajead K, Farnett L, Aguilar C. 1994. Hypertension in the elderly: Implications and generalizability of random trials. *Journal of the American Medical Association* 272:1932.

Ostbye T, Yarnall KSH, Krause KM, Pollak KI, Gradison M, Michener JL. 2005. Is there time for management of patients with chronic diseases in primary care? *Annals of Family Medicine* 3:209–214.

Reincke M. 2000. Subclinical Cushing's syndrome. *Endocrinology and Metabolism Clinics of North America* 29(1):43–56.

Rudnick KV, Sackett DC, Hirst S, Holmes C. 1977. Hypertension in a family practice. *Canadian Medical Association Journal* 117:492.

Schoen C, Osborn R, Doty MM, Bishop M, Peugh J, Murukutia. 2007. Toward higher-performance health systems: Adults' health care experiences in seven countries, 2007. *Health Affairs* 26 (6) w717–w734.

SHEP Cooperative Research Group. 1991. Prevention of stroke by antihypertensive drug treatment in older persons with isolated systolic hypertension. Final results of the Systolic Hypertension in the Elderly program (SHEP). *Journal of the American Medical Association* 265:3255–3264.

Staessen JA, Fagard R, Thijs L, Celis H, Arabidze GG, Birkenhager WH et al. 1997. Randomised double-blind comparison of placebo and active treatment for older patients with isolated systolic hypertension. The Systolic Hypertension in Europe (Syst-Eur) Trial Investigation. *Lancet* 350:757–764.

Staessen Ja, Gasowski J, Wang JG, Thijs L, Den Hond E, Boissel JP. et al. 2000. Risks of untreated and treated isolated systolic hypertension in the elderly: Meta-analysis of outcome trials. *Lancet*355:865–872.

Tu K, Chen Z, Lipscombe LL. 2008a. Prevalence and incidence of hypertension from 1995 to 2005: A population-based study. *Canadian Medical Association Journal* 178(11):1429–1435.

Tu K, Chen Z, Lipscombe LL. 2008b. Mortality among patients with hypertension from 1995 to 2005: A population-based study. *Canadian Medical Association Journal* 178(11):1436–1440.

Vasan RS, Beiser A, Seshadri S, Larson MG, Kannel WB, D'Agostino RB et al. 2002. Residual lifetime risk for developing hypertension in middle aged women and men: The Framingham Heart Study. *Journal of the American Medical Association* 287:1003–1010.

Wolf PA, D'Agostino RB, Belanger AJ, Kannel WB. 1991. Probability of stroke: A risk profile from the Framingham study. *Stroke* 22:312–318. Reproduced with permission from Kannel WB. 1996. *Journal of the American Medical Association* 275: 1571–1576. Copyright 1991, American Medical Association.Young WF. 2007. Primary aldosteronism: Renaissance of a syndrome. *Clinical Endocrinology* 66(5):607–618.

15

Diabetes

The category diabetes has evolved over the centuries as clinical observations and physiological investigations have distinguished between different varieties. The Greek word *diabetes* means literally "a passer through" or "a siphon." The condition was well known in ancient times and recognized by its polyuria and thirst, often associated with emaciation. In 1674, Thomas Willis noted the sweet taste of the urine in some cases, making possible the first major subdivision of the category into mellitus and insipidus varieties.

In his textbook of 1786, however, Cullen was still inclined to regard the insipid form as an anomaly rather than as a separate subcategory. In Osler's textbook of 1892, diabetes mellitus (DM) and insipidus are clearly distinguished. Diabetes mellitus is defined as "a disorder of nutrition, in which sugar accumulates in the blood and is excreted in the urine, the daily amount of which is greatly increased." Acute and chronic forms are mentioned, but it is said that there is no essential difference between them, except that in the former the patients are younger, the course more rapid, and the emaciation more marked. Three variants are described: the lipogenic, associated with obesity; the neurotic, due to injuries or functional disorders of the nervous system; and the pancreatic, in which there is a lesion of the pancreas. Von Mering and Minkowski had already shown that extirpation of the pancreas in dogs is followed by glycosuria, and it was postulated that there was an internal secretion of the pancreas. Osler describes an attempt to separate a clinical variety, analogous to experimental pancreatic diabetes, with a rapid and severe course, usually in young and middle-aged persons.

The isolation of insulin by Banting and Best in the 1920s and its use in treatment prompted the separation of diabetes into three classes: insulin dependent (IDDM), non–insulin-dependent (NIDDM), and other.

Like hypertension, diabetes mellitus is defined by the level of a physiological variable, the blood glucose. Like the level of blood pressure, the blood glucose level is continuously distributed in the population and there is no clear cutoff point between diabetes and normal. The definition of diabetes is, therefore, like that of hypertension, an arbitrary one, depending on the shape of the distribution curve and on the risk attached to various levels of blood glucose (e.g., a plasma glucose level greater than 11.1 mmol/L 2 hours after a 75 g load identifies people at much higher risk of microvacular complications (Gerstein and Haynes, 2001).

Another similarity with hypertension is that glucose tolerance in the same individual varies from day to day and within a 24-hour period.

There is, however, one important difference between hypertension and diabetes. In hypertension, mortality rates increase in a linear fashion with increasing levels of blood pressure. In diabetes, there is strong evidence that the relation between level of blood glucose and mortality is nonlinear. The prospective Whitehall study (Fuller, Shipley, Rose, Jarrett, and Keen, 1983) of 18,403 male civil servants between the ages of 40 and 64 found a doubling in death rate from both coronary heart disease and stroke in men with levels of higher than 96 mg per 100 mL or 5.4 mmol/L, 2 hours after ingestion of 50 g of glucose.

Classification of Diabetes Mellitus

The following classification is that recommended by the Canadian Diabetes Association (2003).

1. Type I diabetes is the result of pancreatic beta cell destruction. Injected insulin is generally required to control hyperglycemia and prevent ketosis. This form is prone to ketoacidosis. Beta cell destruction is believed to be caused by an autoimmune process or viral infection.
2. Type 2 diabetes in which insulin resistance is the main defect, followed eventually by beta cell exhaustion. It ranges from insulin resistance with insulin deficiency to a predominant secretory defect with insulin resistance. This type is often associated with obesity. This category includes latent autoimmune diabetes in adults (LADA) which describes people with apparent Type 2 diabetes who appear to have immune mediated loss of pancreatic beta cells.
3. Gestational diabetes mellitus refers to glucose intolerance with first onset or recognition during pregnancy.
4. Diabetes secondary to other conditions:
   a. Pancreatic diseases such as carcinoma, chronic pancreatitis, and hemochromatosis
   b. Cushing's syndrome, pheochromocytoma, hyperthyroidism
   c. Drugs, such as corticosteroids, estrogens, thiazide diuretics, tricyclic antidepressants, phenytoin, lithium, indomethacin, atypical antipsychotics
   d. Genetic syndromes
   e. Congenital lipodystrophy
5. Impaired fasting glucose (IFG) identifies individuals at higher risk of developing diabetes.

6. Impaired glucose tolerance (IGT) is impaired glucose tolerance without clinical diabetes. A quarter of patients with IGT develop clinical diabetes after 5 years and, two-thirds after 10 years. Collectively, IFG and IGT are known as prediabetes but it is important to emphasize that people in these categories do not have diabetes. Indeed some in the IGT category will revert to normoglycemia.

These categories will change and evolve as knowledge of pathophysiology and natural history of diabetes continues to grow.

Diagnostic Criteria

The diagnostic criteria recommended by the Canadian Diabetes Association are as follows:

1. A fasting plasma glucose (FPG) of greater than or equal to 7.0 mmol/L after fasting for at least 8 hours or
   a. Casual plasma glucose of >11.1 mmol/L + symptoms of diabetes (polyuria, polydipsia, or unexplained weight loss) or
   b. A 2-hour plasma glucose of >11.1 after a 75 gm oral glucose tolerance test (OGTT) (Table 15.1).
2. Metabolic syndrome: this category describes a constellation of risk factors that identifies individuals at especially high risk of cardiovascular disease. These risk factors include abdominal obesity, hypertension, dyslipidemia, insulin resistance, and dysglycemia. The most widely used diagnostic criteria are those of the United States (US) Expert Panel on Detection, Evaluation, and Treatment of High Blood Cholesterol in Adults (Adult Treatment Panel III [ATP III]), which requires the presence of at least three of the five criteria (see Table 15.2). The definition of metabolic syndrome provided by the International Diabetes Federation differs slightly and provides a table of waist circumference that is adjusted for ethnicity (Tables 15.3 and 15.4). The prevalence of metabolic syndrome has been estimated to be between 20% and 25% of the U.S. population and is expected to increase.

Table 15.1   PG levels for diagnosis of IFG, IGT, and diabetes

	FPG (mmol/L)		2hPG in the 75-g OGTT (mmol/L)
IFG	6.1–6.9		NA
IFG (isolated)	6.1–6.9	and	<7.8
IGT (isolated)	<6.1	and	7.8–11.0
IFG and IGT	6.1–6.9	and	7.8–11.0
Diabetes	≥7.0	or	≥11.1

2hPG, 2-hour plasma glucose; FPG, fasting plasma glucose; IFG, impaired fasting glucose; IGT, impaired glucose tolerance; NA, not applicable; OGTT, oral glucose tolerance test

Source: Canadian Diabetes Association Clinical Practice Guidelines, 2003.

Table 15.2 Clinical identification of the metabolic syndrome using NCEP ATP III criteria

Risk factor	Defining Level*
FPG	≥6.1 mmol/L
BP	≥130/85 mm Hg
TGs	≥1.7 mmol/L
HDL-C	
Men	<1.0 mmol/L
Women	<1.3 mmol/L
Abdominal obesity	Waist circumference
Men	>102 cm
Women	>88 cm

*A diagnosis of metabolic syndrome is made when 3 or more of the risk determinants are present.

BP, blood pressure; FPG, fasting plasma glucose; HDL-C, high-density lipoprotein cholesterol; NCEP ATP III, National Cholesterol Education Program Adult Treatment Panel III; TG, triglyceride.

Table 15.3 International Diabetes Federation definition of metabolic syndrome

According to the new IDF definition, for a person to be defined as having the metabolic syndrome they must have

Central obesity (defined as waist circumference* with ethnicity specific values)

plus any two of the following four factors:

Raised triglycerides	≥ 150 mg/dL (1.7 mmol/L) **or specific treatment for this lipid abnormality**
Reduced HDL cholesterol	< 40 mg/dL (1.03 mmol/L) in males <50 mg/dL (1.29 mmol/L) in females **or specific treatment for this lipid abnormality**
Raised blood pressure	Systolic BP ≥ 130 or diastolic ≥ 85 mm Hg **or treatment of previously diagnosed hypertension**
Raised fasting plasma glucose	(FPG) ≥ 100 mg/dL (5.6 mmol/L) **or previously diagnosed Type 2 diabetes** If above 5.6 mmol/L or 100 mg/dL, OGTT is strongly recommended but is not necessary to define presence of the syndrome.

*If BMI is >30kg/m², central obesity can be assumed and waist circumference does not need to be measured.

3. Gestational diabetes: this category refers to glucose intolerance that initially manifests during pregnancy. It identifies those at higher risk of developing diabetes in the future and has been associated with macrosomia in the developing fetus. There is debate about the merits of screening for gestational diabetes with both the Canadian Task Force on Preventative Health Care and the U.S. Preventative Services Task Force giving it a "C" recommendation (i.e. no convincing evidence for or against screening). However,

Table 15.4 Ethnic specific values for waist circumference (IDF)

Country/Ethnic Group		Waist Circumference
Europids*	Male	≥ 94 cm
In the United States, the ATP III values (102 cm male; 88 cm female) are likely to continue to be used for clinical purposes	Female	≥ 80 cm
South Asians	Male	≥ 90 cm
based on a Chinese, Malay, and Asian-Indian population	Female	≥ 80 cm
Chinese	Male	≥ 90 cm
	Female	≥ 80 cm
Japanese**	Male	≥ 90 cm
	Female	≥ 80 cm
Ethnic South and Central Americans	Use South Asian recommendations until more specific data are available	
Sub-Saharan Africans	Use European data until more specific data are available	
Eastern Mediterranean and Middle East (Arab) populations	Use European data until more specific data are available	

*In future epidemiological studies of populations of Europid origin, prevalence should be given using both European and North American cut-points to allow better comparisons.
**Originally different values were proposed for Japanese people but new data support the use of the values shown above.

the American College of Obstetricians and Gynecologists, The American Diabetes Association, The Fourth International Workshop Conference on Gestational Diabetes Mellitus, and The Society of Obstetricians and Gynecologists of Canada (SOGC) all recommend either universal or selective screening. If offered, screening takes place between 24 and 28 weeks gestation and measures the plasma glucose 1 hour after a 50 g load. Levels greater than 10.3 mmol/L are diagnostic.

Incidence and Prevalence

In any arbitrarily defined disorder, prevalence rates will depend on the cutoff point chosen. Taking this into account, it is generally agreed that in Caucasian populations the prevalence rate is between 2% and 6%, with considerable variation depending on country. Up to half of these are known diabetics and half undiagnosed. Type 2 DM accounts for 90% to 95% of all diabetes and is eight to nine times more common than Type 1 DM. Diabetes in childhood and adolescence is uncommon. In the United States the incidence rate up to 20 years of age is about 14 cases per 100,000 persons per year.

The prevalence of Type 2 DM and IGT increases greatly with age, both types being eight times more common past the age of 50 than before 50. Type 1 DM can occur at any age, even in the elderly. Formerly believed to be a juvenile form of diabetes, it is now reported that some cases of Type 1 DM begin after the age of twenty. However, it may not present in the classic acute manner (Zimmet, 1995).

Prevalence rates in some aboriginal peoples are far higher than in Caucasian people. High rates are found in some groups of North American Indians, in Australian aborigines, and in natives of some Pacific islands. In the Ojibwa-Cree Indians of Northern Ontario, diabetes was virtually unknown until the 1940s. It now has an age-adjusted prevalence rate of 23% (Harris et al., 1997). In aboriginal populations with a very high prevalence, Type 2 DM is found in children and adolescents (Harris, Perkins, Whalen-Brough, 1996).

Medalie et al. (1975) studied the development of DM in 8,688 males in Israel past the age of 40. The annual incidence rate was 0.8%, with variation from 0.56% for those born in central Europe, to 1.12% for those born in Asia. The most significant factors associated with the development of diabetes were overweight and peripheral vascular disease. Other significant factors were age; high levels of serum cholesterol, blood pressure, and uric acid; and a low level of education. Total calories in the diet were not a factor. The peripheral vascular disease often preceded the diabetes by several years, and Medalie et al. postulate that the metabolic and vascular changes develop independently of each other.

Garcia et al. (1974) followed 5,209 men and women in the Framingham Study, aged 30 to 62 at entry to the study. In the course of 16 years, 239 people developed diabetes, an annual incidence rate of 0.28%. The mortality rate of the diabetics was three times greater than that in the general population. For cardiovascular mortality, the risk was four- and-a-half times greater in women and twice as great in men. This excess cardiovascular mortality is not fully accounted for by the presence of risk factors such as high blood pressure and high blood cholesterol. Coronary disease accounted for most of the cardiovascular deaths. There was a high risk of intermittent claudication in both sexes.

Using an administrative data set based on hospitalizations and physician visits, Lipscombe and Hux (2007), estimated prevalence and incidence of diabetes in the Canadian province of Ontario between 1995 and 2005 in those over the age of 20. They found that prevalence over this time period increased from 5.2% in 1995 to 8.8% in 2005. Of great concern, the prevalence rate increased to a greater extent in those 20 to 49 years of age, than the population greater than 50, though the latter still had the higher prevalence rate. The annual incidence increased from 6.6 per 1,000 in 1997 to 8.2 per 1,000 in 2003 an increase of 31%. An encouraging finding was the mortality among diabetics fell by 25% from 1995 to 2005.

The increase in cardiovascular mortality in diabetics and IGT diabetics in the Whitehall study (Fuller et al., 1983) remained significant even after adjustment had been made for other risk factors. Between half and two-thirds of the relative risk of cardiovascular deaths was unexplained by differences in these other cardiovascular risk factors. Within the diabetic or IGT diabetic group, the risk factors most strongly related to death from coronary disease were age and blood pressure.

About one-third of all patients with insulin-dependent diabetes develop renal failure, and a quarter of the persons entering end-stage renal programs in the United States are diabetics. Five percent of patients with insulin-dependent diabetes become blind.

Using these population studies, it is estimated that a family physician in Western countries with a practice of 2,500 patients will have approximately 145 diabetic patients (Ostbye et al., 2005), the precise number depending on the country and the age structure of the practice. Some of these will be undiagnosed. If the physician has in his or her practice substantial numbers from high-risk racial groups, the number of diabetics will be higher.

Based on Lipscombe and Hux's findings cited above, a family physician may expect to have 10 to 12 new cases of diabetes each year in his or her practice in those over the age of 20.

Etiology, Pathogenesis, and Natural History

In Type 1 DM, deficiency of insulin secretion due to destruction of the islets of Langerhans is the major abnormality. In Type 2 DM, there is both insulin deficiency and insulin resistance. The association between these factors is not well understood.

The etiology of DM is a complex interaction of genetic and environmental factors. The strength of the genetic factor is very variable. In twin studies, concordance rates for identical twins are 55% for Type 1 and 90% for Type 2 DM. The risk of a sibling of an insulin-dependent diabetic developing diabetes by the age of 20 is about 3% to 5%. The risk varies greatly according to whether the sibling is HLA identical in chromosome makeup. Chromosome studies indicate that there are Type 1 DM susceptibility genes closely linked to HLA DR genes. The high degree of concordance in identical twins suggests that genetic factors play an important role in Type 2 diabetes and that clinical diabetes is unmasked by environmental factors, mainly in genetically predisposed individuals. This unmasking of diabetes by environmental and cultural change explains the recent emergence of diabetes as a common health problem in many groups of Native North Americans, and in the natives of some Pacific islands.

Until recently, Type 1 diabetes has been regarded as a disease of acute onset. Prospective studies have now shown that people may have islet cell antibodies for up to 3 years before the onset of diabetes. It has also been shown that children may have glucose intolerance before developing symptomatic diabetes. The clinical onset of Type 1 DM may be preceded by a latent period during which islet cell antibodies and impaired glucose tolerance provide evidence of islet cell destruction and the clinical course may be slowly progressive rather than acute. Two factors—virus infection and autoimmunity—appear to be important in causing destruction of islet cells. If susceptible individuals can be identified during the latent period, the possibility exists of arresting the destructive process, although numerous large prevention trials to date have been unsuccessful.

Both Type 1 and Type 2 DM are prone to the same microvascular and macrovascular complications leading to heart disease and stroke, retinopathy, nephropathy, and some forms of gangrene and neuropathy. Electron microscopy studies indicate that the microvascular abnormalities occur after the onset of the disease. In the United States, about 20% of diabetic patients hospitalized are admitted for foot complications, and about 50% of nontraumatic amputations are done in diabetics (Litzelman et al., 1993). Vascular insufficiency and neuropathy both contribute to foot problems. The fact that vascular changes often precede the onset of diabetes suggests that the metabolic and vascular changes occur independently. As mentioned above, the relationship between hyperglycemia and the increased mortality from cardiovascular disease is not clearly understood. The mortality rate is not fully explained by the known risk factors.

Up to the present time, the life expectancy of patients with diabetes diagnosed before the age of 30 has been 30% to 50% less than that of the general population. Death has been caused by renal disease in about 40% and by cardiovascular disease in most of the rest. The presence of microalbuminuria predicts renal disease many years later, in both Type 1 and in Type 2 DM.

Until recently, it has been assumed that an adult presenting with diabetes had Type 2 DM if not showing the classical acute onset of Type 1 DM. Recent research suggests however, that some adult-onset diabetics have Type 1 DM with an autoimmune etiology (LADA) (Zimmet, 1995). The typical patient with LADA is over 35, not obese, and presents with what appears to be Type 2 DM. The diabetes is often controlled by diet for a time, until oral agents and possibly insulin are required. There is a high frequency of autoantibodies in these patients.

The typical patient with Type 2 DM has central (upper body) obesity. Many also have hypertension and/or dyslipidemia, either of which may be present for many years before the onset of diabetes. All these factors contribute cumulatively to a high risk of coronary, cerebral, and peripheral vascular disease. Two-thirds of patients with Type 2 DM die of vascular disease. Hyperinsulinemia and GTT are predictors of both Type 2 DM and coronary disease (Zimmet, 1995).

About 80 percent of patients with Type 2 DM are obese at the time of diagnosis. The strongest predictor of Type 2 DM is IGT, as defined earlier in this chapter. About 4.7% of the adult population of the United States has IGT diabetes by these criteria. As already indicated, persons with IGT diabetes are themselves at increased risk of death from cardiovascular disease.

Three randomized trials (UKPDS, Kumamoto Study, Steno Type 2 Randomized Study) have shown that improving glycemic control in Type 2 DM reduces the rate of progression of microvascular complications such as retinopathy, nephropathy, and neuropathy. This reinforces the need for family physicians to establish a screening program in their practice population.

Effects of Treatment

The Diabetes Control and Complications Trial (1993) has shown that intensive treatment of Type 1 DM can substantially reduce the development and progression of retinopathy, nephropathy, and neuropathy in white patients between the ages of 13 and 40. The goals of intensive therapy were preprandial blood glucose between 70 and 120 mg/dL (3.9 and 6.7 mmol/L), postprandial blood glucose levels of less than 180 mg/dL (10 mmol/L), a weekly 3 AM blood glucose level greater than 65 mg/dL (3.6 mmol/L), and glycosylated hemoglobin level of less than 6.05%. Intensive therapy included insulin, three or more injections daily or by continuous infusion. The dosage was adjusted, based on self-monitoring of blood glucose four times a day. Conventional therapy in the control group consisted of one or two daily insulin injections and daily self-monitoring of urine or blood glucose. Intensive therapy was supervised by a multidisciplinary team. Patients visited their study center each month and were in touch by telephone between visits to review and adjust their regimens.

The chief adverse effect of intensive treatment was a two- to threefold increase in severe hypoglycemia. The risk of hypoglycemia increased continuously with lower levels of glycosylated hemoglobin. Similarly, the benefits of therapy increased continuously. There is, therefore, no target level at which benefits are maximized and risks minimized. For each patient, therefore, the target value must be established to minimize the risk. Also, it cannot be assumed that the risk–benefit ratio is the same for children, older adults, and for patients with advanced complications.

Intensive therapy was associated with transient worsening of retinopathy, but the abnormalities often disappeared by 18 months, and the longer-term outcome was a reduction in the risk of progression. Other trials have shown that photocoagulation prevents new visual loss in patients with proliferative retinopathy and macular edema (Clark and Lee, 1995). Vitrectomy is beneficial in patients with visual loss caused by proliferative retinopathy with vitreous hemorrhage, scarring, and retinal detachment.

Angiotensin-converting enzyme (ACE) inhibitors can delay the onset and progression of nephropathy in Type 1 DM and stabilize serum creatinine and albuminuria in Type 2 DM (Clark and Lee, 1995). These benefits are conferred even when blood pressure is normal. Hypertension increases the rate at which diabetic nephropathy progresses; and antihypertensive therapy slows its course.

Tight control of plasma glucose has been shown to reduce the incidence of microvascular complications in Type 2 DM (Ohkubo et al., 1995; UK Prospective Diabetes Study [UKPDS] Group, 1998). This makes it critical that the family physician institute a screening program in order to allow for early identification and treatment of those with diabetes or at increased risk of developing the disease. This requires a degree of practice organization even greater than that needed for detection and control of hypertension.

The Impact of Diabetes on the Individual and the Family

In no disease is successful management more dependent on the attitude of the patient, relationships within the family, and the relationship with the physician. The complex nature of control, the need for frequent monitoring, the dietary restrictions, and the limitations on activity all have an impact on the life of the individual and on other members of the family. The family physician can be a source of great support to patient and family; on the other hand, the physician can be a hindrance to them if he or she fails to understand their problems, mismanages therapy, or neglects to call on available resources.

The following case report illustrates a family's response to diabetes in the two children, the effects of a disruption in the system and the role of the family physician, specialist unit, and community health services in helping the family to regain its equilibrium.

Case 15.1

A 39-year-old married woman had enjoyed good health until she was admitted to the hospital urgently in a manic state with psychotic features. Previously she had been a well-adjusted individual, with no indications of psychotic or medical illness. There had been significant stressors at home and at work in the weeks preceding her admission.

On admission she was agitated, irritable, and verbally and physically abusive, with paranoid delusions, disorientation in time and place, and auditory and olfactory hallucinations. She had refused all food and fluids for a period of 48 hours before admission.

Organic etiology was suspected at the outset and investigation confirmed a diagnosis of hyperthyroidism. The illness pursued a stormy course for a period of 8 weeks before responding to treatment with radioactive iodine. During this time she required continuous care in the hospital.

The patient's husband was a 43-year-old university graduate in an occupation with a heavy burden of professional responsibilities. The couple had two children, a daughter aged 14 and a son aged 7 years, both of them with insulin-dependent DM.

The children's diabetes had been diagnosed over 4 years earlier. Since then, they had received care from a multidisciplinary team based in a children's hospital. Although both parents were involved in educational programs about diabetes, the children's mother quickly assumed total responsibility for the care and management of their disease. The father's duties at work absorbed most of his time and required him to travel extensively. Absences of 4 or 5 days' duration were not uncommon.

The mother faced many challenges. Both children required careful diet to provide sufficient energy to attain and maintain desirable body weight. Types of insulin and injection times had to be carefully planned to coordinate with an acceptable eating pattern. A consistent pattern of insulin, diet, and exercise had to be developed to promote glycemic control. Frequency of feedings had to be adjusted with snacks used between meals and before bedtime to prevent hypoglycemia. Compensation had to be made for irregularities in the established pattern of living such as delayed meals, increased or decreased physical activity, and intercurrent illness. All of these problems were compounded by the difficulties of having to control a 7-year-old boy who by reason of his youth could not be expected to understand the need for such restrictions. The problem of supervising the care of her daughter was complicated by the normal turbulence of adolescence with rebellion and rejection of parental restraint.

When the mother was admitted to the hospital, all of these matters came to be the responsibility of her husband, already distraught over his wife's illness.

Within days of their mother's admission to hospital, both children experienced disturbance of diabetic control. Within a week the boy had developed a monilial rash involving the perineum and perianal area. Defecation caused him excruciating pain and he became very constipated. Subsequently he developed fissure in ano and experienced rectal bleeding.

The girl experienced sleep disturbance immediately following her mother's admission to the hospital, and on several visits to the office, opportunity was provided for her to ventilate anxiety, anger, and frustration surrounding her mother's illness. She developed a skin eruption on her back and an intolerable itch. Within days, the skin lesions became impetiginized, requiring treatment with antibiotics.

The father became profoundly depressed. He fell a prey to morbid fears of becoming disabled physically or mentally, and he developed feelings of guilt about the neglect of his professional responsibilities. Immediate steps were taken to relieve him of some of his burdens. His employer was contacted and a prolonged leave of absence was negotiated. The multidisciplinary team from the hospital placed themselves at his disposal night and day for provision of advice about control of the children's diabetes. Home care was arranged, and a homemaker was provided to prepare meals and carry out domestic duties in the home. A public health nurse visited daily to provide support, and the father attended his family physician's office frequently for advice and counseling.

Over a period of 2 months, the mother's condition stabilized and she was able to return home. Within 2 weeks of her return, the children's diabetic state stabilized, family supports began to be phased out progressively, and within 4 weeks stability returned to the family unit.

It is important that the physician regularly assess the psychological state of diabetic patients, recognizing that depression is twice as common compared to the general population (Garvard, Lustman, Clouse, 1993; Anderson et al., 2001) and is associated with poorer glycemic control (Egede , Zheng, Simpson, 2002). Eating disorders are frequently observed in adolescent and young women with Type 1 DM (Daneman, 2002) and require treatment in a team setting for such problems.

The Child with Diabetes

The literature on diabetes and the family reflects recent changes in thinking about family relationships. In the 1940s and 1950s, investigators tended to think in terms of a one-way, linear relationship between parent and child. The child was viewed as the passive recipient of the parents' management. More recently, the systems view has become dominant. All family members are viewed as interacting with each other in a reciprocal fashion (Hanson and Henggeler, 1984). The parents' behavior toward the child is influenced by the severity of the diabetes and the child's own behavior. The child's behavior and metabolism are, in turn, affected by the parents' behavior, and so on. Other significant relationships also have to be considered, for example with siblings and with the physician. Difficulties with control of the diabetes may result from biological factors and may occur even when compliance is good. If the physician gives the impression that poor control implies poor compliance, he or she is likely to produce guilt feelings in the parents.

Some early studies of the diabetic's family were vitiated by methodological faults. Criteria for assessing family function and control of diabetes were often crude. Most studies were cross-sectional; few followed families over long periods of time, and few have provided good clinical descriptions of the lives of diabetics. The occurrence of diabetes in a child is a major challenge to a family's capacity to cope and adapt. The family characteristics associated with good adaptation are emotional stability, financial security, few interpersonal conflicts, and good communication.

Minuchin, Rosman, and Baker (1978) have shown, in a study on a small number of families, that glucose and fat metabolism in a diabetic child is very sensitive to emotional arousal. Three types of family were studied: those of children in good control without behavior problems, those of children with behavior problems and poor control, and those with frequent ketoacidosis. Free fatty acid (FFA) was measured in all family members during a family interview. The parents were first asked to discuss a family problem (period 1). A therapist then entered the room and focused the problems so that conflict increased (period 2). During this time, the diabetic child watched through a one-way mirror. The child then entered the room and joined the discussion (period 3), after which the family relaxed (period 4).

The seven well-controlled diabetic children showed little change in FFA during all periods. The eight with behavioral problems showed a slight rise in period 3. The children with frequent ketoacidosis (called by Minuchin, psychosomatic children) showed a marked rise over all four periods (Figure 15.1).

Figure 15.2 compares the median FFA level in the parents who, in each family, had the higher FFA response, with the median level in the child diabetics. Parents of the well-controlled children showed little change in FFA level. Parents of those with behavior problems showed a rise in periods 2 and 3. Parents of children with frequent ketoacidosis showed a rise in period 2, followed by a fall in period 3. Minuchin interprets the latter finding as a transfer of stress from the parents to the child, who acts as the family scapegoat. In further studies, Minuchin went on to show that the number of episodes of ketoacidosis was reduced after family therapy.

When learning that their child has diabetes, parents are profoundly shocked. They often have guilt feelings about having done something to cause it, or about hereditary factors. The family physician can help by ascertaining these feelings and by providing information about causation and inheritance.

Two maladaptive parental reactions—overprotection and rejection—are associated with problems in the children. It is not difficult to understand how anxiety can make parents oversolicitous about diet and insulin and unduly restrictive of a child's independence. One manifestation of this anxiety is the practice of waking the child during the night to make sure he or she is not going into hypoglycemic coma during sleep. This may arise from fear that the child will die of hypoglycemia during sleep. At first the child may respond passively to overprotectiveness but is likely to rebel when he or she reaches puberty. Rejection and hostility on the part

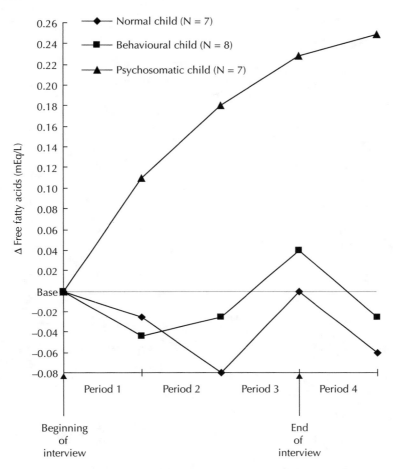

Figure 15.1 Changes in free fatty acid (FFA) levels of diabetic children during family interview. (From Minuchin, Harvard University Press 1978. Reprinted by permission.)

of the parents is associated with serious behavioral problems in the child and poor control of diabetes. The most favorable parental attitude is one of support and flexibility, with recognition of the child's changing needs as he or she grows older.

A child or adolescent with diabetes can never forget for a day that he or she is different from other children. He may go to great lengths to try to conceal his diabetes from friends. Children may need encouragement to be open and frank about their condition. Diabetes makes it especially difficult for adolescents to go through the often turbulent process of becoming independent from parents. Their disease places restrictions on their social life, eating, and use of alcohol, and they often have anxieties about future complications and their prospects for marrying and having children. Problems with diabetic control may be a

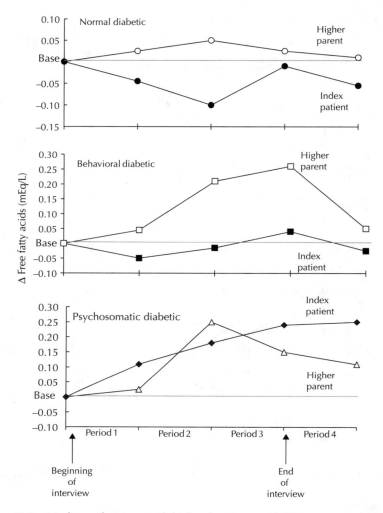

Figure 15.2   Medians of parents with higher free fatty acid (FFA) response and index patient. (From Minuchin, Harvard University press 1978. Reprinted by permission.)

manifestation of adolescent instability and rebellion. Like normal adolescents, however, young diabetics with behavior problems usually settle down as they get older.

Since diabetes is so dependent on frequent monitoring and dose adjustment, it is very vulnerable both to emotional reactions and to self-destructive behaviour. A disturbed patient may deliberately withhold insulin to precipitate ketoacidosis. There is some evidence that many patients with frequent attacks of ketoacidosis are interfering with treatment. Although more common in adolescents and young adults, this can occur at any age.

The family physician can be of great help to child patients and their families who are coping with these problems. Even if the patient is attending a diabetic clinic, many aspects of care are likely to involve the family physician. A diagnosis of diabetes is an indication for an assessment of family function.

The physician will need to ensure that the patient and family are fully informed about all aspects of their disease and that the available resources are appropriately utilized. Each family member should be encouraged to express his or her feelings and given the opportunity to ask questions. As soon as diabetic children are old enough to speak for themselves, they should be seen alone on some occasions. We cannot expect to hear about children's own feelings unless we see them alone. Family assessment and support are especially important when control is poor, where there are behavior problems, and when family crises occur.

The Adult with Type 1 Diabetes

The impact of diabetes on an adult and his or her family depends on the stage in the life cycle at which the diagnosis is made (Anderson and Kornblum, 1984). Whenever it occurs, the sufferer will experience grief, as he or she comes to terms with a chronic disease, loss of health, and diminished expectations. For couples without children, there will be questions about whether they should have children. If the patient is a woman, there will be concerns about the impact of pregnancy on her health, and her capacity to care for an infant. Diabetic parents may fear that they will not live long enough to see the child grow up or remain fit long enough to provide for the child. For patients who develop diabetes before marriage, these issues should have been discussed with the spouse before the decision to marry. Much will depend on how long the patient has had diabetes and the presence of control problems and complications. Parents worry that their child may inherit diabetes. Given the complex inheritance of diabetes, it is difficult to give individualized genetic counseling, but parents may be helped by having whatever information is available. Family planning advice for the diabetic woman is most important. It may be important for a mother that her diabetes started before, not during, her pregnancy. The pregnancy could never, therefore, be considered the cause of her disease.

Diabetes has an impact in several ways on relationships within the family. The diabetic parent's responsibility for self-care often conflicts with the needs of other family members, especially the children. Hypoglycemia produces irritability, which may be hard for children and spouse. The conflicting needs of herself and her child are especially difficult for a diabetic mother with a young infant. If there are frequent episodes of illness, additional responsibilities fall on the spouse or other members of the family.

Like other families where there is a member with a chronic disease, the disease may come to be blamed for every problem. The patient with the disease becomes a scapegoat for all the troubles of the family.

Children of diabetic parents have fears that their parent will die, or abandon them, or that they will inherit the disease. They may also harbor guilt feelings about being responsible for the disease or for episodes of hypoglycemia or ketoacidosis. Children will often not express these feelings unless encouraged to do so. Parents may be completely unaware of them.

How Diabetes Presents in Family Practice

Type 1 DM typically presents as the symptoms of metabolic disturbance: weakness, fatigue, loss of weight, thirst, cramps, frequency of micturition, and visual impairment. In some cases, abdominal pain is the presenting symptom and has to be distinguished from the pain of an acute abdomen. In the only patient I (IRMcW) have seen presenting in this way, the diagnosis was made clear by the strong smell of ketones.

Testing the urine for glucose and ketones is very sensitive and enables the diagnosis to be confirmed on the spot. Ketonuria at the time of presentation, however, is less common than it used to be. A decision must then be made about the initial management. If ketoacidosis is present, immediate admission to the hospital is required. Disasters have occurred because outpatient blood tests have been ordered, thus delaying admission, or because admission has been postponed to the following day. Vomiting is an especially serious symptom in ketoacidosis.

Whether or not patients with Type 1 DM without ketoacidosis are admitted to the hospital will depend on a number of factors, among them severity of disease, age of patient, family factors, and experience of the physician.

Type 1 DM may also present as loss of weight, thirst, and fatigue. Frequently, however, the presenting symptoms are those of the complications of diabetes.

The following are all common modes of presentation:

Pruritus vulvae, vulvitis, or vulval eczema.
Skin sepsis—boils, carbuncles, whitlows, cellulitis, infected eczema.
Leg ulcers.
Pain and paraesthesias in the limbs—symptoms of peripheral neuropathy
Balanitis. The importance of balanitis as a presenting symptom is not widely
   appreciated, although it is mentioned by Osler.
Urinary symptoms. Diabetes may present with a urinary infection, or with frequency of micturition or nocturia due to polyuria. In the elderly, the sudden
   onset of nocturnal incontinence should suggest diabetes.

The following case illustrates how insidiously Type 2 DM can present and how the diagnosis may be missed for years if the urine is not tested:

Case 15.2
A 71-year-old man was found to have diabetes when he presented with thirst, polyuria, and gangrene of the right big toe, which required amputation of the leg. His record showed that 5 years previously he had been treated for balanitis. Three years previously he had pain in both legs. X-ray showed flattening of the lumbosacral disc.

He was treated with a plaster cast and was off work for 4 months. The orthopedic report stated that his leg reflexes were absent and that there was sensory loss on the inner side of the left foot. Later in the same year he was treated for a purulent blister on the finger. There was no record of any urine tests.

Although not certain, it seems likely that this patient had clinical diabetes for several years before he was diagnosed.

Elderly patients sometimes present with drowsiness, confusion, or coma, and dehydration as the result of hyperglycemic nonketotic coma or precoma. The condition resembles a cerebrovascular accident, and the diagnosis may be missed if a blood glucose test is not done routinely in patients suspected of having cerebrovascular accidents.

Gestational diabetes is the one form that should be detected by screening all pregnant women. A test for glycosuria should be done at all prenatal visits and those testing positive should have fasting and postprandial blood glucose tests. Women who are at high risk for gestational diabetes should have blood glucose testing done early in pregnancy, whether or not they have glycosuria. The risk factors are obesity, advanced age, parity of five or more, previous delivery of overweight baby, history of stillbirth or spontaneous abortion, fetal malformation in previous pregnancy, and diabetes in a first-degree relative.

Assessment

If diabetes is suspected on clinical grounds, there is no need to do a GTT in most cases. In the majority, two random plasma glucose (PG) levels above 11.1 mmol/L, or two fasting (PG) levels above 7.0 mmol/L will provide unequivocal confirmation of the diagnosis. The GTT should be reserved for borderline cases and suspected gestational diabetes.

The assessment of a patient with diabetes is a good example of the need for a systems approach. A well-adjusted patient with a supportive family and few environmental stresses is likely to find it relatively easy to attain goals of therapy and maintain control. Patients without these advantages may present several kinds of management problems. Patients from populations with a very high prevalence rate, such as Native North American communities, may face overwhelming difficulties in carrying out treatment, unless some action is taken at the community level. If there are family problems, the patient may be too preoccupied by them to attend to his or her own needs. Lack of family support may make it difficult to adhere to a diet and the absence of symptoms may reduce motivation. The diabetes itself may be used for secondary gain by the patient, thus giving him or her an interest in its continuation. Emotional stresses can have a direct effect on carbohydrate and fat metabolism. Control may also be compromised by self-destructive behavior, such as excessive alcohol and food consumption or deliberate omission of insulin doses.

The patient should therefore be assessed at social/family, personal, and physical levels. If the patient-centered clinical method is used, the patient's own expectations and feelings will be understood. These may well change during

Table 15.5   Assessment of a newly diagnosed patient with diabetes

History	Examination	Laboratory
Special attention to	*Special attention to*	
Symptoms of hyperglycemia	Weight and height	Fasting plasma
Symptoms of long-term	Eyes (fundi and lens	glucose
complications	opacities)	Glycated hemoglobin
Family history of diabetes and	Mouth and teeth	TC, Tg, HDL-C,
cardiovascular disease	Evidence of thyroid	LDL-C
Risk factors for diabetes	disease	Serum creatinine
Risk factors for cardiovascular	Blood pressure	Urine protein, glu-
disease	Heart peripheral	cose, ketones
Relevant medical history	blood vessels	Urine microscopy
(e.g., endocrine disorders)	Peripheral sensa-	Urine for microalbu-
Eating habits	tion and tendon	minuria if NIDDM
Physical activity	reflexes	(or IDDM for
Weight trends and changes	Skin (evidence of	>5 years)
Occupational activity	infections)	TSH is IDDM patients
Patient and family's understanding	Feet (deformities,	ECG if indicated
of diabetes	calluses, nails)	
Patients and family's reactions to	Urine	
diagnosis and management plan		
Family roles and relationships		
Patient and family's coping abilities		
Medications		

the first few months of therapy as the impact of treatment on his everyday life becomes clear. The items that should be covered in the basic assessment are given in Table 15.5.

Treatment

Evidence in Britain, the United States, and Canada suggests that the care of diabetic patients by primary care physicians is often below acceptable standards (Smith, Taylor, and Gordon, 1982; Home and Walford, 1984; Harris, Eastman, and Siebert, 1994, Harris, Ekoe J-M, Zdanowicz, and Webster-Bogaert, 2005). The problem is that practices lack the organization to ensure comprehensive care, follow-up, and the mobilization of resources. One response has been the development of shared care (see Chapter 18, p. 384).

In discussing the results of their qualitative study of patients with Type 2 DM, Murphy and Kinmonth (1995) observed that patients are not passive recipients of medical advice. "They are active interpreters, and at times their interpretations lead them to quite different responses from those advocated by their doctors." In the light of the assumptions that patients were making, their responses were rational, but not always fully informed. For example, some assumed that if they had no symptoms, they were not at risk for complications. Others did not understand that the rationale behind much of the dietary advice was the prevention of cardio-vascular complications.

Patients' responses tend to change over time, as a result of information and experience. Even when well informed, some patients reject the medical model of management in favor of their own model. This was rarely made explicit to their physicians, thus posing a threat to the patient–doctor relationship.

If the practice can be organized for it, there are several advantages for the patient in being followed up by their family doctor. The care of patients' diabetes is not separated from their medical care; the patient is more likely to have contin-uing care from the same physician than in a clinic; the family doctor can involve the family in care and can visit the home if necessary; and the doctor's office is likely to be more accessible than the hospital outpatient clinic.

Taylor and Gordon (1985) described four stages in the management of patients with diabetes:

1. System assessment.
2. Goal setting. The doctor reconciles multiple preferences and integrates these into an ordered set of goals.
3. Management plan. A long-term plan of management is chosen.
4. Tactical implementation. The doctor chooses actions to optimize the manage-ment plan and to monitor its progress.

The initial treatment plan may evolve as a result of negotiation about goals and priorities between doctor and patient. Taylor and Gordon found this to be unusual. More commonly, the patient tries out the doctor's management plan, then decides how much this is acceptable when he or she has assessed its impact on his or her own life's goals and priorities. This trial period may result in a modification of the goals and management plan in a process of adaptation to the illness. The result-ing accommodation may result in less control of the disease than the physician had hoped for. An attempt by the doctor to impose his or her point of view is very unlikely to be successful. If the patient cannot live with the new plan, the only recourse is to try to modify some of the factors limiting the capacity of the patient to comply. Patients who participate in clinical trials tend to be different from the general population in their motivation, commitment, educational level, and free-dom from other diseases. Family doctors, on the other hand, have to apply the results of trials in the general population. In a disease such as diabetes, which calls for a high level of patient participation, the setting of goals will depend on many individual factors.

The following goals of management are important:

1. Prevention of ketoacidosis and avoidance of hypoglycemic reactions in Type 1 DM
2. Weight reduction in obese patients with Type 2 DM
3. Control of hypertension and hyperlipidemia
4. Prevention of blindness, renal failure, and peripheral vascular disease and foot complications

5. Maintenance of optimal body weight in adults and normal growth in children
6. Attainment of blood glucose levels consistently below diabetic levels in Type 2 DM
7. In Type 1 DM, as much reduction of blood glucose level as can be attained without increasing risks from hypoglycemia
8. Early detection of target-organ damage
9. As much responsibility for control as possible taken by the patient
10. Mobilization of support by patient's family

Some of these goals are in conflict with each other. For example, it may not be possible to attain normal blood glucose levels without precipitating hypoglycemic attacks. In each case, the appropriate balance between goals has to be arrived at.

For all types of diabetes, education of the patient and family are of fundamental importance. The patient—and key family members—should have basic knowledge of the pathophysiology of diabetes, the principles of dietary control and foot care, the actions of insulin and oral drugs, monitoring blood and urine glucose, symptoms and management of ketoacidosis and hypoglycemia, control of infections, and maintenance of health. In many areas, the family physician can now make use of educational services provided by diabetic clinics or national diabetic associations. In this event, his role will be to supplement and reinforce this education, especially to family members who may not have been able to attend.

Wherever possible, the family physician should enlist the help of a dietitian. Good dietary control is the key to successful management, and this requires a tailoring of diet to the individual, taking account of weight, age, previous dietary habits, income, and beliefs about food. For Type 2 DM, diet alone is the first step in treatment. The aim is to attain and maintain the ideal body weight for the patient's height and sex. Tables of Body Mass Index (BMI) are readily available and should be used for reference. A rough calculation can made be using the following formula: for females, 100 pounds for 60 inches in height with 5 pounds for each additional inch; for males, 106 pounds for 60 inches in height, with 6 pounds for each additional inch. The total caloric intake can be calculated by multiplying the ideal weight by 10, 15, or 20, depending on the activity of the patient and the need for weight reduction. Patients should follow a healthy diet as recommended for the general population (such as *Canada's Guidelines for Healthy Eating*), including a variety of foods from the four food groups (grain products, vegetables and fruits, milk products, meat and alternatives), attaining and maintaining a healthy body weight, decreasing total fat intake to <30% of calories and ensuring an adequate intake of carbohydrate, protein, essential fatty acids, vitamins, and minerals. Most of the carbohydrate should be in the form of complex carbohydrates with a low glycemic index such as bread, sweet potatoes, and pasta. Refined carbohydrates should be avoided—for example, cake, candy, pies, soft drinks, canned fruits, beer, and wine. Exchange diets give the patient choice and flexibility. Meals should be taken at regular times, and the amount eaten at each meal should not vary much from day to day. An exercise regimen should also be prescribed as even moderate exercise programs result in reductions in morbidity and mortality in both Type 1 and 2 diabetes. If diet and exercise do not produce adequate control (fasting BS <6 mmol), the next step is usually an oral hypoglycemic agent (CDA Guidelines, 2003).

Oral Hypoglycemic Agents

Three groups of oral hypoglycemic agents are available: sulfonylureas (e.g., glyburide, gliclazide), biguanides (e.g., metformin), or alpha-glucosidase inhibitors (e.g., acarbose). Sulfonylureas act by increasing the secretion of insulin and increasing the insulin receptors in peripheral tissues. All sulfonylureas have the same mechanism of action. The difference between the first generation (tolbutamide, chlorpropamide) and second generation (glybaride, glicazide) is one of potency. One important distinction is between short-acting and long-acting sulfonylureas. A long-acting drug is more convenient but should be used only for patients under age 65 with normal renal function. Treatment should be started with multiple low-dose medications then increased if a response is not obtained. If satisfactory control is obtained, then deteriorates, it is probably time to consider insulin. Sulfonylureas are not usually prescribed for obese patients and are contraindicated in severe insulin deficiency, pregnancy, intercurrent illness, and perioperative patients. Insulin is usually required in these patients (Williams, 1994).

Sulfonylureas may potentiate the effect of antidiuretic hormone on the kidney, resulting in hyponatremia and edema. Their action is also affected by interaction with thiazides, chlorpromazine, propranolol, phenytoin, and dicumarol. Dosage may have to be adjusted if these drugs are given concurrently. Alcohol in a patient with liver disease potentiates the hypoglycemic effect. Because of the risks of hypoglycemia, chlorpropamide and glibenclamide should be avoided in the elderly. Diabetic patients with terminal cancer who are on oral hypoglycemic agents are at risk for hypoglycemia if their need for medication is not reviewed as they enter the wasting phase of their disease.

Metformin, one of the biguanide group of drugs, has less hypoglycemic effect than the sulfonylureas and is the drug of first choice in most countries. It is helpful for obese patients with poor dietary control in whom sulfonylureas or insulin might produce weight gain and has been shown to reduce macrovascular complications (UKPDS Group, 1998). Because of the risk of lactic acidosis, metformin is contraindicated in the elderly and in patients with hepatic, renal, or cardiac dysfunction.

A new class of agents is the thiazolidinediones, including, rosiglitazone and pioglitazone which act by increasing insulin sensitivity in peripheral tissues. They have been associated with adverse events including hepatotoxicity, fluid retention, and CHF resulting in the withdrawal from the market in some countries. Their role in the treatment of diabetes is unclear at this time.

Incretins are hormones secreted by the gut postprandially that stimulate insulin, slow gastric emptying, induce satiety, and inhibit glucagon. The two chief forms are glucagon-like peptide-1 (GLP-1) and gastric inhibitory peptide (GIP). Because both of these peptides have short half lives, interest has focused on inhibiting the enzyme (dipeptidyl peptidase 4 or DPP-4) engaged in their breakdown. A DPP-4 inhibitor, sitagliptin, was approved in the United States by the FDA in 2006.

In Type 2 diabetes, when lifestyle changes and oral hypoglycemics are inadequate to achieve target glucose levels, addition of insulin is recommended. Patients need to be reassured that it is the norm for multiple agents, including insulin, to be used to achieve optimal control of blood sugars.

Insulin

Insulin is indicated in Type 1 DM, in gestational diabetes, and in Type 2 DM when hyperglycemia remains or recurs after treatment with diet, with or without oral agents. Insulin treatment is usually best initiated while the patient is going about his or her normal activities. If the patient is admitted to the hospital for this purpose, the balance achieved is very quickly altered when he or she leaves. When insulin is added to oral antihyperglycemic agent(s), a single injection of intermediate-acting or long-acting insulin, or extended long-acting insulin analogue (insulin glargine [Lantus®]), may be added at bedtime (CDA Guidelines, 2003). Insulin pens and vials containing insulin combinations have greatly eased the process of insulin self-administration, even to the extent of enabling blind people to give their own injections. The details of insulin treatment are outside the scope of this book. The issue of control is dealt with in the next section.

Monitoring

How patients monitor their treatment will depend on the type of diabetes. For patients with Type 2 DM, once-daily blood glucose testing at different times is usually sufficient. For Type 1 and gestational diabetes, where tight control is needed, up to four blood glucose tests a day may be required. The urine should be tested for ketones if the blood glucose reaches 20 mmol/L. For patients who are unable to manage blood tests, and whose renal threshold is normal, quantitative urine tests are an acceptable alternative, provided strict control is not an issue.

The frequency of follow-up appointments will depend on the type of diabetes and the state of control. Consultation with or referral to an endocrinologist will depend on the type of diabetes, the needs and wishes of the individual patient, and the experience and resources of the family physician. The care of diabetics who become pregnant and of patients with gestational diabetes should be shared with diabetes and obstetric specialists. A family physician has usually so little experience with diabetes in children that he or she will need the help of a specialist. Unstable diabetics call for close collaboration between family physician and specialist. The family physician deals with the day-to-day management; the specialist advises on strategy and deals with crises such as ketoacidosis.

Foot care is an important, and often neglected, aspect of diabetes management. Shoes and socks should be removed and feet inspected at every visit. Doing this reinforces for patients the importance of caring for their own feet. Patients should be shown how to inspect their feet and trim their toenails. The importance of well fitting shoes should be stressed. Cuts and blisters should be reported to the doctor immediately and aggressively managed. Educational videotapes and pamphlets can be used to support personal teaching. Patients at high risk because of sensory neuropathy can be identified by screening with the Semmes-Weinstein 5.07 monofilament (Rith-Najarian, Stolusky, and Gohdes, 1992). The services of a chiropodist are an important resource for diabetic footcare, but the main responsibility for preventive care and patient education still rests with the physician.

Examination of the fundi through dilated pupils is an essential part of the evaluation of diabetic patients. Patients with Type 1 DM should be screened annually by an ophthalmologist or optometrist from no later than 5 years from the time of diagnosis. Patients with Type 2 DM should be screened by an ophthalmologist or optometrist annually from the time of diagnosis. If these services are not available, there is no reason why screening should not be done by a family physician with additional experience. Proliferative retinopathy—the leading cause of blindness in diabetics—is amenable to treatment by photocoagulation if diagnosed early.

Urinary albumin levels should be measured annually in all patients with Type 1 and Type 2 diabetes. Renal insufficiency develops in 80 percent of patients with Type 1 diabetes who have an albumin excretion rate of 29 mg per day, but in only 4 percent of patients with an excretion rate of less than 29 mg. Standard dipsticks are too insensitive to detect microalbuminuria at this level, but more sensitive products are now available (Clark and Lee, 1995). An albumin to creatinine ratio (ACR) on a random urine sample correlates well with the urinary protein level found in 24-hour urine collections and has largely replaced the latter test in the monitoring of diabetic patients.

The prevalence of hypertension is higher when microalbuminuria is present, and antihypertensive treatment slows the development of nephropathy. ACE inhibitors and calcium channel–blocking agents are best for diabetic patients, with diltiazem and nicardipine the drugs of choice (Clark and Lee, 1995).

At follow-up visits, omissions can be minimized by use of protocols and flowcharts, which remind the physician to do periodic assessments of the heart, peripheral blood vessels, blood pressure, renal function, vision, fundi, and feet. Close attention should be paid to the records kept by the patient, both for what can be learned from them and to encourage him or her to maintain them. Nevertheless, home glucose monitoring has not been convincingly shown to improve control of plasma glucose. HbA1c is the best way to assess control. If attention is exclusively focused on the physician's agenda for the visit, he or she may not be responsive to other items on the patient's agenda (Bartz, 1994). A patient-centered approach leads to improved metabolic control (Stewart et al., 1994).

Diabetic flow sheets in paper or electronic records are extremely useful ways of ensuring that the family physician adequately monitors diabetic patients. These practice tools record key parameters needed for adequate monitoring including fasting glucose, HbA1c, urinary ACRs, lipid profiles, renal function, tests for peripheral neuropathy, and patient education.

Hypoglycemia and Ketoacidosis
Both hypoglycemia and ketoacidosis are important conditions for the family physician. If diabetes is controlled well but not too tightly, hypoglycemic coma should

not be a frequent occurrence. When it does occur, a rapid response to intravenous injection of dextrose can minimize brain damage. For this purpose, intravenous dextrose should always be available in the emergency bag for use in the patient's home or in the office. The bizarre behavior of a patient with hypoglycemia may be mistaken for alcohol intoxication or a psychotic episode. In elderly patients, hypoglycemia may resemble a cerebrovascular accident. When the patient is first seen in coma, the level of unconsciousness may be so light as to suggest hysteria. A key feature of hypoglycemic coma is its rapid onset.

Hypoglycemic attacks in Type 1 diabetics can be reduced to a minimum if the following points are stressed to patient and family: recognizing early symptoms, carrying an emergency supply of lump sugar, wearing a bracelet identifying the patient as diabetic, not missing meals, and decreasing insulin or increasing carbohydrate before vigorous exercise. Access to a glucagon kit is also very helpful in the event of a hypoglycemic episode.

Hypoglycemia is a risk not only for patients on insulin, but also for those on sulfonylureas. The risk is greatest for elderly patients and is greater for long-acting than for short-acting sulfonylureas. The incidence is said to be five times greater for chlorpropamide than for tolbutamide. Glibenclamide can cause prolonged hypoglycemia. Mental symptoms or focal neurological signs in a patient on sulfonylureas should be treated as hypoglycemia until proved otherwise. Patients with severe hypoglycemia should be admitted to the hospital. Sulfonylurea-induced hypoglycemia often requires prolonged treatment (Ferner and Neil, 1988).

For the prevention or early detection of ketoacidosis, the following points should be stressed to patients: for Type 1 DM, test urine for ketones if blood glucose reaches 20 mmol/L or during illnesses; report to the physician if two successive tests are positive; do not miss insulin if feeling ill; report any illness to the doctor, especially if there is vomiting. Patients reporting problems of this kind should be seen immediately, not treated by phone or left overnight. With established ketoacidosis, immediate admission to the hospital is required.

Ketoacidosis can occur in patients with Type 2 DM who are on a sulfonylurea and are abusing alcohol. Lactic acidosis, another form of coma, is a risk in patients with renal or hepatic insufficiency who are on a biguanide.

The Family Physician and the Diabetic Driver

The family physician has a big responsibility for making the patient aware of the risks of driving and for protecting members of the public. Most jurisdictions have some limitations on diabetic drivers. These usually involve a medical examination before issuing a license and further examinations when the license is renewed. The main hazard is hypoglycemia. A diabetic driver who has an accident as a result of hypoglycemia may be charged with driving while under the influence of a drug. Particular care should be taken not to drive in circumstances in which hypoglycemia may occur. At the first hint of hypoglycemia, the driver should stop, draw into the side, and get out of the driver's seat. A supply of sugar should always be available in the car. The problem is that there may not be enough warning to do this. Patients with Type 1 DM who are driving should not be kept under such tight control that hypoglycemia is a high risk. Patients monitoring their own blood glucose should do a test before driving. The licensing authority should be made aware of patients whose control is brittle.

References

Anderson BJ, Kornblum H. 1984. The family environment of children with a diabetic parent: Issues for research. *Family Systems Medicine* 2:17.

Anderson RJ, Freedland KE, Clouse RE, et al. 2001. The prevalence of comorbid depression in adults with diabetes: A meta-analysis. *Diabetes Care* 24:1069–1078.

Bartz R. 1994. Interpretive dialogue: a multi-method qualitative approach for studying doctor–patient interactions. Abstract 133. San Francisco, CA: University of California.

Canadian Diabetes Association Clinical Practice Guidelines Expert Committee: CDA 2003 Clinical Practice Guidelines for the Prevention and Management of Diabetes in Canada *Canadian Journal of Diabetes* 27(supplement 2): S10–11.

Clark CM, Lee DA. 1995. Prevention and treatment of the complications of diabetes mellitus. *New England Journal of Medicine* 332(18):1210.

Daneman D. 2002. Eating disorders in adolescent girls and young adult women with type 1 diabetes. *Diabetes Spectrum* 15:83–105.

Diabetes Control and Complications Trial Research Group. 1993. The effect of intensive treatment of diabetes on the development and progression of long-term complications in insulin-dependent diabetes mellitus. *The New Egland Journal of Medicine* 329(14):977.

Egede LE, Zheng D, Simpson K. 2002. Comorbid depression is associated with increased health care use and expenditures in individuals with diabetes. *Diabetes Care* 25:464–470.

Ferner RE, Neil HA. 1988. Sulphonylureas and hypoglycaemia. *British Medical Journal* 296(6627):949.

Fuller JH, Shipley MJ, Rose G, Jarrett RJ, Keen H. 1983. Mortality from coronary heart disease and stroke in relation to degree of glycemia: The Whitehall study. *British Medical Journal* 287:867.

Garcia MJ, McNamara PM, Gordon T, et al. 1974. Morbidity and mortality in diabetes in the Framingham population: Sixteen-year follow-up study. *Diabetes* 23:105.

Garvard JA, Lustman PJ, Clouse RE. 1993. Prevalence of depression in adults with diabetes: An epidemiological evaluation. *Diabetes Care* 16:1167–1178.

Gerstein HC, Haynes RB, eds. 2001.*Evidence Based Diabetes Care*. Hamilton, London: BC Decker.

Hanson CL, Henggeler SW. 1984. Metabolic control in adolescents with diabetes: An examination of systemic variables. *Family Systems Medicine* 2:5.

Harris MI, Eastman RC, Siebert C. 1994. The DCCT and medical care for diabetes in the U.S. *Diabetes Care* 17(7):761.

Harris SB, Perkins BA, Whalen-Brough E. 1996. Non-insulin-dependent diabetes mellitus among First Nations children: New entity among First Nations people of northwestern Ontario. *Canadian Family Physician* 42:869.

Harris SB, Gittelsohn J, Hanley A, Barnie A, Wolever TMS, Gao J, Logan A, Zinman B. 1997. The prevalence of NIDDM and associated risk factors in Native Canadians. *Diabetes Care* 20:185.

Harris SB, Ekoe J-M, Zdanowicz Y, Webster-Bogaert S. 2005. Glycemic control and morbidity in the Canadian primary care setting (results of the diabetes in Candada evaluation study). *Diabetes Research and Clinical Practice* 70:90–97.

Home P, Walford S. 1984. Diabetes care: Whose responsibility. *British Medical Journal* 289:713.

International Diabetes Federation; IDF Task Force on Clinical Practice Guidelines. www.idf.org

Lipscombe LL, Hux Je. 2007. Trends in diabetes prevalence, incidence and mortality in Ontario, Canada, 1995–2005: A population based study. *Lancet* 369 (9563):750–756.

Litzelman DK, Slemenda CW, Langefeld CD, Hays LM, Welch MA, Bild DE, Ford ES, Vinicor F. 1993. Reduction of lower extremity clinical abnormalities in patients with non-insulin-dependent diabetes mellitus. *Annals of Internal Medicine* 119(1):36.

Medalie JH, Papier CM, Goldbourt U, et al. 1975. Major factors in the development of diabetes mellitus in 10,000 men. *Archives of Internal Medicine* 135:811.

Minuchin S, Rosman BL, Baker L. 1978. *Psychosomatic Families*. Cambridge, MA: Harvard University Press.

Murphy E, Kinmonth AL. 1995. No symptoms, no problem? Patients' understanding of non-insulin dependent diabetes. *Family Practice* 12:184.

National Diabetes Data Group. 1979. Classification and diagnosis of diabetes mellitus and other categories of glucose intolerance. *Diabetes* 28:1039.

Ohkubo Y, Kishikawa H, Araki E, et al. 1995. Intensive insulin therapy prevents the progression of diabetic microvascular complications in Japanese patients with non-insulin-dependent diabetes mellitus: a randomized prospective 6-year study. *DiabetesResearch and Clinical Practice* 28:103–117

Ostbye T, Yarnall SH, Krause KM, Pollak K, Gradison M, Michener JL. 2005. Is there time for management of patients with chronic diseases in primary care? *Annals of Family Medicine* 3:209–214.

Rith-Najarian SJ, Stolusky T, Gohdes DM. 1992. Identifying diabetic patients at high risk for lower-extremity amputation in a primary health care setting. *Diabetes Care* 15(10):1386.

Smith CK, Taylor TR, Gordon MJ. 1982. Community based studies of diabetes control: Program development and preliminary analysis. *Journal of Family Practice* 14:459.

Stewart M, Brown JB, Weston WW, McWhinney IR, McWilliam CL, Freeman TR. 1994. *Patient-centered Medicine: Transforming the Clinical Method*. Thousand Oaks, CA: Sage Publications.

Taylor TR, Gordon MJ. 1985. Developing a unitary model of the clinical management process. In: Sheldon M, Brooke J, Rector A, eds., *Decision-making in General Practice*. London: Macmillan.

UK Prospective Diabetes Study (UKPDS) Group . 1998. Intensive blood-glucose control with sulphonylureas or insulin compared with conventional treatment and risk of complications in patients with type 2 diabetes (UKPDS 33). *Lancet* 352:837–853.

von Mering J, Minkowski O. 1890. Diabetes mellitus nach Pankreasexstirpation. *Archiv für experimentelle Pathologie und Pharmakologie* 26:371–87.

Williams G. 1994. Management of non-insulin-dependent diabetes mellitus. *Lancet* 343:95.

Zimmet PZ. 1995. The pathogenesis and prevention of diabetes in adults. *Diabetes Care* 18(7):1050.

Part III

The Practice of Family Medicine

16

Home Care

At the time of writing (2007–2008) many jurisdictions are unable to recruit enough family physicians for the needs of their patients. Large demands in office practice have often reduced both hospital and home visits. Some practices have discontinued home visits altogether. This expedient is an unfortunate necessity, but must not lead to a permanent cessation of home care by family physicians. Nor should home care medicine become a separate entity, furthering even more the fragmentation of our profession.

Never has there been a greater need for general practitioners to be attending their seriously ill patients in the home. Hospitals are dangerous places for the increasing numbers of the elderly in the population—dangerous due to hospital infections and the rapid destabilization the aged can undergo. Patients with infections, who in former times would have been treated in their homes, are now taken to general practitioners' offices, or to crowded emergency rooms, where diseases can easily spread.

Without a countrywide network of general practitioners, trained to deal with large numbers of patients with infections, we are vulnerable in times of pandemics. There was a time when influenza epidemics were dealt with in this way. In my (IRMcW) first practice in the 1950s and 1960s, these epidemics would lead to a change from our usual office practice. Patients knew they were not to leave their homes. Phone calls would start to pour into the office. The office practice would be contained as far as possible and the partners would divide up the home visits. Patients with complications such as pneumonia would either be transferred to hospital or, if not severe, would be visited daily. It was not unusual for the practice to make 100 home visits in the day.

Fifty years ago, home visits were a major part of the family physician's work. In the intervening years, many factors have combined to reduce their number. Increasing car ownership has made it easier for people to come to the office.

Immunization and antibiotic therapy have reduced the incidence and duration of acute infections, especially in childhood. Technological developments have concentrated the care of serious illness in the hospital. Widespread telephone ownership has enabled physicians to give advice and receive follow-up information over the telephone. Less emphasis is now placed on bed rest for many conditions.

The decline in home visiting has been greater in North America than in Europe although it has occurred, to some extent, on both continents. In Britain, 10% of all contacts between general practitioners and patients take place in the home (McCormick, Fleming, and Charlton, 1995). In the Netherlands, the proportion of patient contacts that were house calls fell from 17% in 1985 to 8.5% in 2001 (Jones, Schellevis, and Westert, 2004) US and Canadian general practitioners did an average of one a day or less (Cave, 1987). A Canadian survey of more than 10,000 family physicians reported that 48.3% stated that they still include house calls in the services they offer to patients (National Physician Survey, 2007). Using billing claims data in the province of Ontario, Chan (2002) found that provision of house calls by family physicians varied by age of practitioner. Fifty seven percent of older, established physicians provided this service, but only 37% of younger physicians did so. Generally, most home care services are provided by nurses. A national survey showed that US family physicians make on the average only 21.2 home visits per year, and 35% do not make any home visits (Keenan et al., 1992). There are also differences in the way practices are organized for home visits. In Europe, it is often still the practice to set aside part of each day for home visits. In North America, some doctors set aside a half day each week for visiting patients with chronic illness. Visits for acute problems, however, are often fitted into a full office schedule.

One effect of the reduction in home visits in North America has been the geographic dispersal of practices. Patients may be accepted into a practice when distance would make home care impossible.

One of the arguments for not attending patients at home is that the quality of care is better if they are seen in the office or the hospital. As far as we are aware, this argument has not been supported by data. In my (IRMcW) own experience, failure to attend patients at home can lead to care of poor quality. Elderly patients with febrile illnesses have been managed entirely by telephone, even though it is not possible to distinguish between influenza and pneumonia without examining the patient. It is not unusual for dying patients to be taken by ambulance to the emergency department to have his pain medication adjusted, when this could easily have been done in the home.

Changes in the health-care system are now increasing the demand for home care. Elderly people—the largest group receiving home care—are an increasing proportion of the population. Admission to the hospital can be destabilizing for elderly patients, as well as exposing them to the risk of cross-infection. The cost of inpatient care has risen; patients are discharged home earlier; and new surgical techniques have reduced postoperative length of stay. Economic pressures have forced reductions in acute care beds, so that physicians are now faced with managing patients with complex illness in the home who would formerly have been admitted to the hospital. Medical technologies in the period 1950 to 1990 have been mainly a centralizing influence, requiring the concentration of patients in intensive care units. Many of the newer technologies now favor dispersal. Self-monitoring of blood glucose and blood pressure can be done in the home; ECG tracings and X-rays can be transmitted across a distance; equipment for home intravenous and subcutaneous therapy has been greatly simplified; and data can be electronically transmitted between home, hospital, laboratory, and office. Finally, many people strongly prefer home care to hospital admission. There is an increasing trend for dying patients to choose to spend their last days at home. Improvements in the medical management of serious disabilities and injuries have increased the number of disabled people of all ages living at home.

These demands have led in many countries to the development of integrated home care programs providing home (domestic) help, home nursing and often physiotherapy and occupational therapy. Many examples of these home care programs exist, their structure and financing depending on local conditions. Sometimes there is a well-defined institutional structure, as in the New Zealand Hospital At Home (Hiddlestone, 1981) and the New Brunswick Extra-mural Hospital (EMH) (Health Care Without Walls: The New Brunswick Extra-Mural Hospital, 2006). The Extra-Mural Program continues to grow and develop. The mission of the Program is

to provide a comprehensive range of coordinated healthcare services for individuals of all ages for the purpose of promoting, maintaining and/or restoring health within the context of their daily lives and to provide palliative services to support quality end of life care for individuals with progressive life threatening illnesses.

The New Zealand Hospital at Home continues to function and in 2005 completed a randomized clinical trial (RCT) of a newly established Hospital at Home (HAH) program in Auckland, New Zealand. A pilot project had suggested that 25% of prospective medical admissions aged over 65 were potential candidates for HAH care.

Two hundred and eighty five people were randomized, with a mean age of 80 years. Patients were either experiencing a health crisis or being discharged early from hospital. Nurses led the HAH team and geriatricians or general practitioners were the physicians.

Significantly more patients treated at home reported high levels of satisfaction as did their relatives, who also had lower scores on the Carer Strain Index. The mean cost per patient was almost twice for patients treated at home, largely due to the HAH program not operating at full capacity (Harris, Ashtan, Broad, Connolly and Richmond, 2005).

The hospice movement has fostered integrated home care services for the terminally ill. Besides nursing, these often include the services of a chaplain and volunteer visitors. In 1992, there were an estimated 1,000 hospice programs in the United States (MMWR, 1993).

The organization of home care services takes various forms, depending on the existing organization of health services and their sources of funding. Each type has its advantages and disadvantages, and the choice should depend on how each model fits with the local context.

In the United States, pressures from funding sources to reduce hospital stays led hospitals to establish their own home care agencies. These are full departments of the parent hospital and are subject to all its standards and regulations. The largest of these (South Hills) was established in Pittsburg (SHHS/HHA) in 1963 and serves nine hospitals. It employs over 300 staff and provides a wide range of professional and support services. Because of its size, 95% of its service providers are direct employees rather than contracted employees. The SHHS/HAA intake team is involved in discharge planning (Frasca, Christy, 1986).

The advantage of this model is its vertical integration of home and hospital services. Discharge planning is enhanced, hospital staff are available for home care problems, readmission can be accomplished without difficulty, and there is continuity in the patient's records. The fact that the agency is an integral part of the hospital makes it a presence for hospital-based physicians and gives them the confidence to entrust their patients to it. Managed care organizations in the United States have attained similar levels of integration.

One of the problems encountered by some community-based hospital-in-the-home programs has been the difficulty of persuading hospital-based physicians to use the service. This may result in a minimal impact on hospital utilization. In small communities, where family physicians follow most of their in-hospital patients, this is unlikely to present a problem. In large urban areas, especially teaching centers, it must be a consideration.

In Canada, the New Brunswick EMH is an example of this model (Ferguson, 1994). This has the legal status of a hospital and operates under the Public Hospitals Act, but is not an outreach service of an acute care hospital. Because the province has no home care program, the EMH is the sole provider of home care. About half the patients are admitted from acute care hospitals. Liaison with acute care hospitals may be made easier in New Brunswick by the fact that the province has no large urban centers and general practitioners usually follow-up their patients in the hospital.

In December 2000, the College of Family Physicians of Canada published a discussion paper on The Role of the Family Physician in Home Care. The paper came out strongly in favor of home care by family physicians, both as the customary "house calls" and also as members of teams providing care in organized "Hospital-in-the-Home" programs. It recommends that the role of the family physician in home care be defined by medical necessity and patient need. Home care was seen as both long-term, low level care and care for patients with acute illnesses attended by multidisciplinary teams.

In 2007, 150 leaders in home care from across Canada were convened by the Public Policy Forum for a roundtable discussion on the future of home care in Canada. The home and community sector was recommended to integrate home care data into the national reporting system, to create common definitions, reconsider funding models, help address human resources, and be accountable.

In 2007, the Canadian Home Care Association (CHCA) published a paper on The Integral Role of Home Care in Improving Access to Care. In a project sponsored by the CHCA it was found that through collaboration and partnership "The family physician gains a greater understanding and awareness of the scope and availability of home care services ... (and) the role of the primary care physician and the needs of the physicians are better understood by the home care team members."

The IPSITH (Integrating Physician Services in the Home) study was conducted by the Thames Valley Family Practice Research Unit, a health systems-linked research unit funded by the Ministry of Health and Long-Term Care of Ontario, with the assistance of the Community Care Access Centre (CCAC) of London and Middlesex.

Its purpose was to compare outcomes between a new home care program integrating general practitioners and nurses, with usual care. The patients involved were all acutely ill.

The infrastructure consisted of family physicians and their own patients, working with an experienced nurse practitioner, as well as a network of laboratories, diagnostics, pharmacies, and oxygen suppliers. The IPSITH process goals were prompt medical assessment, effective communication, close monitoring, and prompt response to crises.

The program was evaluated through a nonrandomized case comparison of the 82 IPSITH patients with the 82 usual care patients. The program included the usual care providers and the patient's family physicians, the CCAC case manager, who had overall supervision for all patients. Forty-four family physicians enrolled in the program and 29 of these enrolled patients. Thirty-nine specialists agreed to provide urgent consultations on request and 18 agreed to see the patient in the home on request.

The illnesses enrolled by the physicians were skin infections (25), respiratory illness (14), dehydration (12), congestive heart failure (10), functional decline, dementia (3), urinary tract infection (4), gastrointestinal disorders (6), and others (8).

The key findings were that IPSITH was successful, and that the role of the nurse practitioner was crucial as a link between physician and patient. All the process goals were met. Patients strongly preferred home to hospital, as did care givers, but less strongly. The physicians were somewhat in favor of home care. Time consumed and remuneration were the main barriers. However, most cases needed less than three home visits, and some none at all. The nurse practitioner minimized the need for doctor visits and was key to the success of the program. The team had better outcomes (fewer emergency room visits, and higher patient satisfaction) than the comparison group.

The Peterborough (UK) HAH started as a community-based organization, separate both from the hospital and from the existing home care services. It was modeled on the Santé Service Bayonne in France. This initial model failed because of integration problems with the existing domiciliary services (Mowat and Morgan, 1982). A Mark II version began in 1980 and was integrated successfully with the existing services (Knowelden, Westlake, Clarke, and Wright, 1988). Most of the admissions are elderly patients with terminal illness. With the exception of the early discharge scheme for orthopedic patients, the HAH has had little impact on hospital practice. Perhaps its community base makes it less visible to hospital-based physicians.

Since the year 2000, British general practitioners have been assessing their responses to the Department of Health's decision to provide community-based alternatives to acute hospital admissions. Primary care trusts (PCTs) are regarded as crucial in development of intermediate care. "Intermediate Care" was coined as a generic term for such innovations as HAH, rapid response to sickness, residential rehabilitation, and supported discharge from hospital. The plan proposes 5,000 extra intermediate care beds, to include community hospitals, nursing homes, and purpose-built facilities. An editorial (Wilson and Parker, 2003) explores general practitioner's attitudes to intermediate care, their participation in schemes and workload issues. Support of general practitioners as members of PCTs are regarded as crucial in development of intermediate care. The National Service Framework (NSF) for older people believes that intermediate care services need to be integrated across services, including primary care.

The Royal College of General Practitioners (RCGP) and General Practitioner Committee of the British Medical Association (BMA), in a joint statement, saw opportunities as integration of care across primary, secondary, and social care boundaries. Threats included inability of general practitioners to deliver, and diversion from their core functions as generalists. A significant increase of general practitioners would be needed.

The editorial continues to observe that little is known as to "grass roots" general practitioners support for intermediate care. One survey found that support varied with the medical condition. Terminal care, chest infections, and stroke were supported by 50% to 60%. Established HAH schemes seem to be popular with general practitioners; one proposed randomized clinical trial had to be discontinued because general practitioners would not deny patients the benefit of the HAH (Turrell, 2001).

General practitioners have been reluctant to register long-term patients in nursing homes; one explanation being remuneration for the shift in workload. Similar variation in uptake by general practitioners was found in a study of attitudes to admitting patients to community hospitals, where they retained medical responsibility (Grant and Dowell, 2002). The main determinant of use involved whether the general practitioner had sufficient time to treat the patient, and how comfortable they were about assuming medical responsibility. The RCGP/BMA paper suggested that many general practitioners chose the discipline to avoid inpatient care. In recent times, general practice has been increasingly focused on chronic disease and prevention.

At the grassroots level, integration can be enhanced by attachment of home care nurses to group practices. This fosters working relationships between nurses and physicians, a factor that is often lacking in large home care organizations.

In home care, the physician is a key member of the team. If the doctor is prepared to be actively involved and to visit the home frequently, a very good relationship can develop with other team members, as well as with the patient and family. If, on the other hand, the physician remains on the sidelines, going only when called, then he or she can very easily become a marginal member of the team. We have seen this happening frequently with terminally ill cancer patients. In the absence of regular visits by the doctor, the main responsibility for care falls on the nurse. The nurse, patients, and family lose confidence in the physician; thus when a crisis occurs, it is not surprising that they seek help from other sources.

Home care means more than doing home visits. It means being prepared to become a member of a team caring for a seriously ill patient at home. It may, in some cases, mean visiting the patient every day, just as the doctor would if the patient was in the hospital. It means going even when there is "nothing to do." Our experience is that when a patient is seriously ill there is never nothing to do. The most important outcome of the visit may be the support given to the patient, the family, and other members of the team.

Reasons for Home Visits

Most patients managed at home require conventional medical and nursing care rather than high-level technology. The four highest volume diagnoses for community home health beneficiaries in 2000 were: diabetes, hypertension, heart failure and chronic ulcer of skin. In 2004, five diagnosis-related groups accounted for the majority of hospital discharges of Medicare patients to home health care: rehabilitation, joint procedure, heart failure and shock, pneumonia and chronic obstructive pulmonary disease. (National Association for Home Care and Hospice, 2008). Cancer patients, another large group, were presumably discharged to home hospice care rather than home health care.

Patients managed at home fall into a number of categories:

1. Unstable chronic illness or acute exacerbations of chronic illness—for example, congestive heart failure, Alzheimer's disease, acute or chronic bronchitis, exacerbations of schizophrenia.
2. Acute episodic illness—for example, influenza, pneumonia, patients immobilized by acute pain, acute psychiatric episodes.
3. Patients discharged from the hospital who still require medical supervision, such as after myocardial infarction, cancer chemotherapy, or respiratory infection. The family doctor should be involved in discharge planning so that the patient returns to a home prepared for his or her arrival and a professional team with a plan for care.
4. Patients discharged from the hospital who require rehabilitation, such as after a stroke, injury, or surgery.
5. Housebound patients with chronic illness or disabilities of many kinds—for example, rheumatoid arthritis, multiple sclerosis, extreme old age.
6. Mothers and newborns discharged from obstetric units, especially those with poor social supports.
7. Assessment of patients to decide on admission to the hospital.
8. Patients with advanced cancer or the end stage of other chronic disease.

Assessment of Patients in the Home

Many aspects of clinical assessment are the same, whether done in the home, the office, or hospital. In some ways however, one can learn more from an assessment done in the home:

1. The home expresses the values and the history of the family.
2. Functional assessment (activities of daily living) can be done in patients' actual environment—their own stairs, toilet, and kitchen.
3. Hazards in the home can be identified and corrected—for example, by placing bars and rails in places where an elderly person is likely to fall.
4. Review of medications can include those in the medicine cupboard and other places, sometimes revealing duplicate prescriptions or incompatible drugs.
5. The impact on the family can be experienced directly. Physical and emotional exhaustion can be identified in caregivers before breakdown occurs.
6. The organization of the household, and its suitability as a place for a patient with complex illness, can be assessed directly.

Home visits can deepen a physician's understanding of a family. This enrichment is difficult to establish by conventional research methods because it is essentially subjective. Gray (1978) tells, for example, of a young woman who showed him a drawer full of baby clothes made for the baby she had lost. We have become aware of long-past bereavements by asking about family photographs in the home. Of course, this kind of information can be obtained from a good family history, but its quality is different. The knowledge is visceral. In an address on the importance of home visiting in child health, Cicely Williams (1973) commented that "practical experience in visiting homes and neighborhoods will provide more understanding in a single glance and five minutes of listening than will volumes of written questionnaires."

Home Care Technology

Advances in technology have made it possible to transfer many therapeutic procedures to the home setting:

• Home parenteral nutrition
• Home enteral nutrition by nasogastric tube
• Drug delivery systems: pumps for administering drugs for diabetes, or cancer pain
• Intravenous (IV) antibiotic
• Blood transfusion
• Respiratory therapy: oxygen concentrators and cylinders, mechanical ventilation, tracheostomy management
• Renal and peritoneal dialysis

In the United States, infusion therapy is the fastest growing sector of home care, with costs increasing from $1.5 billion in 1988 to $2.6 billion in 1990. Programs typically involve a team that may include nurse IV specialists, clinical pharmacists, infectious disease specialists, and social workers. Patients are trained in aseptic technique and recognition of drug reactions. Twenty-four=hour emergency care is a requirement for this service. Home care is not always provided by these programs, in which case patients have to attend as outpatients.

Home parenteral nutrition (HPN) has been made possible by developments such as the long-term indwelling Silastic catheter and has been shown to be cost-effective. Patients usually infuse solutions during a 10- to 12-hour period at night. HPN is organized through hospitals, and a home assessment is carried out to ensure that strict hygiene is observed. Training of patients in the technique takes place in hospital. The main indications for HPN are as follows:

- Short bowel syndrome
- Nutrition combined with cancer chemotherapy
- Inflammatory bowel disease
- Chronic fistula of digestive tract
- Scleroderma of digestive tract

HPN may be a long- or short-term therapy. HPN has been growing rapidly in the United States where companies marketing nutritional support products have become involved in assessing, educating, and treating patients and monitoring the quality of care. Nutritional support teams are well established and typically consist of nurses, physicians, nutritionists, and pharmacists.

Home enteral nutrition (HEN) is also an increasingly common service in the United States. In 1987, almost 8,000 people were receiving HEN, most of them over 65. HEN can be applied to a wider range of patients than TPN and is easier to administer and less costly. Tubes can be changed by patients, caregivers, or nurses. HEN has been estimated to be growing by 25% to 30% annually (Nutritional Support Services Survey, 1987).

Oxygen therapy is widely available at home, either by cylinder or oxygen concentrator, and is commonly prescribed for COPD. Mechanical ventilation in the home is used for respiratory failure caused by spinal cord injury or neuromuscular disease. It can be provided through a tracheostomy, by external pressure to the chest wall, or by intermittent positive pressure through a nasal mask. France has a national home respiratory care program. Twenty-eight regional organizations serve over 50,000 people with respiratory problems, 1,200 of whom, in 1986, required prolonged ventilation assistance; and 12,000 received respirator care for 12 to 24 hours a day. Ventilator-dependent patients and their families are vulnerable people and require well- organized support, with the assurance of a rapid response to crises. There is no margin for error either in the equipment or in the support system (Goldberg and Faure, 1986; Goldberg, 1989, 1990).

Dialysis for end-stage renal disease (ESRD)—either renal or peritoneal (CAPD)—can be carried out in the home. However, home renal dialysis is only possible for the limited number of patients with the necessary home environment and family support.

The Quality of Home Care

The quality of medical care in the home should be as high as or higher than in the hospital. For patients with serious and complex illness, this places special responsibilities on the physician, including the following:

1. Readiness to respond quickly to crises
2. A deputizing arrangement that can provide the same level of service as the attending doctor
3. Maintenance of clinical records that are available to the home care nurse and to deputizing physicians
4. Communication with home care nurses and other team members, and with hospital and community services
5. Maintenance of skills in clinical management, including facility with new technologies—for example, pain control in advanced cancer

Our experience in palliative care has been that family doctors varied in their commitment to home care along a spectrum from proactive to reactive. The proactive took the initiative in visiting the home, forming a management plan, and communicating with nurses. The reactive did nothing unless they were called by nurse or family, did not initiate home visits or calls to nurses, and did not arrange for appropriate deputizing services. The proactive physicians were respected and appreciated by both patients and nurses. The reactive ones forfeited the respect of both.

As the care of patients with serious illness is increasingly transferred to the home, it is difficult to see how physicians without a commitment to home care will be able to fulfill their commitments to their patients or maintain their clinical skills. It is often said that most home visits can be delegated to nurses. Although this is technically correct, family physicians should ponder the consequences of doing so. Visiting patients at home is one of the means by which bonds between a doctor and a family are forged and strengthened. A firsthand knowledge of the family home gives physicians an understanding of the patient and the family that they can get in no other way. Moreover, the great enrichment of the doctor's own working life from caring for patients in their homes must not be underrated. Doctors who cut themselves off from home care risk losing their skills in the management of clinical problems such as congestive heart failure and advanced cancer. From the point of view of the patient, home care can be crucial. Norman Cousins, in his book *Anatomy of an Illness* (1979), has movingly described the peace of mind that comes from being cared for at home, even in serious illness.

During the 14 years of my first practice, I have carried out thousands of home visits (IRMcW). There were few patients whose homes I had not visited. As I drove or walked through the town or the surrounding countryside, I got pleasure from thinking of the stories I had heard or the scenes I had witnessed in the houses I passed. Sometimes there would be sadness, and sometimes guilt at one of my failures. We were able to see our housebound patients because our practice only covered six miles in each direction. In the times when home visits were the norm, it was natural for practices to have geographic boundaries. In North America now there are many practices scattered far and wide. If we are to rebuild home visits as integral to our practices for our housebound patients, we will need to draw geographic boundaries again. Eventually, these geographic practices could form networks enabling health services to deal effectively with global pandemics.

In the meantime, patients joining a practice should be informed if they are outside the boundary for home visits.

Cost of Hospital in the Home

The few randomized controlled trials have not found HAH to be consistently less expensive than in hospital. A large, randomized control trial in the United Kingdom found no major differences in costs between the two arms of the trial for patients recovering from hip and knee replacement and elderly medical patients. HAH care increased costs for patients recovering from hysterectomy and for those with chronic obstructive pulmonary disease. Cost minimization analysis found a mean cost to the National Health Service of 2,516 pounds per hospital at home patient and 3,292 pounds per hospital patient. In this trial all patient groups except those with chronic obstructive pulmonary disease preferred hospital at home care.

At the present time (2008), it appears that the HAH initiatives are on the increase and that many general practitioners are willing to care for their patients in their home provided that they are aided by nurse practitioners and suitably remunerated. The idea of the hospital at home would fit well with primary care groups which are growing in many parts of the world. HAH can provide many kinds of care from short-term illnesses to long-term disabilities and housebound aged, and to the dying. Issues for general practitioners in these models are the need to maintain competence in the field and arrangement for deputizing or being on call.

In all the discussion about the HAH, it is surprising that hospital infections are not mentioned. For the elderly, the HAH should be a protection against this hazard. We need a randomized control trial which compares elderly patients in the hospital at home with hospital care, with particular accounting of patients with hospital-acquired infections.

References

Cave AJ. 1987. Development of an instrument to measure the effects of housecalls. Masters of Clinical Science thesis, University of Western Ontario.

Chan BTB. 2002. The decline of comprehensiveness of primary care. *Canadian Medical Association Journal* 166(4):429–434.

Cousins N. 1979. *Anatomy of an Illness as Perceived by the Patient.* New York: W.W. Norton.

Ferguson G. 1994. *The New Brunswick Extra Mural Hospital (EMH), From Dream to Reality.* New Brunswick Department of Health and Wellness. Frederiction NB.

Frasca C, Christy MW. 1986. Assuring continuity of care through a hospital-based home health agency. *Quality Review Bulletin* 12(5):167.

Goldberg AI, Faure EAM. 1986. Home care for life-supported persons in France: The regional association. *Rehabilitation Literature* 47:3–4, 60–64.

Goldberg AI. 1989. Home care for life-supported persons: The French system of quality control, technology assessment and cost containment. *Public Health Reports* 104(4):329.

Goldberg AI. 1990. Mechanical ventilation and respiratory care in the home in the 1990's: Some personal observations. *Respiratory Care* 35(3):247.

Grant JA, Dowell J. 2002. A qualitative study of why general practitioners admit to community hospitals. *British Journal of General Practice* 52(481):628–630,632–635.

Gray DJ. 1978. Feeling at home. *Journal of the Royal College of General Practitioners* 28:6.

Harris A, Ashtan T, Broad J, Connolly G, Richmond D. 2005. The effectiveness, acceptability and costs of a hospital-at-home service compared with acute hospital care: A randomized controlled trial. *Journal of Health Services Policy* 10(3):158.

Health Care Without Walls: The New Brunswick Extra-Mural Program, 2006. www.gnb.ca/0051/03484/pdfHiddlestone HJH. 1981. Hospital without walls. *World Hospitals* 17:15.

Keenan JM, Boling PE, Schwartzberg JG, Olson L, Schneiderman M, McCaffrey DJ, et al. 1992. A national survey of the home visiting practice and attitudes of family physicians and internists. *Archives of Internal Medicine* 152:2025.

Jones R, Schellevis F, Westert G. 2004. The changing face of primary care: The second Dutch national survey. *Family Practice* 21(6):597–598. Knowelden J, Westlake L, Clarke S, Wright K. 1988. Evaluation of Peterborough Hospital at Home. Medical Care Research Unit, Department of Community Medicine, University of Sheffield.

McCormick A, Fleming D, Charlton J. 1995. *Morbidity Statistics from General Practice: Fourth National Study 1991–1992*. London: Her Majesty's Stationery Office.

MMWR. 1993. Home-health and hospice care—United States, 1992. 42:820.

Mowat IG, Morgan RTT. 1982. Peterborough Hospital at home scheme. *British Medical Journal* 284:641.

National Association for Homecare and Hosptice 2008 www.nahc.org.facts

National Physician Survey (NPS) 2007. www.nationalphysiciansurvey.ca

Nutritional Support Services Survey. 1987. Enteral nutrition. *Nutritional Support Services* 7(12):8.

Williams CD. 1973. Health services in the home. *Pediatrics* 52:773.

Wilson A, Parker H. 2003. Guest editorial: Intermediate care and general practitioners, an uncertain relationship. *Health and Social Care in the Community* 11(2):81–84.

17

Records

Good records are fundamental to good patient care. They are also one of the means by which a physician enlarges and deepens his or her own experience. Just as scientists or naturalists keeps notes about the phenomena they observe, so should physicians record their observations on patients.

In all countries with advanced technology, medical records are in a process of rapid transition from paper to an electronic form. Many features of the "paperless" record system can be quite safely predicted. The longer-term impact of the new information technology on medical practice and the health care system are more difficult to predict. New technologies often have unforeseen consequences.

Records in family practice serve a number of purposes:
1. They provide the physician with readily accessible basic data about the patient. This is called the profile or database. The database should have several components:
    a. Demographic data: age, sex, place of birth, marital status, occupation, family relationships, social status, and ethnic group
    b. Past history: major medical events, such as hospitalizations and surgical operations; major life events, such as bereavements or broken marriages
    c. Past family history: history of familial or genetic problems, major illnesses in family members, present health status, major events in the life of the family
    d. Biological baseline data, such as weight and blood pressure
    e. Data on preventive procedures, such as immunization and screening procedures
    f. Allergies and drug sensitivities
    g. Smoking history and alcohol consumption

    h. List of current medications, both prescribed and nonprescription

    i. Risk factors

2. They provide a continuing clinical record of all illnesses. The data should be accurate, concise, and readily understandable by any physician, not only the writer. The record should include all positive findings, important negative findings, diagnoses and problem labels, results of investigations, management plans, and drugs prescribed. The introduction of the problem-oriented record and the use of flow sheets have been notable advances in clinical record keeping (Weed, 1968).

3. They keep track of the patient's attendances. The frequency of visits often provides an important clue to the origins of illness in individuals and families. The record should make it possible to identify clusters of visits made for different reasons by different family members.

4. They provide data for an organized approach to preventive medicine in individual patients and in the practice population as a whole.

5. They support the physician's own intellectual development. Physicians learn mainly from their own experience and the practice record system is, therefore, a most important source of continuing education. After the doctor has been a few years in practice, the records should be a mine of information on the natural history of disease. Provided the data is in an accessible form, the physician has all he or she needs to stimulate his or her own intellectual growth. One of the fascinations of family practice is following the evolution of illnesses in one's own notes made over long periods of time.

6. If records are of sufficient quality they can provide data for clinical research.

7. Finally, records are an essential tool for practice management and quality assessment.

The Problem-Oriented Record

The problem-oriented system introduced by Weed is particularly well suited for adaptation to family practice. The starting point of a clinical record should be the patient's problems, stated with a minimum of interpretation. These may be in the form of symptoms, social situations, abnormal physical findings, or attitudes. Problems such as "marital conflict" or "denies illness" are listed in the same way as "shortness of breath on exertion." The record should enable one to follow the evolution of a problem through the various phases of formulation, resolution, and management.

For the family physician's purposes, the most important components of the problem-oriented system are as given below:

1. The problem list. This comes at the beginning of the record and forms an index to its contents. All problems are listed, numbered, and dated in the chronological order of their recognition. If the problem is resolved (by surgery, for example), the date of its resolution is recorded. One decision the family physician has to make is whether to record all minor problems, such as individual

respiratory infections. If these are included, the list can become very lengthy, but if they are excluded, one may fail to identify a significant pattern of attendances. One solution is to have a separate list for minor problems. At the end of the problem list is a list of long-term medications and treatments.

2. Progress notes. When notes are made in the body of the record, they are numbered with the index number of the problem being dealt with. This enables the physician to follow the evolution of a problem through the whole record. According to the SOAP format, S stands for subjective data (the patient's complaints), O for objective findings, A for physician's assessment of the problem, and P for the management plan.[1] Following this standard system of record keeping makes it easier to extract significant information from the notes.

Anything that is important in the care of the patient should have a place in the medical record. The problem-oriented record made a step forward by shifting the focus from diseases to problems. But there are still aspects of care that are underrepresented. We have not yet found a way of recording the patient's experience of illness, expectations of care, resources, functional capacities, or feelings. The record is still "doctor centered." The structure of the record has an influence on the clinical process, and items that the doctor is not expected to record will tend to be undervalued.

The Electronic Record System

Computerized data systems[2] make possible many things that were difficult to attain in paper systems (Ornstein, Oates, and Fox, 1992).

The organization of preventive care, with reminders to physicians and reminders to patients.

Monitoring of success in attaining preventive targets, such as immunization rates in the practice population.

Immediate access to items such as patients' list of medications, previous tests and X-ray results, and allergies.

Immediate warnings about drug interactions or drugs prescribed to patients who are allergic to them.

Decision support tools reminding physicians to consider diseases in their differential diagnosis or to include a test in their investigation.

The organization of follow-up for patients with chronic diseases, with reminders to physicians about surveillance protocols.

The horizontal integration of information from different sectors of the primary care system, such as physicians' practices, home care, and community agencies.

The vertical integration of information between the primary care and secondary care sectors, with major implications for communication between family physicians and consultants.

Information can be entered by keyboard or by automated loading of such items as laboratory and imaging results, consultants' letters, and hospital discharge summaries. Voice entry is widely available.

Data can be accessed by entering code numbers or key words. The value of the data obviously depends on the accuracy of coding and the clarity of the record. Records contain many items that are clear to the physician but may be ambiguous to an outside data extractor. For example, the statement "heart: no abnormality" does not indicate how the doctor examined or investigated the heart. Information is reduced when it is recorded (van Ginneken, van der Lei, and Moorman, 1992). The richness of the clinical encounter that is characteristic of family practice becomes shrunk to an alphanumeric code.

One likely effect of the new electronic technologies is that physicians' decisions will be much more open to scrutiny and control by managers and governments. Whether or not this information is used wisely will have important implications for medicine. For example, when such information is combined with adherence to clinical practice guidelines as indicators of quality of care and these, in turn, tied to remuneration, strong forces are engaged. There is a real danger of turning the record into a "prescriptive technology," which is closely tied to compliance with outside standards (Franklin, 1999). It will take vigilance on the part of practitioners to avoid such an undesirable outcome.

References

Franklin U. 1999. *The Real World of Technology*: Revised Edition. Anansi, Toronto.

Ornstein SM, Oates RB, Fox GN. 1992. The computer-based medical record: Current status. *The Journal of Family Practice* 35(5):556.

van Ginneken AM, van der Lei J, Moorman PW. 1992. Towards unambiguous representation of patient data. Proceedings of the Annual Symposium on Computer Applications in Medical Care, p. 69.

Weed LL. 1968. Medical records that guide and teach. *New England Journal of Medicine* 278:593.

Notes

1. See pp. 74–75 for a critique of the terms subjective and objective.

2. For additional reading, see Institute of Medicine, Committee on improving the patient record. 1991. *The Computer-Based Patient Record: An Essential Technology for Health Care*. Washington, D.C.: National Academy Press.

18

Consultation and Referral

One of the most important duties of family physicians is the deployment of all the resources of medicine and society for their patients. Without the continuing care and responsibility of the family doctor, uncoordinated care by fragmented specialties can be both wasteful and dangerous. Effective communication with colleagues—both in medicine and the other health professions—is therefore an essential skill of family practice. A failure of communication can be as harmful to the patient as a missed diagnosis or an error of treatment. The complexity of modern medicine carries with it the risk of divided responsibility, a situation fraught with danger. The system of communication described in this chapter is designed to eliminate divided responsibility and clarify the lines of communication among colleagues.

Consultation

In consultation, the doctor responsible for the patient asks a colleague for his or her opinion about the patient. The term consultant in this context means "a person who is consulted" and implies no particular office. The person consulted may be a specialist, a family physician, or a member of one of the allied health professions. Although the opinion will obviously carry weight, it is not binding. The patient is at no time under the care of the consultant; unless referral follows consultation, the physician requesting consultation remains in charge. Because of their respective roles in the health-care system, most requests for consultation are from generalists to specialists. It is important to recognize, however, that other types of consultation do take place. A family physician may seek the opinion of another family physician who has a special area of interest and expertise. A specialist may seek the advice of the patient's family physician after referral has taken place.

Selection of the consultant most appropriate to the patient's needs is an important responsibility of the family physician. Case 8.5 gives an example of appropriate selection, where the attitude of the consultant played a crucial part in the patient's recovery.

A consultation may be formal or informal. Informal consultations are part of the daily language of medicine—on the telephone, in the corridor, or in the coffee room. Formal consultation is often a crucial episode in the patient's management. It should never be arranged or conducted in a casual manner. The following steps are necessary if the consultation is to be effective:

1. The physician requesting consultation should communicate directly with the consultant. In most cases, the communication should be in writing: either a letter, a note on the hospital chart, or a specially designed form sent by mail or electronic means. When the request is urgent, as in surgical consultation for an acute abdomen, a communication by telephone is an acceptable substitute. The ideal form of communication—not often attainable these days—is for the consultant and the doctor requesting consultation to see the patient together.
2. As a minimum, the letter requesting consultation should list all the significant problems of the patient, state the physician's main findings, the investigations that have been carried out, all medications that have been prescribed, and the purpose of the consultation. The reasons for consultation are many and varied: to help with a diagnostic puzzle, to advise on a specific course of treatment, to give an opinion on the significance of a test result or physical finding, or only to reassure the patient. Unless the consultant knows what question is being asked, he or she may waste time on unnecessary investigations and finish by answering the wrong question.
3. The reason for the consultation should be explained to the patient. It is important that the patient should not see consultation and referral as a rejection—a particular risk with psychiatric consultation.
4. The consultant should write back promptly (or telephone in urgent cases), giving his or her findings and opinion. If the consultant is unable to give an opinion, but thinks that another consultant would be appropriate, he or she should recommend this to the referring physician. The consultant should not refer the patient to another consultant himself or herself.

The patient's influence on the decision to refer appears to be high in most countries where it has been studied (European Study, 1992). A problem may occur when the patient requests a consultation. If physicians are unsure of themselves, they may interpret this as a lack of trust by the patient. Feelings of humiliation may lead the physician to refuse or resist the request or to agree to it with bad grace. A patient's request for another opinion should always be taken seriously, and it should be very exceptional not to agree to it readily. The situation can be avoided if the question of another opinion is first raised and discussed openly by the physician.

Failure to consult can often be traced to two causes: a failure by physicians to appreciate their own limitations and a feeling that consultation and referral are a personal defeat. My own observation of physicians is that a readiness to consult is usually a sign of maturity and self-confidence.

Problems may also arise when the referring physician disagrees with the consultant's opinion. In most medical schools, students are still taught mainly by specialists under conditions that tend to underemphasize the teacher's fallibility. When the young physician goes into practice, the authority vested in teachers becomes transferred to consultants. It then becomes very difficult to accept the fact that the consultant may be wrong, and even more difficult to take whatever steps may be required to protect the patient's interest. The fact is that when referring physician and consultant disagree, each has an equal chance of being correct. The special knowledge and experience of the consultant is balanced by the family physician's knowledge of the patient and his or her illness. Family physicians must, therefore, accept the possibility that consultants may be wrong. Two courses are open. First, the family physician can discuss the disagreement openly with the consultant. When there is no urgency, he or she may refer the patient back for a reconsideration. It is only fair that the consultant should have an opportunity to revise his or her opinion, perhaps in the light of new evidence. If this fails to resolve the issue, the family physician should then advise the patient of the disagreement and offer to obtain a third opinion if the patient so wishes. To reiterate a point made earlier, in consultation the referring physician remains fully responsible for the patient and must take whatever action is in the patient's interests. After referral, when responsibility for the patient is temporarily transferred, disagreements about the patient's care are more difficult to handle. The family physician's continuing responsibility, however, does require that he or she make any disagreement known, verbally and in writing, to the physician responsible for care. Another difficult problem for the family physician is a failure of rapport between patient and consultant. These situations require much tact and sensitivity.

Case 18.1

Following a lumpectomy for carcinoma of the breast a 66-year-old woman became extremely agitated and angry upon being told by her surgeon that she could go home. The patient's family physician, doing routine hospital rounds, encountered a woman who had closed herself up in her hospital room and refused to talk to anyone. By simply sitting and waiting he was able to determine that staying an extra day in hospital would alleviate some of her anxieties. The family physician communicated this to the surgeon who agreed to the extra stay. Weeks later, in talking about her feelings with her family physician, she recognized that she had the same feelings of vulnerability and anger as she experienced many years earlier when her life was threatened by an intruder in her home.

Referral

Referral implies a transfer of responsibility for some aspect of the patient's care. For the family physician, the transfer of responsibility is never total, for he or she always retains an overall responsibility for the patient's welfare. Even if the patient is having major surgery in some distant medical center, the family physician should still be available to patient, family, and surgeon.

The division of responsibility between referring physician and specialist must be clearly defined. This is made easier by defining the different types of referral:

1. **Interval referral.** The patient is referred for complete care for a limited period. The referring physician has no responsibilities during this period except those described above. A common example is the referral of a patient for major surgery or a major medical illness. It is essential to good care that after referral only the specialist should prescribe treatment. The family physician should advise and comment, but not order treatment unless asked to do so. This situation may arise, for example, if a patient develops a respiratory infection, skin rash, or mental breakdown following surgery. In these circumstances it would be natural for the surgeon to ask for the family physician's advice as a consultant with special knowledge of the patient and skill in dealing with common disorders.
2. **Collateral referral.** The referring physician retains overall responsibility, but refers the patient for care of some specific problem. The referral may be long term, as for chronic glaucoma, or short term, as for counseling for a psychological or social problem.
3. **Cross-referral.** The patient is advised to see another physician, and the referring physician accepts no further responsibility for the patient's care. This may occur after self-referral by the patient or even after referral by a family physician. In either case, the practice must be condemned, because it is wasteful of resources, demoralizing for the patient, and alienating for the family physician. If a consultant feels that another specialist's opinion is required, he or she should so inform the referring physician before making any referral himself or herself.
4. **Split referral.** This takes place under conditions of multispecialist practice, when responsibility is divided more or less evenly between two or more physicians, such as one for the patient's diabetes, another for his ischemic heart disease. The danger of this type of care is that nobody knows who has overall responsibility for the patient.

The danger of fragmented care is division of responsibility. This can all too easily lead to what Balint (1964) has called the "collusion of anonymity." This refers to decisions being made about a patient's management without a clear understanding of who is responsible for them. Although teamwork is necessary for good patient care, teams should not make decisions. It should always be clear who is responsible to the patient for clinical decisions.

Understanding the Decision to Refer

In studies of referral, the term referral is used to denote both consultation and referral as defined above. The referral rate is usually expressed as the number of referrals per 100 patient–doctor encounters (office or home). Studies on referral patterns have shown considerable variation among physicians. The 20% of physicians with the highest referral rates refer twice as many patients as the 20% with the lowest rates (Fleming, Cross, and Crombie, 1991; European study, 1992). No association has been found between referral rate and the age and social class mix of practice populations or the case mix among presenting patients. Two studies from the Netherlands have found distance from hospital (Gloerich, Schrijnemaekers, and van der Zee, 1989) and doctor's attitude to defensive medicine (Grol et al., 1990) to be weakly associated with referral rates. A study in 15 European countries showed a strong inverse relationship between referral rates and number of doctor–patient encounters. Low-referring doctors saw more patients in the working week than high-referring doctors. Two studies have reported higher referral rates in doctors who had higher levels of confidence and diagnostic certainty (Reynolds, Chitnis, and Roland, 1991; Calman, Hyman, and Licht, 1992).

It is clear from these descriptive studies that referral is a very complex process and that it is important not to jump to conclusions about associations between referral rates and quality of care. A good deal of quantitative descriptive data has been amassed, and there is a move now to explore the issues by qualitative methods and to base research on some conceptual framework. Dowie (1983) interviewed 45 physicians and found a relationship between higher referral rates and doctors' lack of self-confidence and defensiveness about referral. Muzzin (1991 a,b,c), who interviewed family doctors, consultants, and patients involved in 50 referrals, identified trust among physicians, consultants, and patients as the key to satisfactory referral. Bailey, King, and Newton (1994) applied an analytical framework to the referral decision in a study using both quantitative and qualitative methods. In the qualitative analysis, high referrers were more likely than low referrers to refer despite doubts about the usefulness of the referral (e.g., the effectiveness of treatment), and there was evidence of more uncertainty about decision making among the high referrers. There was no evidence that referral rates were related to patient-centeredness.

The Interface between Primary and Secondary Care

Successful referral depends on good communication among primary physician, consultant, and patient, and good communication is a reflection of the degree of integration among the primary, secondary, and tertiary sectors of the health services. In studying communication problems across these interfaces, it is important to attend to all participants in the process: patients, referring physicians, consultants, nurses, administrators, and staff. Communication problems are rarely the fault of any one person or group. Any solution to the problem will probably need intervention at several points in the communication network.

Wood (1993) and Wood and McWilliam(1996) addressed problems of communication between family physicians and oncologists by qualitative studies of both groups. The identified problem was that patients were followed by the cancer clinic rather than being referred back, even for straightforward conditions such as stage I breast cancer.

The greatest source of dissatisfaction among family physicians was the failure of oncologists to assign them a specific role in follow-up care. Poor communication was identified as the key problem: difficulty of reaching the right consultant, several specialists following the same patient, not enough direct communication by telephone, and lack of information about discharge and follow-up plans. Family physicians also shared some feelings that inhibited their assertiveness in making a role for themselves: lack of self-confidence, fear of a loss of specialist support, inadequate knowledge, and fear of being blamed for not doing enough.

These responses provide an insight into how a problem in one component can affect the function of the whole system. Family physicians who lack self-confidence will tend to withdraw from cancer care, and the very act of withdrawal will reduce their experience and further impair their self-confidence. Their lack of self-confidence will probably be sensed by their patients, who will see cancer or surgical clinics as their source of care. The load on the cancer clinic will increase, and the clinic—believing family physicians are not interested—might hire clinical assistants to help with the workload. Patients might receive subtle (if unintended) messages from the clinic that the family doctor is no longer involved in their care. That message can be conveyed simply by not mentioning the family physician.

The oncologists whom Wood interviewed viewed family physicians as very variable in their commitment to following up their cancer patients and in their knowledge of cancer therapy. Communication was often thwarted by lack of time, difficulty in contacting family doctors, and the rarity of a personal relationship. Oncologists were critical of family doctors for not sending information about tests done or illnesses occurring between visits to the clinic. They valued their relationships with their patients and felt a need to go on seeing some patients who were doing well.

Both family physicians and oncologists expressed a wish for closer collaboration and their suggestions for attaining this were very similar.

At the present stage in the evolution of health services, some progress has been made in horizontal integration at the primary care level. The major challenge in many systems is vertical integration between levels. Information technology is providing new tools for removing some of the difficulties. For other difficulties, however, the route to integration lies in dialogue and mutual understanding among primary care physicians, consultants, patients, and others.

Shared Care

Problems in the communication between primary and secondary care has increased the interest in the different kinds of shared care. Shared care is defined as: "the joint participation of hospital consultants and general practitioners in the planned delivery of care for patients with a chronic condition, informed by an enhanced information exchange over and above routine discharge and referral notices" (Hickman, Drummond, and Grimshaw, 1994).

Hickman et al. are in the process of developing a taxonomy of shared care systems which by 1994 had yielded six categories by questionnaire surveys:

1. Electronic mail, which requires a common database with multiple access points for all participating doctors and nurses.
2. Computer-assisted shared care, in which patients are recalled by a central database either to general practice or to hospital and an agreed data set collected for entry on to a central computer
3. Shared record cards, which can be either patient-held or posted back and forth between generalist and specialist.
4. Liaison meetings, used most frequently in mental health and drug dependency.
5. Regular communication by letter or standard record sheets. Basically a manual version of computer-assisted shared care.
6. Community clinic, where a consultant or specialist nurse conducts clinics in primary care.

Greenhalgh reviewed shared care for diabetes in 1994 commenting that the establishment of a successful shared care system is a complex exercise in change management.

She stresses the need for general practitioners to take ownership of the system. Some form of structured care is necessary. This means registering of patients at the time of diagnosis, recall, reminders, and regular review.

Frequent audits should be mandatory for all shared care systems, and the effects of the system on other parts of the practice be noted. As requirements change over time, the system will also have to change. Until recently, general practitioners were not expected to manage Type 1 diabetes. The increased use of insulin will soon be beyond the reach of the diabetologists. There is no reason why family physicians should not institute and manage insulin therapy.

References

Bailey J, King N, Newton P. 1994. Analyzing general practitioners' referral decisions. II. Applying the analytical framework: Do high and low referrers differ in factors influencing their referral decisions? *Family Practice* 11(1):9.

Balint M. 1964. *The Doctor, his Patient and the Illness*. London: Pitman Medical Publishing.

Calman NS, Hyman RB, Licht W. 1992. Variability in consultation rates and practitioner level of diagnostic certainty. *Journal of Family Practice* 35(1):31.

Dowie R. 1983. *General Practitioners and Consultants: A Study of Out-patient Referrals*. London: King Edwards Hospital Foundation.

The European Study of Referrals from Primary to Secondary Care. 1992. Report to the Concerted Action Committee of Health Services Research for the European Community. Occasional paper 56. Royal College of General Practitioners.

Fleming DM, Cross KW, Crombie DL. 1991. An examination of practice referral rates in relation to practice structure, patient demography, and case mix. *Health Trends* 23:100.

Gloerich ABM, Schrijnemaekers V, van der Zee J. 1989. Referrals in sentinel practices. In: Bartelds AIM, Fraucheboud J, van der Zee J, eds. *The Dutch Sentinel Practice Network: Relevance for Public Health Policy.* Utrecht: NIVEL.

Greenhalgh PM. 1994. Shared care for diabetes: A systematic review. Occasional Paper 67. Royal College of General Practitioners.

Grol R, Whitfield M, Maeseneer J de, et al. 1990. Attitudes to risk taking in medical decision making among British, Dutch, and Belgian general practitioners. *British Journal of General Practice* 40:134.

Hickman M, Drummond H, Grimshaw J. 1994. A taxonomy of shared care for chronic disease. *Journal of Public Health Medicine* 16(4):447.

Muzzin LJ. 1991a. Understanding the process of medical referral. Part 1: Critique of the literature. *Canadian Family Physician* 37:2155.

Muzzin LJ. 1991b. Understanding the process of medical referral. Part 2: Methodology of the study. *Canadian Family Physician* 37:2377.

Muzzin LJ. 1991c. Understanding the process of medical referral. Part 3: Trust and choice of consultant. *Canadian Family Physician* 37:2576.

Reynolds GA, Chitnis JG, Roland MO. 1991. General practitioner out-patient referrals: Do good doctors refer more patients to hospital? *British Journal of Medicine* 302:1250.

Wood ML. 1993. Communication between cancer specialists and family doctors. *Canadian Family Physician* 39:49.

Wood ML, McWilliam CL. 1996. Cancer in remission: Challenge in collaboration for family physician and oncologists. *Canadian Family Physician* 42:899.

19

The Health Professions

Family physicians can gain the maximum benefit for their patients only if they understand the role of each of the health professions. As in medicine, these roles are changing. The purpose of this chapter is to summarize the current roles of health professionals who work in collaboration with family physicians.

Nursing

Nurses in the community work in a number of roles:

1. Home care nurses provide nursing care for patients at home with acute or chronic illness, or after discharge from hospital. On visits, they may provide dressings, injections, monitoring of blood pressure and temperature or other signs, bed or tub baths, treatment of pressure areas, rehabilitation exercises, or any other nursing service. Home nursing may be a single service offered on request from the family doctor or part of an integrated home care service. The best arrangement is for the family physician and home care nurse to work together as a team. Attachment of nurses to practices is a good way of attaining this. Home care nurses may have special training and qualifications in such areas as intravenous therapy, ostomy care, nursing for the terminally ill, newborn care, or geriatric nursing.
2. Public health nurses (health visitors) are concerned chiefly with health education, prevention of disease and disability, and rehabilitation. They may work in prescribed geographical areas or be attached to a family group practice. In some areas, they are based in schools. Their responsibilities include health education for pregnant mothers, either individually or in groups; postnatal visiting at home with guidance on infant care and feeding; anticipatory guidance in child development; family planning advice; preparation of patients and their

families for hospitalization, and follow-up after discharge from the hospital; visiting patients with communicable diseases, including education for patient and family in preventing spread; guidance of patients with chronic disease; assessment of family function and home environment; assisting the physician by observation and appraisal of patients under care at home; and assessing the health status of elderly patients at home.

3. Midwives may work both in obstetric units and in the community, providing prenatal, intrapartum, and postpartum care in collaboration with obstetricians and family physicians.

4. Nurses as members of the primary care team. Increasingly, nurses and family physicians are working together as a team. The day-to-day working relationship can allow the roles of doctor and nurse to evolve according to the local context and their individual skills. The nurse may be available to patients with new clinical problems, responsible for following up patients with chronic diseases such as diabetes and asthma, carrying out screening procedures, or counseling patients with special needs.

5. Specialized roles in nursing. Many nursing specialties have emerged in recent years. Some of these, such as intensive care and oncology nursing, do not have major involvement in primary care. Other specialist nurses work closely with family physicians. The success of shared care depends very much on the liaison role of nurses specializing in such fields as diabetes care and psychiatric nursing. Nurses specializing in palliative care often work closely with family physicians.

Nurses and physicians have a great deal to learn from each other. Physicians can learn from the special expertise of nurses and also from the different perspective the discipline of nursing brings to patient care. As a member of a palliative care team, I learned from nurses how to assess a patient's level of pain and discomfort and how important attention to the smallest detail is in the care of seriously ill patients. To be a helpful colleague to a nurse, a physician has to maintain the clinical diagnostic and therapeutic skills on which the nurse relies. If a palliative care nurse needs help with pain control, the physician will be helpful only if he or she is well informed. In many cases, the key role of the family physician will be to contribute his or her store of knowledge about patient and family, so that decisions about care are in accordance with the patient's values and preferences. For example, it may not be appropriate to mobilize multiple resources for a family that has always been very private and self-sufficient.

The role of nurse-practitioner is now much discussed. The term, however, is used differently in different jurisdictions. In some, a nurse-practitioner is a nurse with additional training in medical diagnosis and management. The role may therefore overlap considerably with the role of physician. This has some potential for causing problems both for nursing and for medicine. If the overlap is small, and the nurse functions as a physician's assistant, the role may become a subprofessional one, and the team may lose the benefit of a nursing perspective. On the other hand, if the overlap is large, nurse-practitioners may replace physicians and are likely to be redefined as physicians at some future time. This is what happened historically when apothecaries became redefined as medical practitioners (see p. 5). Other professionals have much to learn from nursing's unique approach to patient care, and it is important that this not be lost as nurses move into new roles.

Occupational Therapy

Occupational therapy uses activities to help patients regain lost function and develop their abilities. The activities range from everyday tasks such as eating and dressing to creative work and activities involving interpersonal relationships. Occupational therapists are skilled in assessing patients' capacity for work or activities of daily living and in prescribing programs to meet their needs. They have an important part to play in the rehabilitation of patients with such common problems as stroke, amputation, arthritis, multiple sclerosis, and mental disorder. Assessments in the home are particularly important in occupational therapy, for they may lead to appropriate changes in the physical layout of the home. Occupational therapists also work with disabled children to help them develop new skills.

Physiotherapy (Physical Therapy)

Physiotherapists are concerned with the assessment, maintenance, and improvement of bodily function. As with medicine, the view of bodily function as separable from mental function is giving place to a more organismic view of function as an expression of well-being of the whole person. An assessment based on this view includes an examination of the whole body as well as part where symptoms are localized. It also includes attention to the patient's feelings and experiences, bodily flexibility, and breathing (Thornquist, 1992). Mental states are associated with bodily dysfunction, and physical therapy can improve mental well-being, even in schizophrenia (Roxerdal, 1985).

Physiotherapists are trained to be generalists. Some differentiation of role occurs, depending on the graduate's field of work. Most physiotherapists work in three areas: musculoskeletal disorders and injuries, neurological disorders, and cardiopulmonary disorders. Physiotherapists have a major role in rehabilitation. Some develop expertise in more specific fields, such as sports medicine.

Physiotherapists who work in primary care teams have excellent opportunities for the prevention of disability by early intervention and health education. Family physicians can also form useful links with physiotherapists who have special expertise in chronic pain, stress management (relaxation, breathing control), and manipulation.

Medical Social Work

The aim of social work is to help people improve their social functioning. Difficulties with social functioning may arise from acute or chronic physical illness, poverty, mental or physical handicaps, unemployment, or problems with relationships.

The following are all common social work functions: assessing the emotional and social components of illness; obtaining a social history to learn the patient's past behavior patterns and to relate these to current problems; identifying families who are at risk for mental and social breakdown so that preventive measures can be taken; assessing eligibility for assistance programs; establishing liaison with appropriate community resources; individual counseling, such as for unmarried mothers, isolated persons, and patients with problems of personality or relationships; marital and family counseling for problems arising from relationships within the family.

Referrals to a social worker are especially helpful when problems with relationships are an important aspect of a patient's illness or when support from community resources is needed.

Clinical Psychology

Clinical psychologists offer a variety of methods for helping patients and families to identify and solve their problems. The approach taken by any particular psychologist will probably emerge from one of three psychological theories of personality development and human behavior: psychodynamic, behavioral, or humanistic. The main goal of those adhering to a psychodynamic orientation is to bring unconscious conflicts into awareness through exploratory and analytic or interpretative techniques. With the behavioral orientation, problems are approached with a view to correcting behavior patterns assessed either by the individual or by society as maladaptive. The humanistic approach focuses on the self-actualizing forces believed to be inherent in each individual that, when blocked, produce emotional distress or other symptoms of disrupted functioning. A fundamental aspect of this approach is that growth and change occur in the context of certain necessary relationship conditions: unconditional positive regard, genuineness, and empathic understanding.

Any of these therapeutic approaches can be applied to a wide variety of problems and symptoms, ranging from family dysfunction to psychophysiological symptoms, phobias, or other disruptions of functioning associated with anxiety, depression, or breaks from reality. Family physicians are often in the best position to assess the needs and capacities of the patient requiring psychological intervention, and therefore to match the patient with the most appropriate therapist and therapeutic approach.

In addition to providing psychotherapeutic services for the patients of family doctors, the clinical psychologist can serve as consultant to the family physician for a variety of purposes. First, the psychologist will often have some expertise in developmental psychology. Thus, the patient's symptoms or behaviors may be interpretable as a reflection of some developmental crisis. The psychologist can assist in putting the symptoms in perspective, acknowledging their adaptive as well as maladaptive functions. Second, the psychologist can work with the physician in sorting out organic from psychophysiological symptoms and as a consequence minimize intrusive investigation, as well as suggest treatment or management strategies. In addition, the psychologist can facilitate understanding and management of patients' problems in living when the patient will not accept a referral to the psychologist or some other allied professional. Finally, the psychological consultation can be useful in helping the physician to deal with problems in the patient–doctor relationship, and with difficult patients—for example, the uncompliant or superficially compliant patient, persons addicted to drugs or alcohol, or patients and their families who are in the process of dealing with illness or dying.

Behavioral Therapy

Behavioral therapy techniques developed by psychologists have proved useful in the treatment of such diverse conditions as chronic pain, depression, physical disabilities, addictions, psychophysiologic symptoms, and phobias (Bakal, 1979; Russell, 1986). The techniques can be broadly classified as conditioning, biofeedback, cognitive therapy, and relaxation training. Besides being used by psychologists, these can also be used by physicians and physiotherapists.

Conditioning

Behavior is related in two ways to environmental stimuli. Respondent behavior is controlled by preceding stimulus events. An unconditioned stimulus produces a response by direct association, as when a dog salivates at the arrival of food. A conditioned stimulus produces a response by association, as when a dog salivates at the sound of a bell that has previously been paired with the arrival of food. Classical conditioning is the process of learning to respond to conditioned stimuli.

Operant behavior is affected by events following the behavior. If the behavior is followed by reinforcement, the behavior is increased, a process known as operant conditioning. Positive reinforcement is any event that increases the behavior that preceded it. Negative reinforcement occurs when a behavior is increased after withdrawal of a negative stimulus.

Conditioning is used in a number of ways to modify behavior. In counterconditioning, the fear or anxiety produced by the stimulus is replaced by an alternative learned response. A maladaptive behavior may be reduced by removing the reinforcement. For example, an overdependent patient who makes frequent demands for attention will be reinforced in this behavior if the physician responds to it by meeting every demand. If, on the other hand, he provides regular appointments and does not respond to demands between appointments, the behavior will cease to be reinforced and is likely to decrease in frequency. A patient with chronic pain who receives an analgesic on demand will be reinforced in his pain behavior. Regular analgesic medication at set times with no response in between will tend to reduce the behavior.

In aversive conditioning, the response is accompanied by an unpleasant stimulus, as in the administration of Antabuse to alcoholics. Much of what we do to improve compliance with therapy is a form of conditioning. By removing unpleasant side effects, we reduce their aversive effects. To help patients to remember to take their medication, we try to associate it with certain cues, such as keeping the pill bottle by the shaving gear.

Often patients are unaware of the stimuli that produce symptoms or behavioral responses. Their awareness can be increased by asking them to keep a diary recording the events and sensations that precede or accompany the onset of a symptom. The patient thus develops self-knowledge, and the physician becomes aware of the stimuli that have to be either removed or responded to differently.

Cognitive Therapy
This is based on the observation that conditions such as depression and chronic pain are maintained by thought processes such as inappropriate perceptions, interpretations, expectations, and coping responses. A depressed businessman may misinterpret certain cues as indicating that his business is on the rocks. A patient with chronic pain may have developed responses that actually increase the pain rather than relieving it. Cognitive therapy aims to teach the patient different ways of responding and coping.

Cognitive therapy is designed to provide the patient with a conceptual framework for understanding the nature of his or her problem. The patient learns a different way of coping with the problem. Instead of responding to physiological and psychological cues with a panic reaction or anxiety-producing thoughts, the patient uses them to trigger the coping responses for which he or she has been trained.

Relaxation Training
The relaxation response (Benson, 1975) is a physiological and psychological state in which there is decreased activity of the sympathetic nervous system, diminished muscle tension, and mental tranquility. It is induced by sitting or lying in a comfortable position, breathing deeply, systematically relaxing each muscle group in turn, emptying the mind of all thoughts, and repeating a sound or word over and over again. The technique is similar to the practice of meditative prayer practiced in all the major religions. The theory of relaxation training is that it counteracts the fight or flight arousal mechanism, which is an ineffective response to psychological stressors.

Biofeedback
Biofeedback is a technique for giving a person some control over physiological systems that normally function beneath the level of awareness. The method is that of control by negative feedback, an important principle of cybernetics and system theory (see p. 76). Physiological processes such as skin temperature, pulse rate, blood pressure, and skeletal muscle contraction are electronically monitored and displayed to the individual. Although biofeedback has been used successfully in conditions like recurrent headache, it is not clear that the relief of symptoms actually depends on the feedback mechanism. It may work by giving the patient a cognitive coping strategy. All the methods discussed here are ways of giving

patients more control of their own bodies—one of the three conditions considered necessary for the placebo effect.

Case 8.5 provided an example of the application of behavioral therapy principles. In this case the principles were applied by the physicians and physiotherapist, without the involvement of a psychologist. The first physician was reinforcing the patient's panic reaction to chest pain by doing an ECG every time the patient came. The second physician helped to extinguish this behavior by arranging annual visits to a cardiologist and placing a moratorium on ECGs between these visits. The physiotherapist reduced the stimuli leading to panic reactions and reinforced behavior that increased the patient's activity. The family physician used cognitive therapy to help the patient to change her perception of what was happening to her. The doctor also reduced and then discontinued the medication, which was reinforcing the patient's belief in her invalidism.

Dietetics (Nutrition)

Two aspects of a dietitians's work of special importance to the family physician are nutrition education and dietary problems. The dietitian provides instruction to various groups in the community: pregnant women, mothers of young children, and elderly people.

The most common problems requiring dietary counseling are obesity, diabetes, hyperlipidemia, and digestive disorders. Individual or group counseling may be used. Nutritionists also have a key role in enteral and parenteral nutrition.

Pharmacy

With the declining use of mixtures, the role of the pharmacist has changed from dispensing medicines to advising both physicians and patients on the use of drugs. As a consultant to the physician, the pharmacist has an important role in advising on dosage, side effects, contraindications, and drug incompatibilities. For patients, the pharmacist interprets the physician's instructions on how drugs should be taken. In many communities, pharmacists are widely used by the public for advice on treatment of common disorders such as colds, dyspepsia, and enteritis. The rapid development of drug therapy has increased the importance of communication between family physician and pharmacist. If the physician can identify the pharmacists who are filling most of his or her prescriptions, it is helpful if this communication can be at the personal level.

Chiropody and Podiatry

Proper care of feet, especially in individuals with diabetes, is an important part of comprehensive care. Monitoring and responding to early problems is essential to avoid complications such as the diabetic foot.

The title chiropodist is gradually being replaced by podiatrist depending on the country. In some jurisdictions they are legislatively distinct with chiropodists having a narrower scope of practice. Podiatrists in many countries describe their scope of practice as including disorders of the foot, ankle, knee, leg, and hip.

The Team Concept

No one profession can meet all of patients' needs, hence the need to work together in teams. There are strengths, but also pitfalls, in team work. There are also misconceptions about what team work is. We distinguish three types of teams: core, greater, and ad hoc.

The *core team* is a team in which the members work together, day in day out, closely integrated in the performance of a special task. Some common examples are the doctor–nurse teams that operate intensive care units, palliative care units, and family practices. In family practice, the team may include office nurses, public health nurses (health visitors), and home care nurses if they are based in the practice. By working closely together, the team members can develop a strong mutual understanding that can greatly enhance patient care.

To attain this, however, requires close attention to team morale and to communication between members. A group is a team only in name if it does not meet together frequently and regularly. Regular meetings should be held to discuss patients, but some meetings should also be devoted to team function and to the support of its members. Mutual respect is a key principle of team function and this cannot be attained unless each member's views are listened to with respect. Being a member of a true team means being prepared to have one's actions and views challenged—sometimes a difficult thing for physicians to accept. Each team member has his or her own role, but roles do overlap, and there are many decisions in which different team members have a very legitimate stake. In deciding how to manage a patient addicted to tranquilizers, for example, or whether a patient with terminal cancer should be given an antibiotic for pneumonia, both nurses and physicians have much to contribute, even though the physician is the one who writes the prescription. Because decisions are discussed freely and openly, it does not mean that there is blurring of responsibility. Once the decision is arrived at, the responsibility for its implementation should be clearly assigned. Blurred responsibility and fragmentation of care are signs of a poorly functioning team. One of the most important responsibilities of the team leadership is the maintenance of morale, especially a team where there is a high level of work stress. The key to maintaining morale is the care and support given to each team member. When a team has urgent and difficult daily tasks to perform, it is all too easy for the welfare of team members to lose its priority. In a study of intensive care and palliative care teams Vachon (1987) found that stress and "burnout" were much less frequent on teams where the welfare of members was the first priority of the leadership.

The *greater team* is the core team plus additional members who join the team for a specific function, but who are only involved when their services are needed. One of these members may perform the same function on several core teams as, for example, when a social worker in a health center works with several family practice nurse–physician teams. There is a similar need for team meetings, mutual respect, and open discussion. The relationship of these members with the team, however, is somewhat different in that they are less involved on a day-to-day basis and usually have their home in another administrative unit.

The *ad hoc team* is a team assembled for a particular patient and exists only for that patient. *Case 8.5* was an example. The family physician brought together a cardiologist and a physiotherapist to work with the patient on her problem. It was not necessary for the team to meet; it was essential, however, for their activities to be coordinated and for a common purpose to be understood. Without leadership, the result would have been fragmentation of care. In the modern health care system, fragmentation is an all too common problem.

References

Bakal DA. 1979. *Psychology and Medicine: Psychobiological Dimensions of Health and Illness*. New York: Springer.

Benson H. 1975. *The Relaxation Response*. New York: Morrow.

Roxerdal G. 1985. *Body Awareness Therapy and the Body Awareness Scale: Treatment and Evaluation in Psychiatric Physiotherapy*. Department of Rehabilitation Medicine, University of Goteborg, Sweden.

Russell ML. 1986. *Behavioral Counseling in Medicine*. New York: Oxford University Press.

Thornquist E. 1992. Examination and communication: A study of first encounters between patients and physiotherapists. *Family Practice* 9:195.

Vachon MLS. 1987. *Occupational Stress in the Care of the Critically Ill, the Dying, and the Bereaved*. Washington: Hemisphere Publishing Corp.

20

The Community Service Network

Family physicians are accustomed to thinking of themselves as part of the medical network, deploying the services of numerous specialists for the benefit of their patients. Their familiarity with the medical system arises from the hospital-centered education that is the norm in most medical schools. This educational environment, however, does not help them to understand that the physician is only one of many resources within the community for helping people to deal with their interrelated health and social problems. Unless family physicians have good lines of communication with these services and an awareness of what they have to offer, their effectiveness will be severely limited. The purpose of this chapter is to give a general description of the community service network. Although there are differences of detail between different jurisdictions, and between urban and rural communities, all advanced industrialized societies have support systems of the kind described here.

These services are important to family physicians in two ways. First, they can be a source of information about their patients. This applies especially to those two health services that are concerned with people's working lives: the school and industrial health services. Second, they can provide support and help of many different kinds. Family physicians starting in practice or moving to a new area should make every effort to learn about the local network of services, preferably by developing personal relationships with the people they will be dealing with regularly. The medical officer of health and his or her staff are particularly important for the family physician. It is important also to educate practice staff in the need to keep lines of communication open. Nothing is more infuriating for a nurse than to find that when he or she tries to speak to a family physician about one of the physician's patients, the route is blocked by an overprotective nurse or receptionist.

Public Health

Public Health and family physicians are natural allies in developing and maintaining systems for prevention of illness and promotion of health. Establishing and maintaining contact with the local Public Health Department is an important linkage between the family physician and the broader health care system. Very successful models have included a defined Public Health Nurse (PHN) attachment to community practitioners which enhances communication and establishes a continuum of care between family physicians and Public Health. The PHN becomes a member of the core team and provides in-home well baby visits to new mothers, evaluation of the isolated elderly, and teen outreach programs.

Doug Campos-Outcalt (2004) defines five functions that family physicians should fulfill as a part of the Public Health system: (1) implementing recommended preventive services guidelines in their practices; (2) serving as the front line of the surveillance system (e.g., as a sentinel physician); (3) appropriately referring to the Public Health Department (e.g., for prenatal classes or early child care classes); (4) accepting referrals from the Public Health Department (e.g., new patients who do not have a family physician); and (5) interacting constructively with the local health department. He goes on to suggest four levels of Public Health expertise beginning with basic, and progressing through intermediate and advanced, to leadership. Each of these levels has defined knowledge and skills. All family physicians should have basic level expertise, those engaged as sentinel clinicians should have intermediate level knowledge and skills. Those who wish to be involved more deeply as consultants, medical directors, or to serve on Boards of Health require advanced knowledge and skills. Generally those engaged in leadership roles have taken extra degree courses such as a Masters in Public Health (MPH).

Services for Children

All advanced societies have legislation to protect and safeguard the welfare of children. All have either official or voluntary bodies responsible for the welfare of children. These organizations deal with such matters as the following:

Investigations of allegations that children may be in need of protection
Counseling for family problems
Placing children in foster homes, group homes, or institutions
Supervision of children in care
Counseling for expectant unmarried mothers
Adoption
Prevention of childhood problems by community work and education in
    parenthood

Day-care centers are an important source of help for families with preschool children, especially single parent families. Not only can the children be assured of care by competent, trained workers, but parents themselves can also learn about child rearing.

Under this heading should be included services to parents and expectant parents: prenatal groups run by nurses, groups for young parents run by various social agencies, and self-help groups for parents with difficulties.

All societies have agencies for helping mentally and physically disabled children. These usually provide the parents and family doctor with a skilled assessment of the child together with advice and support in his long-term care and education. Agencies also exist for aid to children with specific disabilities such as blindness, deafness, cerebral palsy, muscular dystrophy, cystic fibrosis, and other conditions.

School Health and Guidance Services

School health services were at first concerned mainly with the physical health of schoolchildren. As child health improved, attention shifted toward learning disabilities and behavior disorders that impair learning. Children may be referred to the health and guidance services either by a teacher or by the family doctor. Because school behavior problems often have their origins in family disturbance, the family is usually involved in the assessment. Information provided by the family physician may, therefore, be very helpful to the school. The prescription for the child may include special learning measures, family counseling, and drug treatment for attention deficit disorder.

The presentation of school learning and behavior problems to the family physician is an indication for consultation with the school. Investigation of the problem can then be planned jointly between family doctor and educational services. It is important for the family physician to be aware of the services available within the school system in the area. These may include guidance, psychological services, speech therapy, and special education. Public Health Nurses are often attached to schools, and school physicians may be involved in the diagnosis and management of learning and behavior disorders.

Industrial Health Services

All industrial societies have legislation governing industrial health and safety. Large industrial plants often have their own full-time industrial nurse, working either with or without a visiting medical officer who is often a family physician. The medical officer is responsible for advising the company on the health and safety of the workforce, the prevention of industrial accidents and diseases, and the implementation of legislation on industrial health. The medical officer should communicate with the family physician when a patient is injured or taken ill at work, when the patient is returning to work after illness or injury, or when poor work performance or absenteeism is an early sign of illness.

Successful rehabilitation of a worker may depend on a graduated return to employment or a change of job within the same industry. In either case, collaboration with the industrial medical officer is important. Industrial nurses and medical officers often get to know workers very well and may be the first to identify signs of ill health. The first sign of alcoholism, for example, may be Monday morning absenteeism. Information provided by the industrial nurse may, therefore, be very important to the family physician. An industry may also have its own rehabilitation program for sick or injured workers.

Although communication with industrial health services is important, a word of caution is necessary about communication with employers. The family physician's responsibility is to the patient, not to the employer. Information about the patient should never be provided to the employer without the patient's consent.

Mental Health Services

The earlier discharge of patients from psychiatric hospitals has not only placed more responsibility on the family physician, but also created a need for more community services for the mentally ill. These include "half-way house" accommodation, rehabilitation workshops, follow-up visits, and group therapy by social workers. Special units for alcoholics and drug addicts exist in most communities, in addition to self-help groups like Alcoholics Anonymous.

Many urban communities also have crisis services based on the model of the Samaritans movement in Great Britain. People in despair can call a number where they will be able to talk to trained volunteers. Some services also provide face-to-face counseling for those in despair and contemplating suicide.

Services for the Elderly

All services in the home are important for the elderly—nursing, physiotherapy, occupational therapy. "Meals on Wheels" delivers nutritious hot meals. Day hospitals provide assessment, rehabilitation, recreation, and social activities.

Churches, service clubs, and volunteer organizations provide support services and arrange social activities. Geriatric units provide short-term admissions for patients so that their families can have a break.

Home Care Services

Nurses, occupational therapists, physiotherapists, and podiatrist (chiropodists) all do home visiting. In some areas their services are integrated with homemaker services in a home care program. Integrated home care may be helpful for patients discharged from the hospital, for patients treated at home for acute or chronic illness, and for terminal illness.

Self-Help and Mutual-Help Groups

Many organizations exist for patients with specific diseases, such as cancer, multiple sclerosis, diabetes, arthritis, and chronic obstructive pulmonary disease

(COPD). They may provide wheelchairs, walking aids, transportation, financial aid, support and counseling for families, visitors for patients after mastectomy, amputation, or colostomy, and education for patients and families

Some provide group therapy and support, such as the various organizations that are available for people who are overweight. Others provide group support for the bereaved or for relatives of patients with disorders such as schizophrenia and developmental delay.

Volunteers

Besides the formal network of community services, there also exists in all communities a more informal system of volunteer services. Some of these are extensions of churches, service clubs, and women's organizations. Some exist at the neighborhood level—good neighbors who rally round at times of crisis or need. Knowledge of these resources is very helpful to the family physician. In many communities, volunteer organizations exist to provide such services as providing meals on wheels, visiting the isolated and lonely, transporting patients, and working on hospital units.

Location of Basic Services

A family physician new to a community will find workers administering government support programs in a courthouse, city hall, township office, or other government facility. Children's Aid Societies are a source of information on family and children's services. Libraries have government publications describing universal services complete with addresses of branch offices.

References

Campos-Outcalt D. 2004. Public health and family medicine: An opportunity. *Journal of the American Board of Family Medicine* 17:207–211.

21

Alternative or Complementary Medicine

Alternative, complementary, or unconventional medicine[1] (CAM) is the name given to those medical practices not usually available in mainstream institutions and not usually taught in medical and other professional schools. Although seemingly ambiguous, this definition reflects the history of the relationship of these practices to mainstream medicine, which, after all, only delineated itself scarcely 150 years ago. Those practices outside the mainstream were designated alternative, but as some of them achieve greater acceptance they are considered complementary to conventional medicine and, in some instances, may be fully accepted as mainstream. However, the vagueness of this definition does lead to problems in a number of areas. Some practices that are alternative in one country may, by reason of history and custom, be included in the professional sector of another. Homeopathy in North America is generally considered nonconventional, but in the United Kingdom it enjoys greater acceptance and is best described as spanning the folk and professional sectors of health care. Osteopathy in the United States has status similar to conventional medical doctors. Midwives in many countries have crossed the boundary from alternative to professional sector and provide a significant proportion of maternity care. Such "crossovers" undoubtedly influence both the former "alternative" practices and mainstream medicine. Even in countries with the most advanced systems of medical care and the most effective technology, the use of alternative medicine is widespread. In the United States, a national population survey showed that one in three people used at least one unconventional therapy over a 12-month period. Two-thirds of these did so without visiting a provider of unconventional therapy. Of respondents reporting at least one of the 10 most common medical conditions, 25% used an unconventional therapy, and 10% visited a provider of unconventional therapy. The frequency of use of unconventional therapy among all the conditions studied was highest for back problems (36%), anxiety (28%), headaches (27%), chronic pain (27%), and cancer (24%). Of people reporting a principal medical condition who used an unconventional therapy, only 4% saw a provider of unconventional therapy without also seeing a medical doctor. No respondents saw a provider of unconventional therapy for cancer, diabetes, lung problems, skin problems, high blood pressure, or urinary tract problems without also seeing a medical doctor. Eighty-nine percent of respondents who saw a provider of unconventional therapy during the year did so without the recommendation of their physician, and 72% did not inform their doctor of the use of unconventional therapy (Eisenberg et al., 1993). In Canada 75% of people over the age of 15 used one or more natural health products in 2001 and 12% of those over the age of 12 attended an alternative practitioner in the year before the survey. The most frequent was chiropractor (11%), massage therapist (8%), and acupuncturists (2%). Over time, the use of CAM has increased so that by 1998, total expenditures in the US on alternative therapies was $21.2 billion (Eisenberg, 1998).

Widespread use of alternative therapies in other countries has also been reported (Ministry of Health [Netherlands], 1981; Fulder and Munro, 1985; MacLennan, Wilson, and Taylor, 1996). Comprehensive reports on alternative medicine have been published by the British Medical Association (1993) and the Netherlands Ministry of Health and Environmental Protection (1981). In the United States, the National Institute of Health has established an Office for the Study of Unconventional Medical Practices.

In considering why there is so much interest in CAM, one study in the United States found that those who utilized CAM, felt it aligned more with their values, and about beliefs toward health and life. They tended not to reject conventional medicine, but combined it with CAM (Astin, 1998). For several reasons, family doctors should be well informed about alternative medicine. They should be in a position to advise patients who wish to use alternative therapies. Some unconventional therapies are known to be effective for certain conditions; some are potentially dangerous if used without a diagnostic assessment; some remedies are toxic and others may interact with medically prescribed drugs; many therapies are harmless and, although not supported by good evidence, may give comfort to the patient. Because many alternative practitioners are not members of self-regulating professional bodies, the public has very little protection against charlatans. Family doctors may be in a position to protect patients from harm or exploitation, especially if they have knowledge of local providers. The help that a family doctor can give will be enhanced if there is openness between doctor and patient and if the doctor is perceived as unbiased.

Family medicine has often served as a portal for the entry of CAM practices into mainstream medicine. Many family physicians combine acupuncture and conventional medicine, for example. "Integrative medicine" explicitly exists at the boundary of conventional medical practice and CAM. This relationship should not be surprising considering the overlap in the values shared by both. Family medicine, like some of the CAM practices emphasizes the diagnosis of the patient, not only a disease, seeking to understand the biological, psychological, and social dimensions and their interactions. Even when a patient's health belief system exists outside the mainstream, the family physician affirms its importance if it advances the health of the patient. Like some CAM practices, family medicine emphasizes the development of a cooperative relationship with patients. That there is such an overlap in values has been attributed to the common roots of general practice and some CAM practices in the humoral medicine of Hippocrates (Greaves, 2003). Greaves argues that alternative medicine is a continuation of humoral medicine which emphasizes the need for balance within the body and its parts and recognizes the strong relationship between mental and physical processes. When the biomedical model became dominant in the mid-nineteenth century, humoral medicine and its practitioners were relegated to the 'alternative' category. General practice, although part of conventional medicine, never fully severed its roots in the former humoral tradition.

Alternative to What?

Unconventional therapy is defined in terms of its opposite: conventional or mainstream medicine. However, there are different ways a therapy can be unconventional. Conventional medicine has a number of levels. Its foundation, as in all sciences, is a set of assumptions about what the world is like. These assumptions are neither questioned nor made explicit (Kuhn, 1967). They may take the form of metaphors, such as the metaphor of nature as a machine. At another level, medicine has theories that can be tested experimentally for their coherence and truth. On the practical level, therapies are derived from theories and are subject to testing for their effectiveness. When medicine is at its best all these levels are congruent with each other. Assumptions are reasonable, theories have stood up to empirical testing, and therapies derived from the theories shown by clinical trials to be effective. Often, however, this is not the case. Therapies that should work in theory, do not work in practice; a therapy derived from an inadequate theory may prove to be very effective. The strength of modern medicine is its insistence that a therapy should prove itself experimentally, however well founded its theory.

Some unconventional medicine is an alternative at all these levels. Traditional Chinese medicine is based on a worldview totally different from that of Western medicine. Its theory of disease is at variance with Western science. On the other hand, acupuncture can be evaluated by clinical trial and can be adopted by mainstream medicine without subscribing to the theory from which it is derived. Chiropractic theory has no empirical foundation, but chiropractic manipulation is effective for certain conditions. Hypnosis was for a long time rejected by mainstream medicine because of its theory of animal magnetism. Now, hypnosis is recognized as an effective therapy in some circumstances, and the theory of animal magnetism has been abandoned. Some alternative paradigms and theories have deep roots in the tradition of Western medicine. The various movements in medicine that come under the term holistic, for example, have roots in the Hippocratic tradition.

In medical education there has been an increasing recognition of the need to include some exposure of medical students to CAM (Wetzel, Kaptchuk, Haramati, and Eisenberg, 2003). In a survey of medical schools in the United States, it was found that among 53 responding institutions (out of 73), most provided only a minimal amount of contact hours. Topics that tended to be emphasized were acupuncture (76.7%), herbs and botanicals (69.9%), meditation and relaxation (65.8%) spirituality/faith/prayer (64.4%), chiropractic (60.3%), homeopathy (57.5%), and nutrition and diets (50.7%) (Brokaw, Tunnicliff, Raess, and Saxon, 2002).

Categories of Alternative Medicine

Alternative medical practices come in a bewildering variety. The British Medical Association Report listed 116 therapies. Most of these fall into one of the following categories:

1. Ancient medical traditions such as Chinese medicine: a complete paradigm, theory, and range of therapeutic practices.
2. Shamanistic healing in traditional societies that retain their links with the past. Although using herbal medicines, the shaman is distinguished by an initiation that is believed to confer power over the spirit world. The healing process often involves altered states of consciousness and includes members of the patient's family and community.
3. Folk medicine: lore handed down through generations, often about medical properties of plants. Some modern drugs and practices had their origins in folklore—for example, smallpox vaccination, quinine, digitalis, ergotamine, colchicine.
4. Alternative paradigms and practices with recent roots in Western societies: homeopathy, osteopathy, chiropractic, anthroposophic medicine, naturopathy.
5. Nutritional therapies, ranging from herbal medicines to dietary regimes.
6. Body therapies, including many kinds of massage.
7. Spiritual healing, either within the mainstream religions or by individuals claiming to have special powers.
8. Individual therapies, either borrowed from other traditions or developed autonomously: acupuncture, biofeedback, hypnotherapy, meditation, imaging.

The availability and use of these different therapies varies from one country to another. In the United States, osteopathy has become so close to conventional medicine that osteopaths are often regarded as equivalent to medical doctors. Chiropractic is prominent in the United States and Canada, and in several Canadian provinces chiropractic services are covered by medicare. Naturopathy is widespread in Germany. Homeopathy is practiced by significant numbers of medical doctors in several European countries.

One useful taxonomy of unconventional healing practices is provided by Kaptchuk and Eisenberg (2005). In this taxonomy, there are two very broad divisions: CAM and parochial unconventional medicine. The largest division, CAM, is then subdivided into professional systems (chiropractic, acupuncture, homeopathy, naturopathy, massage, and dual-trained physicians), popular health reform (mega-vitamins, nutritional supplements, botanicals, macrobiotics, organic food, vegan diet), New Age healing (esoteric energies, crystals and magnets, spirits and mediums, reiki, qigong), mind–body (Deepak Chopra, Bernie Siegel, Course in Miracles, Silva Mind Control, biofeedback, hypnosis, guided imagery, relaxation response, cognitive-behavioral therapy), and non-normative (chelation, antineoplastons, pleomorphic bacteria cancer therapy, iridology, hair analysis). Parochial unconventional medicine has three divisions: ethno-medicine (Puerto-Rican spiritualism, African-American rootwork, Haitian voodoo, Hmong practices, Mexican-American curonaderismo), religious healing (Pentecostal churches, Catholic charismatic renewal, Christian Science), and folk medicine practices (copper bracelets for arthritis, chicken soup for the common cold, red string for nosebleed). To this taxonomy some would add a category called the popular sector which includes self-medication, advise from pharmaceuticals, advise from family, friends and self- help groups (Helman, 2001).

Common Alternative Practices

The frequency with which alternative medicine is used makes it advisable for family doctors to have a basic knowledge of the common practices, their claims, their benefits, and their risks. Some of them are better thought of as complementary to conventional medicine rather than alternative to it. Evaluating the usefulness of various CAM therapies is difficult for the practitioner due to the relative lack of high quality evaluative studies. This is to some extent rooted in the different epistemologies of many CAM practices and conventional medicine. The latter places highest value on randomized control trials and replicability, and is rooted in a reductionist framework. CAM practitioners would argue that a broader framework is necessary and credence given to different types of knowledge if we are to fully understand and help our patients. Most family physicians would agree. There are useful references available for the practitioner and some of these are listed at the end of the chapter. Websites have the advantage of being more frequently updated and easier to access than textbooks.

Manipulation

Manipulation can be effective in relieving spinal pain or pain resulting from mechanical or degenerative causes in the vertebrae. One mechanism of pain relief, common to manipulation, acupuncture, massage, and transcutaneous electrical nerve stimulation, is thought to be the release of enkephalin by selective stimulation of mechanoceptors. There is no evidence that spinal manipulation acts in any other way than the relief of pain (Maigne, 1984; British Medical Association, 1986).

As part of the Rand study of the appropriateness of spinal manipulation (Shekelle et al., 1991), the literature on its effectiveness for low back pain was critically reviewed. The conclusions of the group were as follows.

Spinal manipulation and bed rest are both efficacious for acute low back pain (less than 3 weeks' duration) without neurological findings or sciatic nerve root irritation (sciatica). Manipulation possibly confers significant short-term benefit in pain relief.

For acute low back pain with sciatica, manipulation may offer short-term pain relief, but the literature is insufficient. For acute pain with minor neurological findings, with or without sciatica, the literature is either insufficient or conflicting.

In a recent review of 39 randomized clinical trials (RCTs) it was found that spinal manipulation was more effective in alleviating pain and improved the ability to perform everyday activities when compared to sham treatments but was no more effective than conventional medical therapies (Assendelft, et al., 2004). Massage therapy, especially acupuncture massage has some efficacy in alleviating subacute and chronic low back pain. This effect has been observed to continue for many weeks and months after cessation of therapy (Cochrane, 2004).

For subacute low back pain (3–13 weeks), the literature is conflicting on the use of manipulation when there is no sciatica and absent neurological signs. The majority of studies suggest there may be some short-term benefits. For patients with sciatica and minor neurological findings, the literature is limited, but probably supports the use of manipulation.

For chronic low back pain, there is conflicting evidence on the value of manipulation when there is no sciatica and absent neurological signs. For patients with minor neurologic findings, but no sciatica, one trial has reported significant benefits from manipulation at 6, 12, and 24 months.

The main contraindications to manipulation are rheumatoid neck, basilar insufficiency (drop attacks, vertigo) vertebral myelopathy, coagulation disorders, including patients on anticoagulants, and any vertebral disease carrying a risk of spinal cord compression (osteoporosis, spinal metastases).

Homeopathy

Introduced in Germany by Hahnemann in the late eighteenth century, homeopathy[2] was in strong disagreement with the prevailing allopathic medicine, with its purgings and bleedings. It is based on the theory that like cures like, that ailments are cured by minute doses of the drug that in larger doses produces the same symptoms. An individual diagnosis and regimen is established for each patient. Homeopathic remedies are made by serial dilutions and shaking (succussion), a process thought to increase the potency of the drug.

Because serial dilutions may remove all traces of the drug, any effects of homeopathic medicines cannot be explained in terms of current medical knowledge. A metanalysis of 89 randomized or placebo-controlled clinical trials published in 1995 found an overall positive effect with an odds ratio of 2.45 in favor of homeopathy (Linde et al., 1997). It appears therefore that the results cannot be explained in terms of the placebo effect.

Naturopathy

Naturopathy focuses on the healing powers of the body—the ancient medical principle of *vis medicatrix naturae*. The aim of therapy is to strengthen the patient's own powers of healing by attention to diet, rest, relaxation, and by use of stimuli to activate the healing process. The diagnosis is made of a patient, not of a disease—an interesting parallel with premodern medicine when diagnosis often had the same connotation.[3]

Naturopaths view health as having three components: structural, biochemical, and emotional. The diagnosis is made after a long history and physical assessment. Naturopaths are generalists who use a wide variety of therapeutic modalities, including nutrition, homeopathy, botanical medicine, hydrotherapy, massage, manipulation, and traditional Chinese medicine.

By focusing on the "host," naturopathy follows an ancient medical principle, and one that has been neglected by modern medicine. Medical doctors may adopt some of the naturopathic principles while continuing to use the conventional approach to diagnosis and treatment (Boon, 1996).

Herbal Medicine
Medicines prepared from plant materials are used in many traditional societies and in ancient systems of medicine such as the Chinese. They are now widely consumed in Western countries in the form of teas, powders, tablets, or capsules. They may be bought over the counter in pharmacies or prescribed by a herbalist after an assessment of the patient. Because the medicines are prepared from plants, they contain a mixture of substances rather than a single active ingredient.

In Canada, one in 10 people is reported to be taking some form of natural medicine, including herbal remedies. The most popular herbs are garlic, eschinacea, ginseng, alfalfa, and devil's claw root (Institute for Clinical Evaluative Studies [ICES], 1996).

It is not possible here even to summarize the properties of the many herbs in common use. Good reference sources are available and may be kept in the practice library.[4] Because of the possibility of toxic properties and interaction with prescribed drugs, the physician should know if the patient is taking herbal medicines. This information is unlikely to be volunteered. Most herbs are harmless when taken in the recommended dose, following the guidelines in Table 21.1. The fact that some herbs are toxic need not be used to scare patients into avoidance of all herbal remedies.

Because herbal remedies are derived from plants, many people believe incorrectly that they can have no harmful effects. Not only are there some well-known toxic effects of specific herbs, but preparations sometimes contain potentially toxic additives that are not listed on the label. Patients should be advised, therefore, to obtain their medications from qualified professional herbalists or from ethical manufacturers (see Table 21.1).

Some herbs are hepatotoxic and may cause either acute hepatic necrosis or chronic hepatitis and cirrhosis (see Table 21.2). A number of herbs contain the hepatotoxic pyrrolozidine alkaloids. Renal failure has been reported in women receiving Chinese herbal medicine at a weight-loss clinic (ICES, 1996). Amygdalin (Laetrile), used for cancer, may cause cyanide poisoning.

Herbal medicine may interact with orthodox drugs. Taking ginseng and a monoamine oxidase inhibitor may cause headache and insomnia. Psyllium-seed

Table 21.1   Advice for patients on the use of herbal products

If you are going to take herbs, see a practitioner formally
   trained in botanical medicine.
Buy herbal remedies from trusted and reliable sources.
   Avoid herbs in which the purity and quality are suspicious,
   especially imported herbs.
Most herbs, like drugs, should be avoided during pregnancy
   and lactation and should not be given to small children.
Consider drug/herb interactions.
Start with low dosages and beware of the dosages: two
   pills from the same bottle may have completely different
   strengths.
To avoid possible chronic effects, do not use herbal remedies
   for long periods.
If you are unwell, discontinue use immediately and seek
   medical advice.

Source: Reproduced with permission from Getting Acquainted With
Herbs: Weeding Fact From Fiction in *Informed: Information For
Medical Practitioners from the Institute for Clinical Evaluative Sciences
in Ontario* (ICES) 1996: V2(2):2.

Table 21.2   Some hepatotoxic herbs

Chaparral
Comfrey
Germander
Mistletoe and skullcap
Margosa oil
Maté tea
Gordolobo yerba tea
Pennyroyal
Jin by huan

Source: From Koff, 1995.

products can decrease the absorption of lithium. Evening primrose oil, when taken
with phenothiazines, may increase the number of seizures. Garlic increases the
effect of warfarin. Liquorice may upset control of hypertension by causing hypokalemia and salt retention. Karela, used in curries, can destabilize diabetic control
by causing hypoglycemia. Lily of the valley contains cardiac glycosides and can
potentiate digitalis. Horse chestnut, ginger, and ginkgo can potentiate coumadin
(Penn, 1986; Ernst, 2005). Other drugs with these properties are described in the
sources listed at the end of this chapter.

Nutrition
After years of neglect, nutrition is now assuming greater importance in medical education, practice, and research. Cancer of the breast, colon, and pancreas

appears to be associated with the high-fat, low-fiber diet in Western countries. Coronary heart disease regresses in patients who adhere to a low-fat, high-fiber diet and go through a lifestyle change (Ornish, 1992). There is now much public interest in the potential role of diet in preventing or even arresting cancer.

Outside conventional practice and research, claims have been made for dietary therapies in the form of complete nutritional regimens or the intake of megadoses of vitamins. The macrobiotic diet consists of whole grain cereals, vegetables, and fruits, but no animal products. Vitamins and other elements may be added. There is some evidence that this diet may increase survival in advanced pancreatic and prostate cancer (Carter et al., 1993). Conventional nutritionists have considered the macrobiotic diet inadequate, and it is certainly not sufficient for children. However, older patients do not have the same needs, and it may be this feature of the diet that can slow the growth of a tumor while maintaining normal tissue (Wiesburger, 1993). Because we have little else to offer many patients with advanced cancer, we have reason to support those who wish to try the macrobiotic diet, though the evidence so far does not justify using it as a standard therapy. Those using megadoses of vitamins, however, should be warned about the toxic effects of high doses of vitamins A and D.

The upsurge of interest in nutritional aspects of disease, and the discovery of a scientific basis for some unconventional therapies, may lead to a new era of nutritional therapies based on both biochemical research and clinical trials.

Hypnosis

After being rejected by orthodox medicine for many years, hypnosis is now accepted as a therapy for certain conditions and as a way of inducing analgesia and anesthesia. Its main therapeutic uses are for anxiety states, phobias, chronic pain, addictions, and post-traumatic stress disorders. It should be practiced only by physicians, psychologists, and dentists who are in a position to use it as part of a comprehensive management plan after a full clinical assessment. The effect of hypnosis is not so much to remove the symptoms as to enhance the patient's control over his or her reactions.

Meditation

Meditation, a practice in the major spiritual traditions, is now used as a therapeutic method. Medicine has borrowed the technique, without absorbing the doctrines with which it is associated. The essence of meditation is the concentration of attention on what is going on at the present moment in our minds and bodies. Anyone trying to do this for the first time is surprised by how difficult it is to keep the attention focused. One's mind is constantly wandering from one thought and feeling to the next. By systematically reducing tension in the body, attending to one's breathing, and constantly bringing the mind back to a single point of attention, a state of calmness and relaxation is induced. Relaxation produces physiological changes (the relaxation response) and a decrease in arousal (Benson, 1975). Meditation is taught as a way of reducing stress and anxiety and as a response to chronic pain (Kabat-Zinn, 1990).

Acupuncture

Acupuncture based on the principles of traditional Chinese medicine is practiced in China and other parts of Asia but to a lesser extent in other parts of the world. In Western countries, a modified form is practiced, based on a scientific explanatory model rather than the Chinese theory of meridians. Its main application is for pain relief in musculoskeletal disorders, joint pain, and chronic headache (Ernst, 2005). Provided proper aseptic techniques are observed, there is little risk, though some cases of internal injury have been reported (British Medical Association, 1986).

Holistic Medicine/Integrative Medicine

Dissatisfied with the dominant paradigm of medicine, some physicians have developed an approach to practice based on traditional principles of Western medicine: a respect for the *vis medicatrix naturae*, a diagnosis of the individual patient as well as the disease, attention to the whole context of illness, and the formulation of a regimen for each patient as a way of restoring and maintaining health. Returning to these basic principles does not mean rejecting the conventional approach to diagnosis and treatment whenever this is appropriate.

Some of the alternative therapies described above may be included in holistic practice. It is likely that we will see increasing interchange between mainstream and alternative medicine, with serious attempts to validate alternative practices empirically. There are increasing numbers of scientific journals devoted to the subject, for example, *The Journal of Alternative and Complementary Medicine*.

References

Assendelft WJJ, Morton SC, Yu EI, Suttorp MJ, Shekelle PG. 2004. Spinal manupulative therapy for low back pain. Cochrane Database of Systematic Reviews, Issue 1.

Astin JA 1998. Why patients use alternative medicine: Results of a national survey. *Journal of American Medical Association* 279:1548–1553.

Boon H. 1996. Canadian naturopathic practitioners: The effects of holistic and scientific world views on their socialization experiences and practice patterns. Ph.D. dissertation, Faculty of Pharmacy, University of Toronto.

Benson H. 1975. *The Relaxation Response*. New York: Morrow.

British Medical Association. 1986. *Alternative Therapy: Report of the Board of Science and Education*. London: British Medical Association.

British Medical Association (BMA) 1993. *Complementary Medicine: New Approaches to Good Practice*. London: BMA

Brokaw JJ, Tunnicliff G, Raess BU, Saxon DW, 2002. The teaching of complementary and alternative medicine in U.S. Medical Schools: A survey of course directors. Academic Medicine 77(9):876–881.

Carter JP, Saxe GP, Newbold V, Peres CE, Campeau RJ, Bernal-Green L. 1993. Hypothesis: Dietary management may improve survival from nutritionally linked cancers based on analysis of representative cases. *Journal of the American College of Nutrition* 12:209. Cochrane database.

Eisenberg DM, Kessler RC, Foster C, Norlock FE, Calkins DR, Delbanco TL. 1993. Unconventional medicine in the United States. Special article. *New England Journal of Medicine* 328(4):246.

Eisenberg DM, Davis RB, Ettner SL, Wilkey S, Van Rompay M, Kessler RC 1998. Trends in alternative medicine use in the United States, 1990–1997: Results of a follow-up national survey. *Journal of American Medical Association* 280:1569–1575.

Ernst E. 2005. The Evidence for or against common complementary therapies. In: Lee-Treweek G, Heller T, Spurr S, MacQueen H, Katz J, eds., *Perspectives on Complementary and Alternative Medicine: A Reader.* London and New York: Routledge, pp. 293–297, chapter 33.

Fulder SJ, Munro RE. 1985. Complementary medicine in the United Kingdom: patients, practitioners, and consultations. *Lancet* 2:542.

Greaves D. 2003. *The Healing Tradition: Reviving the Soul of Western Medicine.* Oxford, San Francisco: Radcliffe Publishing.

Helman CG. 2001. *Culture, Health and Illness.* New York: Arnold, chapter 4.

Institute for Clinical Evaluative Sciences in Ontario. 1996. Getting acquainted with herbs: Weeding fact from fiction. *Informed* 2(2):1.

Kabat-Zinn J. 1990. *Full Catastrophe Living: Using the Wisdom of your Body and Mind to Face Stress, Pain and Illness.* New York: Bantam Doubleday Dell.

Kaptchuk TJ, Eisenberg DM. 2005. A taxonomy of unconventional healing practices. In: Lee-Treweek G, Heller T, Spurr S, MacQueen H, Katz J (Eds.). *Perspectives on Complementary and Alternative Medicine: A Reader.* London and New York: Routledge, chapter 2.

Linde K, Clausius N, Ramirez G, Melchart D, Eitel F, Hedges LV et al. 1997. Are the clinical effects of homoeopathy placebo effects? A meta-analysis of placebo-controlled trials. *Lancet* 350:834–843.

Koff RS. 1995. Herbal hepatotoxity: Revisiting a dangerous alternative. *Journal of the American Medical Association* 273(6):502.

Kuhn TS. 1967. *The Structure of Scientific Revolutions.* Chicago, IL: University of Chicago Press.

Maigne R. 1984. Legislation and administrative regulations on the use by licensed health service personnel of non-conventional methods of diagnosis and treatment of illness.

MacLennan AH, Wilson DH, Taylor AW. 1996. Prevalence and cost of alternative medicine in Australia. *Lancet* 347:569.

Ministry of Health and Environmental Protection. 1981. *Alternative Medicine in the Netherlands: Summary of the Report of the Commission for Alternative Systems of Medicine.* Leidschendam, the Netherlands: Ministry of Health and Environmental Protection.

Ornish D. 1992. *Dr. Dean Ornish's Program for Reversing Heart Disease.* New York: Ballantine.

Penn AG. 1986. Adverse reactions to herbal medicines, in BMA. Shekelle PG, Adams AH, Chassin MR, Hurwitz EL, Park RE, Phillips RB, Brook RH. 1991. *The Appropriateness of Spinal Manipulation for Low-Back Pain.* Santa Monica, CA: RAND.

Wetzel MS, Kaptchuk TJ, Haramati A, Eisenberg DM 2003. Complementary and alternative medical therapies: Implications for medical education. *Annals of Internal Medicine* 138(3):191–196.

Wiesburger JH. 1993. Guest editorial. A new nutritional approach in cancer therapy in light of mechanistic understanding of cancer causation and development. *Journal of the American College of Nutrition* 12(3):205.

Notes

1. There is no universally agreed name for what has been called alternative, complementary, or unconventional medicine. The term complementary seems to be replacing alternative. It has the advantage of conveying the relationship between mainstream medicine and other healing practices.

2. For additional reading, see the chapter on homeopathy by Heather Boon in *Nonprescription Drug Reference for Health Professionals*, Premier Edition, published by the Canadian Pharmaceutical Association, Ottawa, 1996.

3. Naturopaths are licensed in Ontario, Manitoba, Saskatchewan, and British Columbia, and in the latter are covered by Medicare. Licensed naturopaths must complete a 4-year full-time graduate program at the Canadian College of Naturopathic Medicine or one of the three naturopathic colleges in the United States.

4. For example, the *British Herbal Pharmacopoeia* and a similar publication used in Germany, the *Nonprescription Drug Reference for Health Professionals*, published by the Canadian Pharmaceutical Association; and The Desktop Guide to Complementary and Alternative Medicine: An Evidence Based Approach. Ed. Edzard Ernst. Mosby, 2001.

Useful websites:

National Center for Complementary and Alternative Medicine
Medline plus-Alternative Medicine. A service of U.S. National Library of Medicine and the National Institutes of Health.

22

Practice Management

A family doctor's effectiveness depends not only on clinical skills, but also on managerial ability. Poor practice management can lead to poor patient care, public dissatisfaction, and demoralization of the doctor and his or her staff. This chapter will concentrate on the central management question of family practice: the allocation of limited resources to meet needs and demands for care in such a way as to respect the values of family medicine. The word limited is used advisedly. Even in the most affluent societies, resources are insufficient to meet every need and every demand. Every family physician must, therefore, be involved in the process of assessing needs, establishing priorities, and allocating resources. The management process is illustrated in Figure 22.1. As indicated on the flow chart, the process is a cyclical one, feedback from the evaluation leading to reexamination of objectives, priorities, and practice procedures.

Formulation of Objectives

In the first instance, objectives are determined by the values of the physician and the expectations of the patients. Prominent among them will be values of family medicine such as accessibility of the doctor, availability of the service, personal care, continuity of care, and preservation of the patient–doctor relationship. Quality of clinical work and work satisfaction for the staff are values that all practices will share. To these may be added personal values, such as a satisfying personal and family life for the physician. Other objectives may relate more specifically to the prevention and management of disease. The result will be a list of practice objectives, of which the following are examples:

1. Patients requesting appointments for acute problems will be seen on the same day. This immediately raises the question "What is an acute problem?" Because policies will be implemented by the practice staff, they will need guidelines.

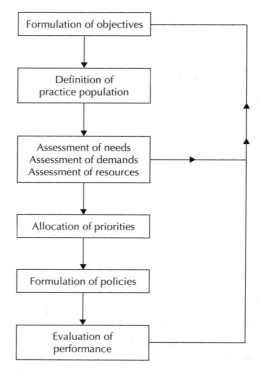

Figure 22.1   The management process.

For instance, in some practices of our acquaintance, a patient who calls about a breast lump is considered to have an acute problem and should be seen on the same day.

2. Patients requesting appointments for nonurgent problems will be seen within 2 weeks.
3. During office hours, patients will be seen by their personal physician.
4. Average time spent by patients in the waiting room will be no longer than 15 minutes.
5. Patients asking to speak to the doctor will receive a call from him or her on the same day.
6. All adult patients will have their blood pressure taken every 5 years.
7. Patients under treatment for hypertension or diabetes will be seen at least once every 3 months.

It will soon become apparent that some of these objectives are conflicting. How are patients with acute problems to be seen if all appointments for the day are filled by people with nonurgent problems? Should a patient see his or her own doctor if all that doctor's appointments are already taken, even if a partner is available? If objectives conflict, they must be put in some order of priority. It may, for example, be considered a higher priority for acute problems to be seen on the same day than for the patient always to see his or her own doctor.

One response to this conflict is advanced access or same day booking systems which seek to balance patient needs with physician capacity. This approach came from the application of queuing theory and principles of industrial engineering as applied to the practice setting (Murray and Berwick, 2003; Mitchell, 2008). In this model, patients are offered an appointment with their physician on the same day, thus ensuring accessibility and continuity of care. This is consistent with the basic tenets of good family practice. To achieve this degree of organization requires commitment from the practitioner, but has been shown to be possible in many countries including the United States (Murray, Bodenheimer, Rittenhouse, and Grumbach, 2003), Canada (Mitchell, 2008), and the United Kingdom (Pope et al., 2008), at times with local adaptations. Advanced access improves patient and physician satisfaction, reduces urgent care visits (O'Hare and Corlett, 2004), and improves patient care (Solberg et al., 2006). When objectives have been thus formulated, they are then made into practice policies. These will include allocation of responsibilities among staff members. For example, what incoming calls does the receptionist pass on to the nurse or to the doctor? How many appointments are left free each day for acute problems? Who checks to see whether patients have had a blood pressure taken? Who is responsible for taking blood pressures? Who checks whether patients have come for follow-up visits? Under what circumstances may patients have repeat prescriptions? How are these to be authorized?

Defining the Practice Population

Any assessment of needs requires a definition of the population for which the practice is responsible. In prepaid systems, this is readily available because patients register with the practice. Defining the population in fee-for-service systems is more difficult but is still eminently feasible. The list is compiled by going through the practice records and entering all patients who have used the practice regularly. Because more than 90% of a practice population attend at least once during a 5-year period, this list of patients who have attended does give an almost complete picture of the population at risk. Of course, the list will be inaccurate because it will contain some patients who have moved or changed doctors. However, the purpose of the list is management, not research, so a high degree of accuracy is not required. An alternative method, also feasible under the fee-for-service system, is to enter into a contract for continuing care when a new family joins the practice. Assessment of needs can be more refined if the defined population is listed in the form of an age–sex register. The compilation of a practice register by manual methods is a laborious and time-consuming procedure, and it must be emphasized that although it is a desirable objective, a practice register is by no means essential for the next stage of the process. Electronic health records have greatly simplified this step.

Assessment of Unmet Needs

Two types of unmet needs[1] can be identified:

1. Needs of which the patient is unaware. It is well known that demands for service are not the same thing as an expression of needs. Community health surveys have shown the existence of many unmet needs even when good primary care services are available. The following are common examples:
   a. Disabilities that elderly patients do not recognize as treatable disorders.
   b. Well-validated preventive procedures, the need for which may not be known to the patient, such as immunization, Pap smear, or hypertension screening.
   c. Mental illnesses such as depression, in which apathy or lack of insight inhibit the patient from seeking care.
2. Needs that the patient feels have not been met by the health care system.

Patient satisfaction, adequacy of preventive care, and unmet needs for common specific problems may be assessed by a brief questionnaire presented to a sample from each age group, drawn either from the practice records or from an age–sex register. The results enable the physician to identify specific areas in which the practice is failing to meet needs. Another method of assessment is to carry out periodic surveys of specific subgroups of the population that are felt to be at high risk of having unmet needs. Groups that may be at risk are the aged, single parent families, families of patients with chronic disabilities, and immigrant groups.

Assessment of Demands

Demands on resources can be divided into those generated by patients and those generated by the physician.

Patient-generated demands can in turn be divided into the following main categories:

Telephone consultations
Office visits for acute conditions
Office visits for nonurgent problems
Request for home visits
Office visits for preventive care
Requests for repeat prescriptions
Emergency and night calls
Visits for prenatal and well-baby care

Physicians generate demand for their services by asking patients to make follow-up appointments and by calling them in for preventive procedures.

Demands can be readily assessed by doing periodic surveys of incoming telephone calls, requests for appointments, home visits, repeat prescriptions, and so on. Greater detail can be obtained by recording such information as problem label or diagnosis, drugs or other treatment prescribed, investigations ordered, or referrals made. For management purposes, it is not necessary to record this information continuously. It is quite sufficient to do it for all patients for a week at a time or for a sample of patients over a similar period.

Assessment of Resources

The resources of the practice include the physical plant, the communication system, the physicians, the staff, the attached personnel, and the hospital and community resources that can be deployed by the practice.

Evaluation of Performance

The next stage is evaluation to determine whether or not the objectives have been achieved. Different types of evaluation are needed for different objectives. Donabedian (1966) has described three types: evaluation of structure, process, and outcome. Structure refers to the physical facilities and qualifications of staff and is more relevant to external audit than the kind of internal evaluation we are discussing here. Outcome evaluation means the assessment of the results of care: recovery from illness or disability, relief of symptoms, functional capacity, and satisfaction with care. Although outcome is the ultimate criterion of good care, outcome evaluation poses certain problems. Outcome is often determined by factors that are outside the practice's control: social and economic conditions, for example. In chronic conditions such as hypertension, the outcome may be many years distant. Provided a process criterion can be related to a successful outcome, this is a satisfactory substitute for outcome evaluation. For example, it is reasonable to use control of hypertension as a process criterion because this is known to prevent unfavorable outcomes of hypertension. For similar reasons, the proportion of the practice population screened can be used as a process criterion.

Most types of evaluation useful to the family physician are assessments of process. One exception is the assessment of satisfaction with care. Because results of treatment are known to be related to patient satisfaction, this is an important aspect of evaluation in family practice.

Three main strategies of evaluation are available to the family physician:

1. A direct approach to the patient.
2. Periodic assessments of practice procedures: documentation of incoming telephone calls, calculation of average time spent in the waiting room, and assessment of delay in obtaining appointments for acute and nonurgent conditions.
3. Audit of records. This can be used to monitor such aspects of performance as management, prescribing, referral, and use of investigations.

Reconsideration of Objectives and Policies

Almost certainly, the evaluation will reveal that some objectives are not being achieved. Certain questions must, therefore, be asked:

1. Are the objectives realistic?
2. Can the demands be changed? We often tend to assume that the demands on a practice are a given. There are certainly limits to the degree they can

be influenced. We should bear in mind, however, that there are two ways of changing demand. Education of patients may affect not only the nature of demand but also its distribution. Instruction by booklets and slide-tape shows of the self-management of simple problems may reduce the demand for care for conditions such as upper respiratory infection. Prenatal and postnatal classes for mothers may reduce the number of calls for babies. Patient education by word of mouth or by practice brochure can reduce the number of inappropriate demands, such as out-of-hours calls for repeat prescriptions. Doctor-initiated demands are also subject to change by reviewing policies on follow-up visits and for preventive services. For example, should annual physical assessments be encouraged or can resources be used more effectively?

3. Are the resources of the practice being used to their maximum effect? How much time is being wasted? Is the doctor's time being used to the best advantage, or is it badly distributed? Is enough of the day being allocated to office appointments? Is time being wasted by poor patient flow, mislaid records, instruments not being readily available, or communication in the office being inefficient?

4. Are the staff members fully aware of the practice policies and are they carrying them out? Being the first to receive incoming calls, the key staff person in the operation of the practice is the receptionist who can only function effectively with a clear understanding of what is expected.

Common Defects in Practice Management

1. Too many incoming calls for the number of telephone lines. Patients with acute problems may have difficulty getting through because of continuous busy signals.

2. Inadequate telephone answering services for out-of-hours calls. A commercially operated answering service may be inadequately supervised. There may be unacceptable delays between calls being received and relayed to the doctor.

3. Patients having to wait 2 or 3 days for appointments for acute conditions such as sore throat or urinary infection. In these circumstances, it is no wonder that patients use hospital emergency departments.

4. Patients unable to get through the barrier of the receptionist or nurse to speak to the doctor. This may be due to the receptionist's excessive shielding of the doctor from the demands of patients.

Unless the physician adopts a critical approach to the management of the practice, he or she may remain in complete ignorance of the existence of these deficiencies in his or her own practice.

The Decision-Making Process

Once a practice team reaches a critical size, it becomes necessary to define the decision-making process in a way that is clear to all its members, including both health-care professionals and staff. Practice meetings should be held regularly, with a formal agenda and minutes. A practice constitution can define such matters as the right to attend meetings and receive minutes, voting procedures, the roles of officeholders, and the representation of attached personnel.

It is important for morale that all members feel that they have some part to play in the decision-making process, especially in those decisions that affect their own lives. Because the medical members of the practice team are often the owners of the practice and employers of the staff, involvement of the other members in decision-making calls for sensitive management and open communication.

When the physicians are partners sharing the ownership, relationships within the physician group itself are crucial and call for similar procedures for policy decisions, income distribution, and management of resources.

The Impact of Managed Care

Managed care is the term used for integrated systems for the provision of health services, such as health maintenance organizations (HMOs), preferred provider organizations (PPOs), and Independent Practice Associations (IPA). Managed care is also used to denote the range of controls used by such organizations to control the practices of physicians and to limit the options of patients. Examples of such controls include entry to the system only through primary physician "gate-keepers," mandatory second opinion before elective surgery, formal utilization review, and mandatory approval of certain discretionary services.

Driven by the need for cost containment, managed care has become ubiquitous in the United States with 90% of insured Americans reported to be in some form of managed care. Such plans are rapidly replacing the indemnity insurance plan as the predominant system for organizing and financing health care (Weiner and de Lissovoy, 1993). Under an indemnity insurance plan, the sponsor (e.g., an employer) purchased services through insurance companies that acted as intermediaries between purchaser and consumers. Consumers were free to choose providers of services, physicians practiced with few constraints, and insurance companies paid the bills. The insurance companies accepted the financial risk but could pass on any increases in cost to the sponsor in the form of higher premiums.

What distinguishes managed care plans is that there is a "party that takes responsibility for integrating and coordinating the financing and delivery of services across what previously were fragmented provider and payer entities" (Weiner and de Lissovoy, 1993). The prototypical managed care institution is the HMO. Health maintenance organizations are committed to providing care for enrollees who prepay a premium. The organization assumes the financial risk and transfers some of this to the primary care physicians, who are often paid by capitation fee (a regular payment for each patient enrolled in their practice, irrespective of whether or not the patient has received services).

There are four types of HMOs. In a staff HMO, the physicians are paid mainly by salary. In a group HMO, a multispecialty group practice is the major source of care for enrollees. Network HMOs provide services to enrollees through two or more group practices. In an IPA, individual physicians or small group practices contract to provide care for enrollees. The primary care physicians may be paid by capitation or by fee-for-service with a risk-sharing provision. The physician may also treat patients outside the HMO on a fee-for-service basis.

In a preferred provider organization, consumers have the choice of using the preferred physicians who are members of the plan or physicians who are outside it. Benefits act as incentives for consumers to use the preferred physicians. The latter agree to managed care strategies and are usually paid a discounted fee. The physicians in the plan benefit by having patients channeled to them.[2]

Financial risk is defined as "variance in expenditure" (Weiner and de Lissovoy, 1993). The degree of variance depends on the number of enrollees and their health status. If numbers are small, one patient requiring expensive treatment can greatly increase the risk for the payer. Managed care organizations may transfer some or all of the risk to physicians. Primary care physicians, for example, may agree to a budget or capitation payment and take responsibility for provision of all necessary services, including in-hospital and specialist care. Such transfer of risk can take place within government-funded services. In the British National Health Service, fund-holding practices are assigned capitation payments and are responsible for buying services from hospitals and specialist services. In the United States, Medicare payments are based on fees for diagnosis-related groups (DRGs). The fee paid is an average of all patients with the same diagnosis. When the physician's own income is included in the budget or capitation fee, a conflict of interest may clearly arise. The transfer of risk to primary care groups involves physicians in levels of management far beyond those experienced in private fee-for-service practice. This demands management skills and may add to the stress of practice. On the other hand, it can provide an opportunity for creative innovation in the provision of services.

Advances in information technology have made it possible for managers to maintain close surveillance of physicians' activities, including time spent with patients, prescribing costs, referral rates, and compliance with guidelines. If too rigid, these may have deleterious effects on physicians' morale, with negative consequences for patient care.

The term *managed competition* is used to describe competition between managed care plans in a market regulated by government. In the British National Health Service, for example, the government has created an internal market in which providers compete for contracts with payers.

References

Donabedian A. 1966. Evaluating the quality of medical care. Part 2. *Millbank Memorial Fund* 44:166.

Mitchell 2008. Same day booking: Success in Canadian family practice. *Canadian Family Physician* 54:379–383. Murray M, Berwick DM 2003 Advanced access: Reducing waiting and delays in primary care. *Journal of American Medical Association* 289:1035–1040.

Murray M, Bodenheimer T, Rittenhouse D, Grumbach K 2003. Improving timely access to primary care: Case studies of the advanced access model. *Journal of the American Medical Association* 289(8):1042–1046.

Nutting PA. 1986. Community-oriented primary care: An integrated model for practice, research, and education. *American Journal of Preventive Medicine* 2(3):140.

Nutting PA, Connor EM. 1986. Community-oriented primary care: An examination of the U.S. experience. *American Journal of Public Health* 76(3):279.

O'Hare CD, Corlett J. 2004. The outcomes of open-access scheduling. *Family Practice Management*. www.aafp.org/fpm. February.

Pope et al. 2008. Improving access to primary care: eight case studies of introducing advanced access in England. *Journal of Health Services and Research Policy* 13:33–39.

Solberg et al. 2006. Effect of improved primary care access on quality of depression care. *Annals of Family Medicine* 4:69–74.

Toon PD. 1994. What is good general practice? Occasional paper 65. Royal College of General Practitioners.

Weiner JP, de Lissovoy G. 1993. Razing a tower of Babel: A taxonomy for managed care and health insurance plans. *Journal of Health Politics, Policy and Law* 18(1):75–103.

Wright RA. 1993. Community-oriented primary care. *Journal of the American Medical Association* 269(19):2544.

Notes

1. The systematic assessment of health-care needs in the practice population, identification of community health problems, modification of practice procedures, and monitoring the impact of changes is known as Community-oriented Primary Care (COPC) (Nutting, 1986; Wright, 1993). In the United States, COPC has been implemented mainly in not-for-profit primary care organizations. The application has so far been limited in scope. Implementation difficulties include the cost of health surveys, the lack of epidemiological skills, and the problems of reallocating resources in organizations already working at full stretch.

COPC is said to require a new kind of hybrid practitioner with competencies in primary care, prevention, epidemiology, ethics, and behavioral science. As Toon (1994) has observed, these roles may be conflicting, leading to tensions in the individual physician and in the practice, especially if it is a small one. There are, however, some exemplars, notably Dr. Tudor Hart in his South Wales practice. In those organizations that have implemented COPC, there has been at least one physician with an unusual commitment to it (Nutting and Connor, 1986). Whether COPC can work successfully on a larger scale has yet to be demonstrated. Even if it proves to be impracticable in its present form, the principles could still be applied in different ways, such as by collaboration between a number of practices and a public health unit.

2. For an excellent guide to the often confusing nomenclature of managed care, see Razing a tower of Babel: A taxonomy for managed care and health insurance plans (Weiner and Lissovoy, 1993).

Part IV

Education and Research

23

Continuing Self-Education

Each case has its lesson—a lesson that may be, but is not always, learnt, for clinical wisdom is not the equivalent of experience. A man who has seen 500 cases of pneumonia may not have the understanding of the disease which comes with an intelligent study of a score of cases, so different are knowledge and wisdom.

Sir William Osler, 1905

Any observer of physicians cannot help noticing the wide variation in their capacity for self-education. At one end of the scale is the physician who learns something, however little, from every patient and every illness. At the other is the physician who goes on making the same errors time after time, year after year, with little intellectual or personal growth. What is the difference between them? The good learner, it may be said, will be an assiduous reader of journals and will be seen often at postgraduate courses, thus keeping abreast of medical progress. This may be true, but our observation is that the bad learner may also be a reader of journals and a frequent attendee of courses. The difference between them is that the good learner has grasped the truth that the main source of development as a physician lies not in some distant center of learning but in the day-to-day experience of his or her own practice. Hours spent listening to lectures or bent over medical journals will be of little help unless the physician has reflected deeply on his or her own experience. To say this is not to underrate the value of these modes of learning. Both of them have an important place in the continuing education of the physician, but they are not sufficient in themselves.

The necessary conditions for continuing self-education are illustrated in Figure 23.1. To learn from experience, physicians must obviously know what their experience is. They should know the outcome of their actions both in the short term and in the long term. They should have some standard against which to measure their performance and must have the capacity for accepting criticism.

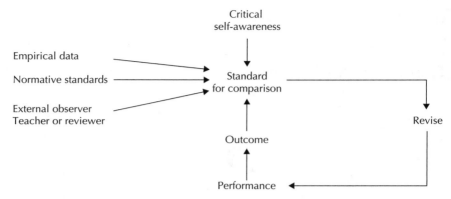

Figure 23.1   The learning process.

and, if necessary, making changes in methods of practice. Information on the physician's methods of practice and their outcome should be available in the practice records. Too often, however, it is hidden in the records. The information has to be not only available but also accessible. It is not enough for physicians to base their actions on the last two or three cases seen; they should be able to review all their cases of diabetes, hypertension, otitis media, depression, or whatever condition is being studied. The electronic medical record has made this much easier to attain.

When physicians review their cases, they will have some questions in mind. How did the patients present? What were the early symptoms? Could the diagnosis have been made earlier? Did the treatment achieve its objectives? They will also be judging their results against certain standards. Two kinds of standards may be used: empirical and normative. Empirical standards are derived from statistical averages obtained from similar settings. These enable the physician to compare activities such as prescribing, referral, or follow-up with those of other physicians. Normative standards are derived from traditional sources of orthodox medical standards. When medical audit is used as an educational process, it is best for the physician or the group to begin by defining their own standards for the specific problem or disease being studied. The development of these standards is an educational process in itself because it involves a review of the literature, a review of empirical data, and often discussions with consultants. Once the standards are defined, the records are then reviewed and data collected. Almost certainly, the results will show that the physician's performance falls short of his or her own standards. The physician or group must then decide whether the standard is realistic; if it is, they should take steps to improve their performance. Repeat of the audit after an interval will show whether the required changes have occurred.

Reviewing their own experience gives physicians some insight into their own learning needs. Additional insight can be obtained by following one of the self-assessment programs made available by educational bodies. Having done this, physicians are ready to learn from others.

Reading

Many family physicians feel overwhelmed by the volume of reading material that is available to them, much of it arriving in the mail unsolicited. Some physicians react by reading very little, others by reading so much that their coverage of the literature may be very superficial. Both of these errors can be avoided by designing a reading program based on the following principles:

To keep up-to-date with developments in medicine, it is not necessary to read a large number of journals. Through their editorials and review articles, good general journals such as the *New England Journal of Medicine, The Lancet, Journal of the American Medical Association, Canadian Medical Association Journal*, and the *British Medical Journal*, provide a continuing review of progress across the whole field of medicine.[1] A subscription to a journal in this category will keep the physician up to date. Sackett, Haynes, and Tugwell (1985) recommend that physicians change their focus from core knowledge to core clinical problems. In scanning the literature, physicians search for articles that will help them with the core clinical problems in their own practice. They also advise physicians to develop the skills of critical appraisal, so that they can select the key articles on the subject.

Some of the most rapid changes are in the field of drug therapy. Reading one journal such as the *Medical Letter*, which provides authoritative reviews of new drugs, will keep physicians up-to-date in this field, as well as making them aware of side effects and drug interactions.

Reading at least one journal of family medicine will keep physicians abreast of progress in their own field (e.g., *Annals of Family Medicine, Journal of the Royal College of General Practitioners, Canadian Family Physician*).

Information technology has made a large and growing body of information readily accessible. The electronic medical record system can become an educational tool through such means as decision support programs. The problem of dealing with the huge volume of information now available has been ameliorated by the production of guidelines by authoritative bodies, and by meta-analysis of evidence from clinical trials.[2]

Other Educational Resources

In many areas, a wide choice of courses is available. Many of these are in the traditional lecture format and aim to provide information. Other kinds of courses are aimed at developing skills. Physicians who wish to learn a particular skill—such as reading ECGs or doing sigmoidoscopies—can arrange to spend time in a clinical center where they will gain this experience.

Teaching is a valuable learning experience because it forces the teachers to examine their own methods of practice. Research is valuable because it involves the exploration of one aspect of family medicine in depth. Travel is of value because it exposes the physician to other attitudes and other ways of doing things. There is no need to go far afield. A visit to a neighboring practice, or a half-day sitting-in with a colleague in his or her office, can provide much food for thought.

In the past, family physicians have been slow to realize how much they have to learn from each other.

Self-Knowledge

Important change requires critical self-knowledge. As Popper and McIntyre have observed (1983), we learn from our errors. Without self-knowledge, however, we have a great capacity for hiding our errors from ourselves, especially those arising from countertransference. Belonging to a group of colleagues that meets regularly to discuss each other's experience can be both a support and an opportunity for learning about ourselves. The more secure members of the group feel with each other, the more they will feel able to confide in each other.

For family physicians, being well informed and up-to-date is necessary but not sufficient. Good family practice depends also on relationships, and the maturing of a family physician is a matter of educating the emotions as well as the intellect.[3] Learning in this sense is often a matter of going through some personal change. Learning to be patient-centered is a case in point. This is not simply a question of learning some communication skills or following a set of rules. Practicing patient-centered medicine is a different way of being a physician, and unless this change has taken place, no technique will be effective.

Impatience with inefficiency in medical practice, and with the apparent reluctance of doctors to change their ways in response to new knowledge, has resulted in attempts to control physicians' behavior by external constraints. As Deci and Flaste (1995) have observed, external controls may produce compliance, but they also produce defiance, and this may negate all the efforts to produce change. True and lasting change in medical practice and medical education has to come first in the hearts and minds of physicians themselves.

References

Deci EL, Flaste R. 1995. *Why We Do What We Do: The Dynamics of Personal Autonomy.* New York: Putnam & Sons.

Osler W. 1905. On the educational value of a medical society. In: *Aequanimitas with Other Addresses to Medical Students, Nurses and Practitioners of Medicine.* Philadelphia, PA: Blackiston's Son.

Popper K, McIntyre N. 1983. The critical attitude in medicine: The need for a new ethics. *British Medical Journal* 287:1919.

Sackett DL, Haynes RB, Tugwell P. 1985. *Clinical Epidemiology: A Basic Science for Clinical Medicine.* Boston, MA: Little, Brown.

Notes

1. Most journals are now available online.

2. The Cochrane collaboration is a worldwide effort to base medical practice on evidence from the meta-analysis of clinical trials. The project is named after Dr. Archie Cochrane, a pioneering British epidemiologist.

3. There is a growing awareness of the importance of emotional education and of its neglect in our culture. See, for example, Margaret Donaldson's *Human Minds: An Exploration*. London: Penguin Books, 1992; Daniel Goleman's *Emotional Intelligence*. New York: Bantam Books, 1995; Edward Deci and Richard Flaste's *Why We Do What We Do: The Dynamics of Personal Autonomy*. New York: Putnam, 1995; and Aldous Huxley's last book, *Island*, is an earlier and prophetic example of this genre.

24

Research in Family Practice

This chapter describes how general practice has contributed to medical knowledge and how family medicine as a discipline has developed its own body of knowledge. It also discusses some of the methodological issues raised by research in the discipline.

The Scientific Development of Family Medicine

Although medicine should be regarded mainly as a science-based technology, it is founded on a descriptive body of scientific knowledge accumulated by physicians over the centuries. Like other sciences, medicine has developed two interrelated conceptual systems: an analytical schema to classify its subject matter, and an explanatory schema to describe the origins and destinies of these categories. The analytical schema is our system for classifying diseases; the explanatory schema is our theories about how these diseases are caused.

The methods used in building our analytical schema are those of the naturalist: observing, recording, classifying, analyzing (Ryle, 1936). The physician observes the natural phenomena of illness in the same way that the field naturalists observe the flora and fauna of their neighborhoods. Many of the early physician-scientists were naturalists in this broad sense. The country doctor, Edward Jenner (1749–1823), for example, was made a member of the Royal Society for his discovery of how the female cuckoo invades another bird's nest (usually a hedge sparrow's)and makes room for her offspring by throwing the young sparrows out of their nest.

Jenner was in practice in the eighteenth century, a time when general practice was beginning to take form, under the name of surgeon apothecaries (Loudon, 1986). His greatest discovery was vaccination for the prevention of smallpox. At least as early as the eighteenth century, healthy children were exposed to smallpox because the mortality (10%), was much less than the mortality during an epidemic. Those who recovered from smallpox were immune for the rest of their lives.

The concept of immunization, therefore, started with two proto-ideas (Fleck, 1979): one, the idea of immunity after survival from smallpox; this was general in the population; the other was the idea of immunity after smallpox in dairy workers in rural areas. Jenner began to study the illnesses of cows, taking an artist with him onto the farms, so he could have accurate drawings of cowpox pustules. Then, for the first time, the concept reached the mind of a scientist (Jenner) with proven powers of observation and the determination to pursue his investigation in the face of skepticism and ridicule.

Twenty years passed before Jenner carried out his crucial experiment. A boy in a gazebo in his garden was inoculated, first with material from a cowpox pustule, then later, with smallpox. He was ready to submit his paper for publication. Jenner had many followers, but also many critics. Many of these failed to replicate this experiment. They had inoculated material from a pustule, but not from a smallpox pustule. How fortunate that Jenner was such a meticulous observer. In other hands, the whole project might have been abandoned—dismissed as another old-wives tale.

Another observation throws light on Jenner's character. While doing a post-mortem examination on a man who had severe angina, his knife cut through some hard material. At first he thought it was a piece of plaster, fallen from the ceiling, then he realized it was a calcified artery from the heart. In those days it was not customary to dissect these arteries, and the cause for an angina was unknown. Normally he would have reported his finding, but his friend Hunter was suffering from angina, and he did not want to give Hunter additional anxiety. Eventually Heberden was credited for the discovery.

William Withering (1741–1799) was similar to Jenner in many ways. He was trained in Shropshire by a surgeon, then went to study medicine in Edinburgh and to graduate as a MD. Back in Shropshire, he set up practice and worked as a physician in the Staffordshre Infirmary. Like Jenner he became interested in a plant which a "wise woman" of Shropshire had told him was good for the dropsy. Withering knew that Leonard Fuchs (1501–1566) used the foxglove and, being a distinguished botanist, was able to put Digitalis on a scientific footing. His study of dosage and of side effects was very important in the use of Digitalis. Jenner and Withering were able to use their skills in observing, recording, classifying, and analyzing, to advance the progress of medicine.

The Nineteenth Century

Our greatest exemplar of the naturalist method was the Scottish general practitioner James Mackenzie. His life story and his writings on research methods in general practice and on medical education are a rich source of ideas and inspiration (Mair, 1973). Mackenzie was born in Scotland in 1853, graduated from Edinburgh in 1878, and soon afterward entered general practice in Burnley, a cotton-manufacturing town in Lancashire. It was there, during the following

20 years, that he carried out the studies that were to lay the foundations of modern cardiology.

Like so many before and after him, Mackenzie was mystified by his inability to diagnose so many of the illnesses he encountered in general practice. His medical education had not prepared him to deal with the illnesses of general practice. Blaming himself for his lack of knowledge, he searched the textbooks for answers—but in vain. The knowledge he sought did not exist. In his book, *The Future of Medicine* (1919), Mackenzie wrote

...from the patient's statement can be acquired information that is absolutely essential to the recognition of disease, especially in the early stages. It would not be exaggerating to say that the failure of medicine to detect disease in its early stage is due to the fact that the sensations of patients have never been adequately investigated. Even when I had recognized the importance of this mode of investigation I found the greatest difficulty in eliciting the sensations, and in understanding the mechanism of their production...there is in the patient's sensations a field of enormous value...

Mackenzie's Research

Mackenzie had bequeathed to us two principles of clinical research. The first was "record your patient's symptoms." The second was "follow your patient indefinitely." By the study of our patient's symptoms you will learn their meaning ("wait and see"). By following your patients you will learn the prognosis of their diseases. How can we follow our patients if they leave our practice? With our patient's cooperation we can arrange to follow them for a confidential report on their health.

One of MacKenzie's discoveries was auricular paralysis (now called atrial fibrillation). He described the discovery in a letter to a friend.

I had been watching a patient with mitral stenosis since 1880, as I was trying to find out when the mitral stenosis appeared, and the changes that occurred in its development. This patient had shown for many years a presystolic murmur, pulsation in the jugular vein and in the liver, due to the systole of the auricle. The heart had been regular...except for the occasional extra-systole. In 1898 she suddenly became very ill with breathlessness, cyanosis and a weak, rapid, irregular pulse. After some weeks the heart slowed down, and records taken showed a complete disappearance of all signs of auricular activity, and in place of a negative venous pulse there was now a positive venous pulse, and on auscultation the presystolic murmur had disappeared and the pulse had now become persistently irregular (Mair, 1973).

This account of Mackenzie's discovery of paralysis of the auricle shows what a single practitioner, following a single patient, can achieve by careful observation. There is no reason why a general practitioner should not do this today, either with single patients or with series of patients collected because of their similarity with each other.

The example shows that discoveries may not appear all at once. A discovery which comes "out of the blue" perhaps when a physician is not thinking of his problem, may require a combination with another idea. Sometimes the person who brings the ideas together is not the person who makes the original discovery.

Mackenzie managed without complicated statistics: counting was all he needed. Nor did he need randomized controlled trials. Clearly they have their important uses, but they also have their drawbacks, especially for general practitioners. They are very expensive, so much so that only a few of those eligible can be accommodated. Because they are expensive, they have to be shortened, often too short to adequately test the efficacy of a new drug or treatment. There is still room for observational studies. If our journals reject all but randomized controlled trials, patients will miss the benefits of those discoveries which, otherwise, will never be brought to light.

It is ironic that Mackenzie became famous for something that he regarded as an incidental aspect of his work: his invention of the polygraph. Then, as now, both public and profession were more impressed by gadgets than by the clinical observations without which they would have been useless. His disciples, the new generation of cardiologists, embraced the new technology but, to Mackenzie's disappointment, failed to appreciate the importance of prolonged clinical observation to discover the natural history of disease. Mackenzie was by no means opposed to investigative medicine or the use of the laboratory; on the contrary, he made frequent use of both. But he never wavered in his belief that the basic science of medicine is clinical observation, and that general practice is the best place to learn the natural history of disease.[1]

There is, unfortunately, very little evidence that Mackenzie's example is being followed today. It is rare to read a description of clinical observations made over a long period of time by the author himself. More commonly, the author has extracted data from records made by other physicians, often not the result of disciplined observations. If there is systematic follow-up at all, it is usually for a short period of time.

Many reasons could be given for this neglect of our traditional methods. Ours is a restless and impatient age. To wait 10 years before publishing one's results would earn few grants and little credit in a medical school. Some physicians may think that the last word has been written on the natural history of disease. Yet we still fall into traps because of our ignorance.

When we encounter a disease we do not recognize, we should ask ourselves if it might be one of those diseases that are forgotten. Ludwick Fleck had taught us how long it may be before a scientific idea becomes a fact, perhaps centuries. "Thoughts pass from one individual to another, each time a little transformed." (Fleck, 1979, p. 39). A "thought collective" is a "community of persons mutually exchanging ideas or maintaining intellectual interactions..." providing "the special 'carrier' for the historical development of any field of thought."

Before there can be a scientific fact, there must be an agreement with societal assumptions. "The futility of work that is isolated from the spirit of the age is shown strikingly in the case of that great herald of excellent ideas Leonardo da Vinci, who nevertheless left no positive scientific achievement behind him" (Fleck, 1979, p. 45).

Alexander Fleming is a case in point. The *Penicillium notatum* which grew by accident on his Petri dish, and killed the staphylococci, might have been thrown away. Fleming had for many years been in search of such an antibiotic. He published his finding, but was ignored. The chemists he worked with were unable to produce a mold that would remain constant in the human body. Eventually, Fleming and his work were forgotten for 12 years. In the early years of the World War II, Florey, an Australian medical scientist, formed a team in Oxford with Chain, a German chemist, and brought Fleming's work back from oblivion. After 12 years, Chain supplied the process which Fleming's work required.

"The great field for new discoveries", wrote William James, "is always the unclassified residuum. Round about the accredited of every science there ever flows a sort of dust cloud of exceptional observations, of occurrences minute and irregular and seldom met with, which it always proves more easy to ignore than to attend to" (Koestler, 1970). There is no greater field for the unclassified residuum than general practice.

The Twentieth-Century Family Medicine Research: Principles and Themes

Research activities in the discipline of general/family practice have advanced greatly in the latter half of the twentieth century. These activities have exemplified the principles of the discipline as they have become more clearly articulated. We will illustrate some of these principles through the examples of well-known investigators in the field.

Franz Huygen was a practitioner near the town of Nijmegen in the Netherlands. The area of his practice had become socially isolated by the devastation of World War II, resulting in a relatively stable population for whom he was the sole practitioner. His meticulous records of illnesses, organized by families and his insightful observations of human behavior published in his book, *Family Medicine: The Medical Life History of Families*, (1978) were important elements in leading family physicians to recognize the importance of family and social context in illnesses and recovery. This principle, the recognition of context, and the unique perspective of family physicians in understanding and studying its influence on patients, has remained an enduring part of research in the discipline.

Michael Klein (Klein, 1988; Klein, Gauthier, and Robbins, 1994) trained initially as a pediatrician, but practicing as a very active family physician/obstetrician in Montreal, challenged the biomedical orthodoxy of his day that dictated that all deliveries required an episiotomy. Through his research, he was able to show that for routine vaginal deliveries, episiotomy actually resulted in more postpartum pain and prolonged recovery than simply repairing any perineal lacerations should they occur. This research has greatly reduced the number of unnecessary episiotomies and allowed faster recovery of new mothers. The principle of challenging the biomedical orthodoxy remains a part of research in family medicine.

Moira Stewart and her colleagues at the Centre for Studies in Family Medicine at The University of Western Ontario used mixed methods research, combining both qualitative and quantitative methodologies to study and validate the patient-centered clinical method. Mixed methods research of this type is becoming the norm in family medicine and other disciplines. The principle that it retains is the combination of standard quantitative methods with recognition of the importance of subjective experience as illuminated through qualitative methods.

Ann Macaulay (Macaulay et al., 1997, 1999), working with first nations communities near Montreal uses participatory and action research methodologies to investigate issues of importance to the community that she serves. The principles illustrated in these approaches to research are family medicine's commitment to marginalized populations and social change.

The Headache Study Group (1986) is an example of a practice-based research network (PBRN), groups of family practitioners who work together to pose questions relevant to their practices and gather the necessary information to address those questions. Practice-based research networks demonstrate the principle of practitioners engaged as participants in the field. They have gradually grown in numbers and sophistication to become important contributors to our base of knowledge.

Of course there are many other prominent and important researchers in family medicine that one could mention. The cases described are simply meant to be illustrative of the key themes and principles found in family medicine research in the twentieth century.

Clinical Discoveries

Seeing illness in its earliest stages, family physicians are in an excellent position for making new clinical discoveries. These may begin as observations, insights, or hunches which can develop over time into important new findings. Physicians practicing full time are rarely in a position to carry the necessary research to a conclusion. Clinical discoveries do not begin as research. They are not planned in advance like traditional forms of research such as those in university departments. They arise in the course of practice. Clinical discoveries are iterative. A certain clinical observation attracts the doctor's attention. He or she takes notes and looks out for other cases, with each case adding more information. As time goes on the observations coalesce, and the physician may have an intuitive insight. Such insights are often not the result of logic: they are, perhaps, a key observation which has been overlooked by others. Roentgen's discovery of X-rays is a case in point. His finding had been ignored by many others. Alexander Fleming's discovery was a single observation: the accidental effect of mold in a Petri-dish containing bacterial culture. His paper was published, but ignored. James Mackenzie was attracted, early in his career by the significance of the pulsations in the jugular pulse. Mackenzie wrote, "Others had studied the subject before, and , beyond recognizing some of its features, left the matter as one of no practical importance. On the other hand, I used it as a stepping stone for a further advance, and by this means the mechanism of regular heart action was revealed" (Mackenzie, 1919, p. 128).

In Mackenzie's time there were no journals of family medicine. He was, however, able to publish his discoveries step by step in the existing medical journals. Now there are many peer-reviewed journals of family medicine and General Practice. Many articles on research have been published, but very few from practicing physicians reporting their discoveries. It has been suggested that the editors and reviewers are judging these discoveries by the criteria of traditional research.

The *Annals of Family Medicine* (McWhinney, 2008; Stange, 2008) has now introduced a new category called *Clinical Discoveries*, which will be reviewed and evaluated according to four criteria: plausibility, support from the basic sciences and appropriate literature, clarity of concepts, and reproducibility of the procedures.

Types of Descriptive Research in General Practice

Although distinguished original work has been done, and continues to be done, in family practice, some of the descriptive research by family physicians has been vitiated by serious faults. Two of these will be mentioned. The first is the collection of information without a clearly formulated question. Even in descriptive research, some question must be asked before the study is begun. Suppose, for example, that a physician wishes to study the natural history of infectious mononucleosis. What facts about the disease does she wish to establish or verify? Does she want to establish its incidence and the predictive value of the early symptoms and signs? Does she want to find out the mean duration of the illness? Does she want to describe the frequency of complications? The questions she wishes to ask will determine the observations to be made and the criteria used in making them. How, for example, will patients be admitted to the study? How will the physician ensure that milder cases are not excluded? Will all patients with sore throat be screened for the disease? What criteria will be used to determine recovery from the illness? Unless such questions have been well formulated, the data will be incomplete.

The second fault is a failure to standardize observations and to define criteria for diagnosis or admission to the study. For example, it is of little help to know that a certain percentage of patients presenting with cough and fever had bronchitis unless we know what criteria were used for diagnosing bronchitis and how well the observers were trained and standardized. Attention to this kind of detail does not require a sophisticated knowledge of research methods. It requires mainly a scrupulous regard for accuracy of observation—the mark of the true naturalist.

Several types of descriptive research can be identified. First are studies of the natural course and outcome of illness: the illness studied may be a well-defined disease category, such as herpes zoster, or a symptom, such as headache. Strictly speaking, the natural history of illness means the outcome of the illness when untreated. When the illness is highly responsive, it is no longer possible to study the true natural history. There are still, however, many diseases that are not greatly modified by treatment. There is also much to be learned from the study of diseases that are responsive to therapy. The action of the treatment on the disease may be to produce a new form of the disease that has its own natural history. In otitis media, for example, the treatment of the acute illness with antibiotics was followed by the emergence of serous otitis. In this kind of study, the denominator is the total number of patients with the disease or symptom. In a study of headache, for example, the denominator is all patients presenting with headache, and the numerator is different subgroups of this population with special features associated with particular outcomes.

The second type of descriptive research involves studies of incidence and prevalence. Information about the incidence and prevalence of symptoms and diseases is used by family physicians in estimating diagnostic probabilities. Studies in general practice have corrected some of the erroneous information on incidence and prevalence that have arisen from studies on selected populations. Incidence and prevalence are usually expressed as rates per thousand of the population at risk. The incidence rate is the number of new cases of the problem or disease seen per thousand of the population in 1 year. The prevalence rate is the total number of cases per thousand of the population at one point in time (the point prevalence) or in the course of a period of time (the period prevalence). For acute illness, the incidence rate is the more useful figure; for chronic illness, the prevalence rate is more useful. Care must be taken in extrapolating incidence and prevalence figures from family practice to the general population. One practice may not be representative of the total population. A more representative population can be obtained, however, by using a large number of practices. Because the recording of incidence depends on whether or not the patient consults, episodes of illness not presented to the family physician will be excluded. Incidence and prevalence studies in family practice are based on the number of patients consulting for the disease or problem in question (the consultation rate). Several types of denominator are used to calculate this rate. In registered practices, the practice population can be used; in practices with no registered population, the denominator may be the number of patients consulting during the year, a population arrived at by counting the practice records or the number of office visits during the year. None of these denominators is entirely satisfactory. The registered practice population may include people who have left the area but have not registered with a new doctor; a population obtained by counting practice records excludes people at risk who have never consulted, and may include some patients who have moved; patients consulting in 1 year are only about 70% of the total practice population. Nevertheless, incidence and prevalence studies in family practice do give a much more complete picture of illness than studies done in hospitals, which rarely have a denominator population. Many examples of incidence and prevalence studies could be cited. Some of these have been done by individual practitioners, such as Hodgkin (1978) and Bentsen (1970). Others have been combined studies, such as the British National Morbidity Study carried out by the Royal College of General Practitioners, the National Ambulatory Care Study in the United States, and the National Morbidity and Interventions in General Practice Survey conducted by the Netherlands Institute of Primary Care.

Determination of the sensitivity, specificity, or predictive value of symptoms or tests make up the third type of descriptive research. To determine these values, certain data must be collected. The sensitivity of a symptom or test is the percentage of all people with the disease who have the symptom or positive test:

$$\text{Sensitivity} = \frac{\text{True positives}}{\text{All people with the disease}} \times 100$$

Suppose that we wanted to discover the sensitivity of palpable spleen in the early stages of infectious mononucleosis. We would need to record in every case the presence or absence of a palpable spleen. The result would then be calculated as follows:

$$\text{Sensitivity} = \frac{\text{Patients with palpable spleen and infectious mononucleosis}}{\text{All patients with infectious mononucleosis}} \times 100$$

The positive predictive value of a symptom or test is the percentage of people with the symptom or positive test who have the disease, that is, who are true positives:

$$\text{Predictive value} = \frac{\text{True positives}}{\text{All positives}} \times 100$$

Suppose that we wanted to discover the predictive value of sinus tenderness for acute sinusitis in patients with headache. We would need to record the presence or absence of sinus tenderness in every patient with headache. We would also have to ensure that sinus tenderness was elicited and recorded in the same way by all observers and that sinusitis was diagnosed according to uniform criteria. The result would be calculated as follows:

$$\text{Predictive value} = \frac{\text{All patients with sinus tenderness and sinusitis}}{\text{All patients with sinus tenderness}} \times 100$$

The fourth descriptive research category is natural history studies using controls. A descriptive study may reveal an association whose significance is not clear. A study of coronary heart disease (CHD), for instance, may show that coronary disease appears to have a higher prevalence in people who have moved into the area than in natives. To demonstrate that the observed significance is not due to chance we must do a controlled study. Two methods are available. First, in a cross-sectional study, a random sample of the practice population would be surveyed at one point in time. Suppose that 10% of natives and 40% of immigrants had coronary heart disease:

	CHD	No CHD	Total
Natives	10	90	100 (10%)
Immigrants	40	160	200 (20%)

An χ_2 test applied to these figures would show that the difference is significant at the $P = 0.05$ level. Second, in a case–control study, for every case of CHD a control, matched for age and sex, would be chosen. Both would be asked their origins:

	Natives	Immigrants	Total
CHD	10	40	50
No CHD	20	30	50

An χ_2 test applied to these figures would show that the difference is significant at the $P = 0.05$ level.

Research in the Technology of Family Practice

Much of medical research is now devoted to the development and evaluation of tools and methods—preventive, diagnostic, and therapeutic. The prototype of this research is the randomized controlled trial (RCT). At one time, it was thought that effective therapeutic methods would be deducible from the theory of disease developed by experimental medicine. The results soon showed that our theoretical knowledge is incomplete. New diagnostic methods and therapies may be derived from scientific theory, but they still require testing empirically. The RCT was developed for this purpose.

Much progress has been made in the description and development of the diagnostic, therapeutic, and preventive methods of family practice. In many instances, this process has involved the formalizing of skills that had long been practiced at the intuitive level. One result has been a theory of family practice designed to explain the family physician's approach of diagnosis, therapy, and prevention. The early chapters of this book are an attempt to expound this theory.

For the evaluation of its methods, family medicine uses the technique of the RCT. It is also applicable to the organizational tools of family practice—record-keeping systems, management systems for case finding or for controlling chronic disease, and functions of the health-care team. Drugs require testing in family practice as well as in hospital. Because the patient population is so different, it may be misleading to extrapolate from one population to another. For example, there have been very few trials of antidepressants in family practice.

The Problem of Abstraction

Science produces generalizations by making abstractions[2] from the world of concrete experience. The problem is that the higher the level of abstraction, the more the rich texture of the world of experience is flattened out and rendered unrecognizable. This applies especially when the things abstracted are only those that can be quantified.

In the preface to *The Varieties of Religious Experience*, William James (1958) wrote, "a large acquaintance with particulars often makes us wiser than the possession of abstract formulas, however deep." A large part of medical knowledge is made up either of particulars or of generalizations at a low level of abstraction.

This is the knowledge gathered over years of observation in the form of case histories or series of cases. Much of it was made useful without quantification, or with quantification of a very elementary kind.

This way of contributing to medical knowledge is still valid. When family physicians see the results of some quantitative studies done in family practice, they are sometimes struck by how little they reflect the actual experience of being a family doctor. Perhaps it is a bald statement of results of a morbidity study, no doubt very useful at the planning level, but so far from the concrete world as to have very little application to day-to-day practice.

The same applies to many behavioral studies. The generalization "communication difficulties increase with cultural distance" is probably of less value than the observation that feelings like anger and gratitude are not openly expressed by Native North Americans. Of course, power of generalization is sacrificed when knowledge is more concrete. The latter item of knowledge is useful only to physicians who care for Native patients. To take another example, it has been shown that self-perception is directly related to control in juvenile diabetics: the worse the self-percept, the worse the control. A less abstract item of information is that many juveniles are so ashamed of their diabetes that they try to hide it from their friends. Which of these items is more helpful to a physician counseling a juvenile diabetic?

Some of the most important questions facing family medicine are very unlikely to be answered by research that involves a high level of abstraction and quantification. A method must be found that preserves the richness and explores the meaning of the family practice experience. How, for example, do family physicians work with families? How do patients experience illness? Qualitative research methods have been developed to answer questions about the meaning of experience.

Family medicine is not alone in trying to find its way in research. The human sciences generally are engaged in the same debate, prompted by the aridity of so much of the work done by the experimental method. The human sciences differ from the natural sciences in some fundamental ways. For one thing, human events do not repeat themselves in exactly the same way. This does not mean that we cannot learn from studying human events. It does mean, however, that understanding rather than prediction is the objective in human research. One cannot study persons like objects. The very act of studying people changes them by altering their perceptions of events and of themselves. In a controlled trial of a system for detecting and managing hypertension in general practices, the control practices changed almost as much as the experimental practices. Both were performing much differently at the end of the study than the beginning. This does not mean that the results were of no value. The purpose of human research is often to produce change. It does suggest, however, that the experimental method has limited value in human affairs. It is this capacity for change that makes prediction invalid: whatever is predicted as a result of human research can be deliberately rendered void by the subjects themselves.

Randomization of human subjects is often impossible. Controlled trials of educational projects are made difficult because students selecting a new program are compared with students not selecting it. One can never then be sure that differences are due to the program and not due to the personal factors that led students to choose it. Again, this does not mean that educational research is of no value. In medical education, there are many examples of carefully designed demonstration models from which much has been learned.

Qualitative research is concerned with the meaning of actions and events.[3] There are no empirical tests for establishing meaning. Engel (1980) gives, as an example of human research, the gesture of "giving up." This gesture can be observed, described, and recorded, but its meaning cannot be deduced from the observation. It is not that we cannot establish the meaning; it is that we have to use other methods. We may find the meaning by entering into a dialogue with the patients about their feelings, we may do it by studying the context of the gesture in a number of patients, or we may understand the meaning intuitively because this act of communication is part of our own language; or we may use all these ways of understanding the gesture. Having verified the meaning in this way, we have a valuable contribution to knowledge, even though it may not be applicable to the whole human race. Other cultures may have different gestures for giving up.

Qualitative research is intensive and time-consuming. The depth required in person-to-person interviews limits the number of people who can be interviewed. Those who have been educated in conventional quantitative methods sometimes ask how it is possible to generalize from such small samples. The answer is that the purpose of qualitative research is not to generalize but to enrich our understanding. A study based on interviews with only 12 women who had spontaneous miscarriages can enrich our understanding of the experience and make us more sensitive to patients' feelings, even though it cannot be generalized to all women (Manca and Bass, 1991).

There is no antithesis between quantitative and qualitative research. Which method is chosen depends on the question asked. The same study may include some questions answerable by quantitative, others by qualitative, methods.[4]

The Problem of Validation

In the search for a different research paradigm, we face the same problems of validation as other human sciences. Empirical science has well-established criteria of validation. What are the criteria in human science? How do we know that the changes we have made are responsible for the outcomes observed? How do we know that in explaining and interpreting human events we are not deceiving ourselves? In this review of means of validation in human inquiry, I am indebted to Reason and Rowan (1981), who describe eight processes of validation:

1. Personal preparation by the investigator. As Schumacher (1977) observed, the understanding of the knower must be adequate to the thing known. One cannot understand a psychological state without the capacity to experience it, or understand a social situation without entering into the experience of those involved. Preparation of this kind requires self-knowledge and the ability to deal with countertransference.

2. Systematic interpersonal development by the co-investigators, with the same purpose of enhancing self-knowledge.
3. Having one member of the investigator group whose role it is to act as devil's advocate by challenging conclusions reached by the group. This is a protection against self-deception by the whole group.
4. The cyclical process of testing, revising, and retesting one's conclusions, often many times (the hermeneutic cycle). This includes feeding back the results to the subjects and refining them in the light of their comments. Conclusions are suspect if they do not make sense to the subjects of the study.
5. Putting together knowledge from different levels of knowing. Gregory Bateson (1979) remarked that extra depth is given to knowledge by juxtaposing descriptions obtained in different ways. Developing different modes of human inquiry does not mean abandoning more orthodox modes.
6. A systematic effort by the investigators to refute their own conclusions.
7. Putting together the conclusions with other evidence from different sources and different methods of inquiry: a validation criterion known as triangulation.
8. A thorough description of the context of the inquiry (thick description).

Much remains to be done in working out modes of inquiry that will do justice to the rich texture of family practice. The process does not necessitate abandoning more conventional modes of inquiry. We will still continue to use experimental and quantitative methods for their proper reasons. We believe, however, that it is time to move away from our almost exclusive concentration on these disciplines.

References

Bateson G. 1979. *Mind and Nature: A Necessary Unity*. New York: E.P. Dutton.

Bentsen BG. 1970. *Illness and General Practice*. Oslo: Universitetoforlaget.

Engel G. 1980. The clinical application of the biopsychosocial model. *American Journal of Psychiatry* 137:535.

Fleck L. 1979. *Genesis and Development of a Scientific Fact*. Chicago, IL: University of Chicago Press.

Fry J. 1961. *The Cattarrhal Child*. London: Butterworths.

Headache Study Group of the University of Western Ontario. 1986. Predictors of outcome in headache patients presenting to family physicians: A one year prospective study. *Headache* 26:285.

Hodgkin K. 1978. *Towards Earlier Diagnosis in Primary Care*, 4th edn. Edinburgh: Churchill Livingstone.

James W. 1958. *The Varieties of Religious Experience: The Gifford Lectures on Natural Religion Delivered at Edinburgh in 1901–1902*. New York: New American Library.

Klein MC, Gauthier RJ, Robbins JM et al. 1994. Relationship of episiotomy to perineal trauma and morbidity, sexual dysfunction, and pelvic floor relaxation.*American Journal of Obstetrics and gynecology* 171(3):591–598.

Klein M. 1988. Episiotomy and the second stage of labour. *Canadian Family Physician* 34:2019–2025.

Koestler A 1970. *The Act of Creation*, The Danube Edition. London: Pan Books Ltd,, p. 191.

Macaulay AC, Paradis G, Potvin L et al. 1997. The Kahnawake Schools Diabetes Prevention Project: intervention, evaluation, and baseline results of a diabetes primary prevention program with a native community in Canada. *Preventive Medicine* 26(6):779–790.

Macaulay A C, Commanda LE, Freeman W et al. 1999. Participatory research maxmises community and lay involvement. *British Medical Journal* 319(7212):774–778.

Mackenzie J. 1919. *The Future of Medicine*. London: Oxford University Press.

Mair A. 1973. *Sir James Mackenzie, M.D., General Practitioner, 1853–1925*. Edinburgh: Churchill Livingstone.

Manca D, Bass MJ. 1991. The miscarriage experience. *Canadian Family Physician* 37:1871.

McWhinney IR. 2008. Assessing clinical discoveries. *Annals of Family Medicine* 6(1):3–5.

Pickles WN. 1939. *Epidemiology in Country Practice*. Bristol: John Wright.

Reason P, Rowan J. 1981. Issues of validity in new paradigm research. In: Reason P, Rowan J, eds., *A Source Book Of New Paradigm Research*. Chichester: John Wiley.

Ryle J. 1936. *The Natural History of Disease*. London: Oxford University Press.

Schumacher EF. 1977. *A Guide for the Perplexed*. New York: Harper and Row.

Stange KC. 2008. Clinical discoveries: A new feature of the Annals. *Annals of Family Medicine* 6:175–176.

Notes

1. Mackenzie's philosophy of medicine and medical education are expressed in his book *The Future of Medicine* (1919). William Pickles' *Epidemiology in Country Practice* (1939) and John Fry's *The Catarrhal Child* (1961) are also excellent examples of descriptive research in general practice.

2. For a fuller discussion of abstraction, see pages 84–85.

3. For descriptions of qualitative research methods, see Crabtree BF and Miller WL, eds. 1992. *Research Methods for Primary Care: Doing Qualitative Research*. Newbury Park, CA: Sage Publications Inc.

4. For examples of qualitative research in this book, see Veale, page 20, Miller, page 141, Jones and Morrell, page 185, Murphy and Kinmonth page 352, Woodward, page 305, Muzzin, page 383, Dowie page 383, Bailey et al., page 383, and Wood, page 383, Woodward, Broom, and Legge, page 305 and 306.

Index